Obstetrics

by Ten Teachers

under the direction of

Stanley G. Clayton

Edited by
Stanley G. Clayton
T. L. T. Lewis
G. Pinker

Thirteenth edition

Edward Arnold

© Edward Arnold (Publishers) Ltd. 1980

First published 1917 under the title *Midwifery*
by Edward Arnold (Publishers) Ltd.,
41 Bedford Square,
London WC1B 3DQ

Second edition	*1920*	*Tenth edition*	*1961*	
Reprinted	*1921, 1923*	*Reprinted*	*1963*	
Third edition	*1925*	*Eleventh edition*	*1966*	
Reprinted	*1927, 1928*	(renamed *Obstetrics*)		
Fourth edition	*1931*	*Reprinted*	*1970*	
Fifth edition	*1935*	*Twelfth edition*	*1972*	
Reprinted	*1937*	*Reprinted*	*1975, 1976, 1978*	
Sixth edition	*1938*	*Thirteenth edition*	*1980*	
Seventh edition	*1942*	*Reprinted*	*1982*	
Reprinted	*1944, 1946*	*First published in paperback*	*1982*	
Eighth edition	*1948*	*Reprinted*	*1982*	
Reprinted	*1949, 1952*			
Ninth edition	*1955*			
Reprinted	*1957*			

British Library Cataloguing in Publication Data

Obstetrics. – 13th ed.
  I. Clayton, *Sir* Stanley George
  II. Lewis, Thomas Loftus Townshend
  III. Pinker, George Douglas
  618.2   RG524

ISBN 0-7131-4365-7
ISBN 0-7131-4415-7 Pbk

Filmset in 10/11 Plantin
by Reproduction Drawings Ltd, Sutton, Surrey.
Printed in Great Britain
by Butler & Tanner Ltd, Frome and London

Contributors

Director

Sir Stanley Clayton, MD, MS(Lond), FRCP, FRCS, FRCOG.
Emeritus Professor of Obstetrics and Gynaecology, University of London: Honorary Consulting Surgeon, King's College Hospital, Queen Charlotte's Hospital and Chelsea Hospital for Women.

Contributors

J. Michael Brudenell, MB BS(Lond), FRCS, FRCOG.
Obstetric and Gynaecological Surgeon, King's College Hospital; Gynaecological Surgeon, Queen Victoria Hospital, East Grinstead.

Geoffrey V. P. Chamberlain, MD(Lond), FRCS, FRCOG.
Obstetric and Gynaecological Surgeon, Queen Charlotte's Hospital and Chelsea Hospital for Women.

Denys V. I. Fairweather, MD(St. Andrew's), FRCOG.
Professor of Obstetrics and Gynaecology, University College Hospital Medical School.

John C. Hartgill, FRCS (Ed), FRCOG.
Obstetric and Gynaecological Surgeon, The London Hospital.

Joseph M. Holmes, MD(Lond), FRCOG.
Obstetric and Gynaecological Surgeon, University College Hospital.

Thomas L. T. Lewis, CBE, MB, BChir(Cantab), FRCS, FRCOG.
Obstetric and Gynaecological Surgeon, Guy's Hospital, Queen Charlotte's Hospital and Chelsea Hospital for Women.

George D. Pinker, MB, BS(Lond), FRCS(Ed), FRCOG.
Obstetric and Gynaecological Surgeon, St. Mary's Hospital; Gynaecological Surgeon, The Middlesex Hospital; Honorary Consultant Surgeon, Royal Women's Hospital, Melbourne.

David W. T. Roberts, MA, MChir(Cantab), FRCS, FRCOG.
Obstetric and Gynaecological Surgeon, St. Mary's Hospital and the Middlesex Hospital.

Marcus E. Setchell, MA, MB, BChir(Cantab), FRCS, FRCS(ED), MRCOG.
Obstetric and Gynaecological Surgeon, St. Bartholomew's Hospital.

Ronald W. Taylor, MD(Liverpool), FRCOG.
Professor of Obstetrics and Gynaecology, St. Thomas's Hospital Medical School.

By invitation the chapters on neonatal care have been written by:

Roderick J. K. Brown, MB, BChir(Cantab), FRCP, DCH.
Consultant Paediatrician to the Middlesex Hospital, Queen Elizabeth Hospital for Children, London, and the Hackney Hospital.

and the chapter on psychiatric disorder in pregnancy and the puerperium by:

Margaret E. Christie-Brown, MD, BS(Lond).
Consultant Psychotherapist, Queen Charlotte's Hospital and Chelsea Hospital for Women.

Preface

This book first appeared in 1917 under the title '*Midwifery by Ten Teachers*'. Through thirteen editions all the contributors have been active teachers and examiners in the London Medical Schools, and their shared experience is presented to the reader.

There have been many changes in the list of contributors in this edition. We are sorry to lose Mr Donald Fraser, Dr Edward Hart, Mr Ian Jackson and Mr Robert Percival on their retirement, and Professor Charles Douglas and Professor Philip Rhodes on their translation to posts outside London. We welcome Mr J. M. Brudenell, Mr G. V. P. Chamberlain, Professor D. V. I. Fairweather, Mr J. C. Hartgill, Mr M. E. Setchell and Professor R. W. Taylor as new contributors. Dr R. J. K. Brown has been responsible for the chapters on neonatal care, and Dr Margaret Christie-Brown for the chapter on psychiatric disorders. To maintain continuity Sir Stanley Clayton has remained as Director, with Mr T. L. T. Lewis and Mr J. D. Pinker as Editors.

During the last 40 years there have been two revolutions in obstetric practice, and we believe that we are now enjoying a third. In the first the general adoption of lower segment Caesarean section permitted safe intervention during labour, often in the fetal interest; in the second puerperal sepsis was held in check. In the present third phase many new methods of assessing the state of the fetus have been introduced, prolonged labour has been prevented by the proper use of oxytocin, and better relief of pain has been achieved with extradural anaesthesia. Maternal and perinatal mortality have never been lower in Britain, although further improvement can yet be achieved.

We have given a full description of the newer methods of obstetric management but have taken care to retain all that was good in earlier practice. In obstetrics the number of facts that the student has to memorize is mercifully less than in some other disciplines, yet in no subject is it more important to have a proper understanding of the principles on which critical decisions must depend. The entire text has been revised with this in mind and much of it has been rearranged. The help our paediatric colleagues give to our work is acknowledged in a rewritten section on neonatal care.

It is our hope that this book will serve not only as a suitable introduction to obstetrics for the undergraduate student but that it will also provide a basic text for those who wish to continue obstetric work after qualification.

We thank Professor Stuart Campbell for ultrasonographs, and Mrs Audrey Besterman for several new figures.

S.G.C., T.L.T.L., G.D.P.

Contents

1

Introduction

It might be claimed that obstetrics, the branch of medicine that deals with parturition, is the primal and most ancient medical art. The term obstetrics, derived from the Latin word for midwife, is of relatively recent introduction; until the late nineteenth century the word midwifery was generally used.

The aim and hope of obstetric practice is to ensure that every pregnancy ends with a healthy mother and a healthy baby, and at the same time to alleviate any discomforts and anxieties of pregnancy and the pain of labour. While we have gone some way towards achieving this goal, a few maternal deaths and a number of stillbirths and neonatal deaths, some of which are preventable, still occur, as the later chapter on vital statistics will show.

All medical students do some practical obstetric work during their training, and many of them enjoy this because it gives them, sometimes for the first time, a degree of personal responsibility for the care of mothers and their babies, with a close view of a most important aspect of family life. The time given to obstetrics in the crowded curriculum is now very short, but during it the student should try to observe the progress through pregnancy, labour and the puerperium of as many patients as possible, rather than merely rushing in at the last moment to attend their deliveries.

Many doctors find great satisfaction in the practice of obstetrics, but the newly qualified doctor cannot regard himself as adequately trained for this responsibility; for those who wish to practice obstetrics after qualification further postgraduate training is essential. If only a proportion of doctors are ultimately going to practice obstetrics it may be asked why it is still retained in the undergraduate curriculum. The answer is simple. No doctor without some knowledge of obstetrics (and gynaecology) could pretend fully to understand the problems of his female patients. In addition, emergencies in pregnancy and labour occasionally call for immediate medical help, which can sometimes be life-saving, and every doctor must be able to render first aid until expert help can be obtained.

Until the early years of the present century most deliveries took place in the home, with only the help of an untrained woman. A few hospitals for maternity cases (usually called lying-in hospitals) were founded in the eighteenth century. For the most part they dealt with abnormal cases, but with slow and unreliable communications these hospitals could only serve the needs of a small and local fraction of the population. The same consideration limited the availability of expert obstetricians, who were only to be

1

found in the larger cities. The extent of domiciliary practice was such that every doctor had to possess some rough and ready knowledge of the art, often gained by bitter experience under these difficult conditions. The midwife of those days was largely self-taught; much of her knowledge was handed down from mother to daughter, and little came from books.

Modern obstetrics is very different, with proper antenatal care, with disappearance of those cases of protracted labour which were formerly so disastrous, with emphasis on methods of monitoring the health of the fetus during pregnancy and labour, and relief of pain by epidural analgesia. A few die-hards may decry modern practice, preferring to leave everything to nature, but obstetric audit shows that modern methods produce improved maternal and fetal results.

There are many fascinating aspects of the long history of obstetrics, such as the story of Caesarean section, the invention by Chamberlen of the obstetric forceps, the introduction of chloroform by Simpson, the establishment of antenatal care by Ballantyne, the recognition of the infective nature of puerperal fever by Semmelweis, the discovery of the rhesus factor, the isolation of ergometrine by Chassar Moir, the pioneering work of Donald in the use of ultrasound—and much more besides which will appear in subsequent chapters.

The provision of good obstetric care for the women of Britain calls for more than obstetric skill among specialists; the ordinary services must be well organized and provided with adequate numbers of properly trained staff.

A few of the landmarks in the development of the midwifery services in this country may be listed:

1726   Establishment of the first Chair of Midwifery in Scotland.
1739   Foundation of Queen Charlotte's Lying-in Hospital, the first specialist obstetric hospital.
1807   Diploma for midwives granted by the Obstetrical Society in London.
1881   Foundation of the Midwives' Institute to raise the statue of midwives.
1886   Obstetrics made compulsory during the training of doctors, after a prolonged and energetic campaign by the Worshipful Society of Apothecaries.
1902   Passage of the Midwives Act which created the Central Midwives Board.
1918   Passage of the Maternity and Child Welfare Act which empowered Local Authorities to provide antenatal clinics.
1929   Foundation of the College of Obstetricians and Gynaecologists, soon to be granted a Royal Charter.
1948   Establishment of the National Health Service, with free provision of all maternity services.

2
Ovulation, menstruation, fertilization and embedding of the ovum

In health, throughout the years between puberty and the menopause, the lining of the body of the uterus is shed and discharged together with some blood through the cervix and vagina at fairly regular intervals of about one month. This external menstrual discharge is the outward sign of the activity of the menstrual hormones on the endometrium.

The menstrual cycle is commonly of 28 days, but it is perfectly normal for it to be anything between 21 and 35 days. The release of the ovum is preceded by a period of growth of the *Graafian (ovarian) follicle*, and after ovulation the follicle becomes the *corpus luteum*. These cyclical changes in the ovary are brought about by gonadotrophic hormones secreted by the anterior lobe of the pituitary gland. The cells of the follicle and corpus luteum also secrete hormones, oestrogen and progesterone, which cause cyclical changes in the endometrium, in myometrial and tubal contractility, in cervical secretion, in the vaginal epithelium and in the breasts.

Under the influence of the ovarian hormones the endometrium reaches its maximum development in the late part of the menstrual cycle, so that if the ovum liberated at mid-cycle is fertilized and carried down the Fallopian tube it will reach the cavity of the uterus when the endometrium is thick and hyperaemic, forming a prepared bed into which the fertilized ovum (zygote) can burrow and continue its development.

If the ovum in a particular cycle is not fertilized the activity of the corpus luteum and production of its hormones stops, and then the endometrium except for its basal layer breaks down and is discharged in the menstrual lochia. On the other hand, if the ovum is fertilized some of its chorionic cells produce another gonadotrophic hormone (chorionic gonadotrophin) which maintains the activity of the corpus luteum for a time. In addition the chorionic cells produce oestrogen and progesterone in steadily increasing amounts. Thus, during pregnancy, oestrogen and progesterone, coming either from the ovary or from the trophoblastic cells of the chorion of the zygote, maintain and carry on the growth of the endometrium, which is now described as the *decidua* of pregnancy.

3

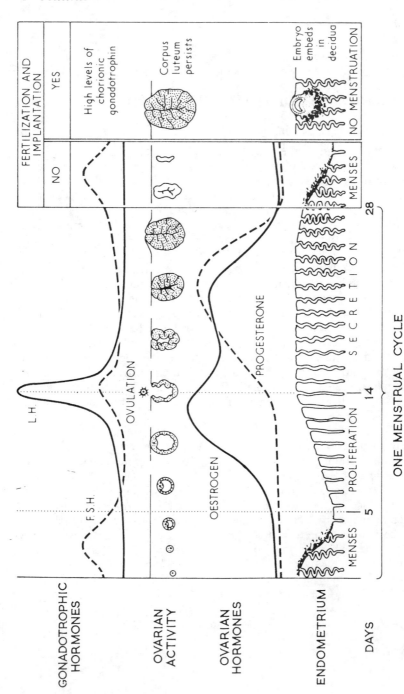

Fig. 2.1   Diagram to show events in the menstrual cycle and early pregnancy.

Ovulation

In the human embryo, as early as the 4th week of life, germ cells migrate by amoeboid activity from the wall of the yolk sac to an area of mesenchyme on the posterior wall of the coelom. These invading cells form the primordial germ cells, some of which proliferate to give rise to numerous primary oöcytes. The oöcyte is a large round cell, with a relatively large nucleus which is rich in chromatin. The primary oöcytes become surrounded by a single layer of smaller flattened cells which are derived from the surface epithelium. (This epithelium was named the germinal epithelium because it was originally thought that the primitive germ cells were derived from it).

Each system consisting of an oöcyte and the surrounding flattened cells is described as a primordial Graafian follicle, and at birth the ovary contains more than 800 000 follicles. In each menstrual cycle several follicles start to mature, but for some reason that is not understood one outstrips the others, and in most cycles only one follicle reaches full development, although some cases of multiple pregnancy are due to ripening and fertilization of more than one ovum in one cycle.

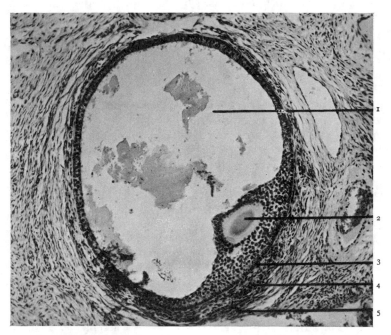

Fig. 2.2 Ripe Graafian follicle: 1, liquor folliculi; 2, oöcyte; 3, granulosa cells; 4, theca interna; 5, theca externa.

The Graafian (ovarian) follicle

During maturation of the follicle the flat cells that surround the primordial ovum multiply and become rounded and arranged in several layers, and are now called *granulosa cells*. Their growth is eccentric, so that the ovum comes to lie at one side of the mass of granulosa cells, and eventually a clear fluid appears among these cells, so that a follicle is formed with the ovum placed to one side of this. (See Fig. 2.2). The clump of granulosa cells that is directly related to the ovum forms a hillock (the cumulus) that projects into the cavity of the follicle, and at this stage the ovum is surrounded by a clear membrane, the zona pellucida, within which it can rotate. The granulosa cells that are immediately related to the zona pellucida become arranged in a radial fashion described as the *corona radiata*. The ovum itself enlarges slightly during maturation of the follicle, chiefly by increase in the volume of the cytoplasm, and reaches a diameter of about 0.15 mm.

The cells of the ovarian stroma which surround the granulosa cells also proliferate and become swollen by the accumulation of lipid. These cells form the *theca interna* and play an important part in the formation of the corpus luteum at a later stage. The ovarian stroma cells outside the theca interna become somewhat compressed by the growth of the follicle and form the *theca externa* (Fig. 2.2).

As the follicle increases in size it approaches the surface of the ovary, where it is seen as a transparent vesicle which varies in size, but may reach a diameter of 10 mm. The follicle eventually projects from the surface of the ovary, and at about the mid-point of the cycle it ruptures and the ovum, still surrounded by the corona radiata, is discharged into the peritoneal cavity. The part of the cycle before ovulation is called the *follicular phase;* and the part after ovulation (when the corpus luteum is present) is called the *luteal phase.* Although ovulation most commonly occurs between the 12th and 15th day of the cycle, there is some variation in healthy women, and this is important in determining the duration of pregnancy. Ovulation has a closer relation to the expected (following) period than to the preceding period; or in other words, there is more variation in the length of the follicular than of the luteal phase.

Ovulation is under hypothalamic-pituitary control (see p. 8) which may sometimes be influenced by the higher centres of the brain. In some mammals ovulation is initiated by coitus, and it is possible that coitus, particularly when attended by strong emotional reaction, may occasionally have this effect in some women. This might explain the fact that at all stages of the cycle pregnancy sometimes appears to have followed a single coitus. The alternative explanation that either the ovum or the sperms may survive for some time in the genital tract is less acceptable, and the available evidence suggests that unless the ovum is fertilized with 36 hours after ovulation it will not survive, and sperms do not appear to retain their fertilizing ability for longer than 24 hours.

Corpus luteum

After ovulation the walls of the follicle collapse and are thrown into folds, and there is usually a little haemorrhage into the empty cavity. The granulosa cells become swollen by the accumulation of yellow lipid, and are now termed *granulosa-lutein cells*, while similar changes occur in the

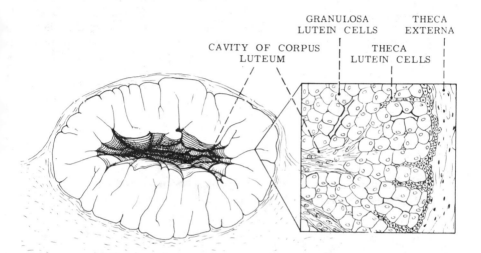

Fig. 2.3 Corpus luteum.

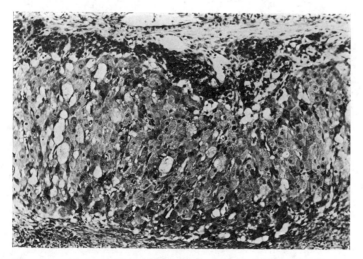

Fig. 2.4 Microscopical section of corpus luteum. The cavity is below and the dark theca-lutein cells are seen above the large lutein cells.

theca interna, the cells of which are now termed *theca-lutein cells*. (Figs. 2.3, 2.4.) The central coagulum soon becomes organized by the invasion of capillaries. The mature corpus luteum is bright yellow in colour and is usually larger than the follicle from which it developed, reaching a diameter of 1 to 3 cm. If the ovum that was discharged from the follicle is not fertilized degenerative changes (luteolysis) begin in the corpus luteum at about the 22nd day of the cycle. By the time that the next menstrual period begins the luteal cells show fatty degeneration, and ultimately the cells lose their outlines and nuclei. During subsequent weeks the whole structure becomes replaced with white connective tissue, and is then described as a corpus albicans. This is eventually absorbed, and finally the site of the follicle is only represented by a small scar.

On the other hand, if the ovum from the follicle is fertilized and pregnancy follows, then the corpus luteum persists and enlarges further, maintaining its hormonal activity for about 12 weeks until its function is taken over by the placenta.

Hormones controlling the growth and activity of the follicle and corpus luteum

Two gonadotrophic hormones, *follicle stimulating hormone* (FSH) and *luteinizing hormone* (LH), control the ripening of the follicle, ovulation and the formation and maintenance of the corpus luteum. In turn the secretion of these gonadotrophic hormones by the anterior lobe of the pituitary gland is controlled by *releasing hormones* from the hypothalamus. It is uncertain whether there are separate releasing hormones for FSH and LH. Only LH releasing hormone has been isolated, and this appears to control the release of both FSH and LH.

Development of the follicle occurs under stimulation by relatively low concentrations of FSH and LH. There is increasing secretion of oestradiol 17β from the follicle, and when this reaches a certain level it causes, by a 'feed-back' mechanism, a spurt of LH releasing hormone from the hypothalamus, and a surge of LH is released by the pituitary gland. About 24 hours after this LH surge ovulation occurs.

After the ovum is released the process of luteinization begins and the corpus luteum then secretes progesterone (and continues to secrete oestrogen). If fertilization does not occur luteolysis takes place, and the levels of oestrogen and progesterone fall (see Fig. 2.1). If the ovum is fertilized the chorion produces *chorionic gonadotrophin* which is responsible for the prolongation of the activity of the corpus luteum during the first trimester of pregnancy. Further details of these hormonal interreactions can be found in *Gynaecology by Ten Teachers*, pp. 34 and 43.

Formation of decidua

Under the influence of the ovarian hormones the endometrium undergoes cyclical changes. If fertilization occurs the greatly thickened endometrum becomes the decidua of pregnancy, if it does not the endometrium breaks down in the process of menstruation.

During the *follicular (proliferative) phase* of the menstrual cycle, under the influence of oestrogen produced by the Graafian follicle, the endometrium becomes more vascular, the cells of the glandular epithelium and stroma proliferate, and the endometrium becomes thicker with long straight glands. In the *luteal (secretory) phase*, when the corpus luteum produces both oestrogen and progesterone, the gland cells become tall and columnar and pour out their secretions of glycogen and mucin into the lumina of the glands. The glands become convoluted (Fig. 2.5) and the

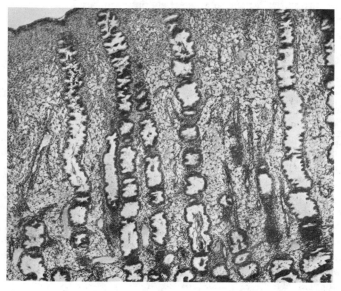

Fig. 2.5 Photomicrograph of endometrium at the end of the secretory or progestational phase of the menstrual cycle.

stromal cells swell. These changes do not affect the deepest parts of the endometrial glands and the stromal changes are most marked in the superficial layer, resulting in a great contrast between the basal layer of endometrium with straight glands, the spongy intermediate layer with distended convoluted glands, and the superficial compact layer. The arterioles have a spiral arrangement, and there is a great increase in vascularity. All these changes are in preparation for the possible reception of the fertilized ovum, and if the ovum is fertilized the changes in the endometrium persist and are accentuated, and the greatly thickened endometrium is now called the *decidua of pregnancy*.

Maturation of the ovum

The nuclei of human body cells each contain 46 chromosomes, and this number is maintained throughout successive divisions of the cells. The chromosomes are responsible for the transmission of all the inheritable qualities. The reproductive cells, the ovum and the spermatozoon, differ from the ordinary body cells in that they each contain only 23 chromosomes. When fertilization occurs and the ovum and spermatozoon unite the total of 46 chromosomes is re-established, the male and female cell each contributing half of the total, so that some inherited qualities are derived from the father and some from the mother. The number of chromosomes in the germ cells is reduced during the maturation of the cells by a special type of cell division called *meiosis*. In ordinary mitosis of body cells each chromosome divides into two, and the two halves of each chromosome separate and pass into the two daughter cells. In the reducing division of germ cells the chromosomes first become arranged in pairs, and then one member of each pair passes to each daughter cell, so halving the number of chromosomes in the mature germ cells.

The ovum undergoes the first maturation division when it is still in the ovary. The primary oöcyte divides by meiosis into two cells of unequal size, a large secondary oöcyte and a small polar body; the latter comes to lie in the perivitelline space within the zona pellucida. After this meiotic (reducing) division the secondary oöcyte only contains 23 chromosomes. The division of the secondary oöcyte, which takes place in the uterine tube, is a mitotic division. At this division a second polar body is extruded, but the final mature ovum still contains 23 chromosomes.

In the case of the spermatozoon a similar reducing division takes place by meiosis when the primary spermatocyte divides into two equal secondary spermatocytes, which each contain 23 chromosomes. By a further mitotic division each of these divides to form two spermatids, so that the original primary spermatocyte gives rise to four spermatozoa, each with 23 chromosomes.

The adult cells of a normal female contain two X chromosomes, and after meiotic division each ovum will contain one X chromosome. The adult cells of a normal male contain one X and one Y chromosome; when meiotic division occurs these separate so that each secondary spermatocyte contains either an X or a Y chromosome, and eventually there will be two types of spermatozoa, those with an X chromosome and those with a Y chromosome. During fertilization, if conjugation of an X sperm and an X ovum occurs, the final combination will be XX, and give rise to female genetic structure; but if conjugation of a Y sperm and an X ovum occurs the final combination will be XY, and give rise to male genetic structure. There are recognizable sexual differences in the nuclei of adult cells, particularly seen as a small club shaped projection of chromatin in the nuclei of polymorphonuclear leucocytes, and as a peripherally placed mass of chromatin (Barr body) in other cells in the female. This is believed to be the inactive X chromosome of the cell.

Transit and fertilization of the ovum

The mechanism by which the ovum reaches the lumen of the Fallopian tube has been much discussed. The ciliated cells of the fimbriae at the abdominal ostium of the tube set up a flow of fluid which has been shown to be capable of carrying small particles from the recto-vaginal pouch into the tube. The fimbriated end of the tube is probably brought into close contact with the ovary at the time of ovulation, although the mechanism of this is uncertain. Once the ovum has reached the cavity of the tube it is carried downwards by the ciliary action. The tubes show peristaltic movements, but the importance of these in moving the ovum down the tube is less certain.

Successful fertilization depends on coitus occurring at the correct time in the cycle and an adequate quality of the semen. Semen consists of spermatozoa and seminal plasma, a fluid which contains, among other things, enzymes, fructose and prostaglandins. During coitus ejaculation of the semen occurs and the sperms are deposited in the region of the cervix. At the time of ejaculation the sperms are not motile, and they only become so when the semen has undergone liquefaction. Fertilization of the ovum normally takes place in the ampullary portion of the Fallopian tube, and spermatozoa reach the tube between a few minutes and 3 hours after coitus. The transit of the spermatozoa results partly from their own motility, and partly from uterine and tubal peristalsis, the stimulus for which may be seminal prostaglandins. The fructose in seminal fluid is an essential nutrient for spermatozoa, and the enzymes are responsible for the coagulation and liquefaction of semen, and assist the sperm to penetrate the cervical mucus and the corona radiata around the ovum.

Sperm are attracted to the ovum by chemotaxis, and after coitus many spermatozoa can be found in the tubes. Several may penetrate the zona pellucida, but as soon as one sperm makes its way into the ovarian cytoplasm the ovum separates from the zona pellucida and becomes impervious to further penetration. The head of the spermatozoon represents the nucleus of the male cell, and it fuses with the nucleus of the ovum to form the segmentation nucleus, whose complement of 46 chromosomes is again complete. The fertilized ovum is carried down the tube by ciliary and peristaltic action, and reaches the uterine cavity 5 to 6 days after ovulation.

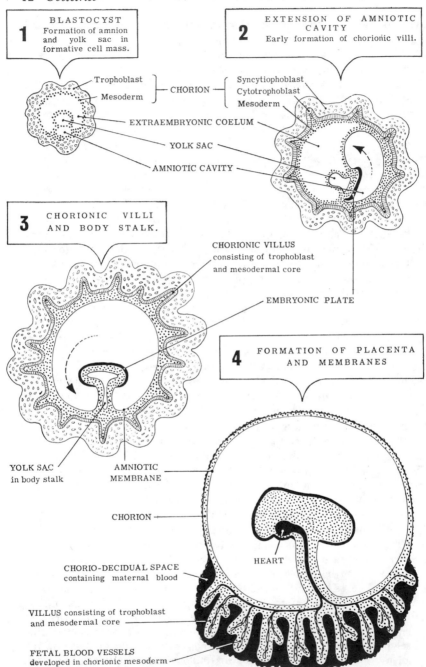

Fig. 2.6 Diagrams to show the formation of the placenta and fetal membranes.

Early development and embedding of the blastocyst

After the formation of the segmentation nucleus the zygote starts to divide, and soon a solid clump of cells called the morula is formed. A cavity appears among the cells of the morula so that it becomes vesicular, and it is then termed the blastocyst. This stage of development is reached while the zygote is still in the Fallopian tube.

The outermost cells of the blastocyst form the trophoblast. This has the power of eroding and digesting the surface epithelium of the decidua, and the fertilized ovum sinks into the thickness of the decidua, lying in a cavity in the stroma between adjacent endometrial glands. The glands are distorted and pushed aside by the enlargement of the growing ovum. The aperture through which the ovum entered the decidua is sealed over with a plug of fibrin. Maternal blood vessels are invaded and eroded by the trophoblast, and extravasation of maternal blood occurs around the ovum.

The structure of the blastocyst is indicated in the diagrams. (See Fig. 2.6.) The inner cell mass, from which the embryo will develop, is seen projecting into the blastocyst, and two small cavities appear in the cells of the inner cell mass, from which the amniotic cavity and the yolk sac develop. The diagrams indicate the progressive extension of the amniotic cavity, which comes to surround and envelop the embryo, and ultimately the amniotic membrane covers the body stalk up to the point at which it becomes continuous with the embryonic ectoderm at the umbilicus.

Very soon the trophoblast, while it is eroding into the maternal decidua, becomes arranged in projecting masses, at first in a labyrinthine formation, but later arranged as villi, which grow and branch. Maternal blood vessels are opened by the cytolytic action of the trophoblast, so that maternal blood lies in the intervillous spaces, and the embryo starts to secure its nutrition from this. The trophoblast becomes differentiated into two layers. There is a thick outer layer of syncytio-trophoblast, in which the nuclei are scattered in a mass of cytoplasm that has no evident division into separate cells. The inner layer of cyto-trophoblast (Langhans' layer) is thinner, and consists of a single layer of rounded cells.

The blastocyst is lined with extra-embryonic mesoderm, and it will be seen from the diagrams (Fig. 2.6) that this is continuous with the mesoderm of the embryo itself. The extra-embryonic mesoderm is continuous with the central tissue of the villi, so that each villus has an outer covering of trophoblast and a central mesodermal core. Lacunae appear in the mesoderm and gradually become joined to form a pattern of primitive blood vessels, extending through both the body of the embryo and the extra-embryonic mesoderm. By this arrangement the placental circulation is ultimately formed; the fetal heart not only pumps blood through the tissues of the fetus itself, but also through the tissues of the placenta.

The combined layer of trophoblast and underlying mesoderm is termed the chorion, and the villi are the chorionic villi. Within the chorion is the amniotic membrane that bounds the amniotic cavity.

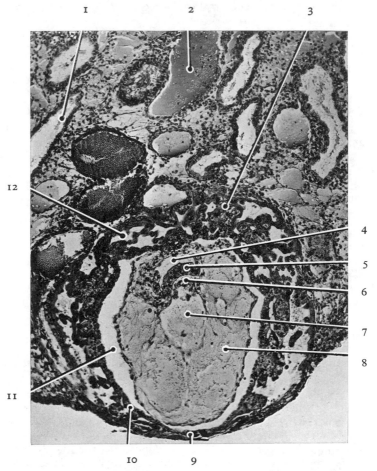

(By permission of Prof. W. J. Hamilton)

Fig. 2.7   Section of human embryo of 10 to 11 days development. 1, Uterine gland. 2, Maternal blood-vessel. 3, Syncytio-trophoblast. 4, Amniotic cavity. 5, Embryonic ectoderm. 6, Embryonic endoderm. 7, Primitive yolk sac (exocoelom). 8, Extra-embryonic mesoderm. 9, Operculum. 10, Cytotrophoblast. 11, Artificial space between the cytotrophoblast and the extra-embryonic mesoderm. 12, Lacuna of trophoblast.

The ovum embeds in the stratum compactum of the decidua and produces a slight projection into the uterine lumen, the most frequent site of implantation being the upper and posterior part of the uterine cavity. According to its relations to the embryo three parts of the decidua are distinguished.

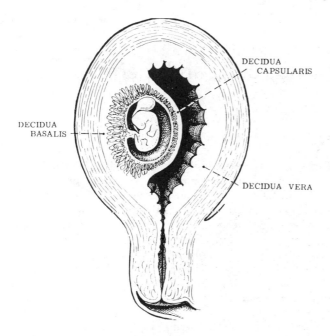

Fig. 2.8 Uterus containing an embryo of about nine weeks.

Decidua basalis. This is the portion of the decidua which lies between the embryo and the muscular wall of the uterus. It bounds the deeper half of the implantation cavity, and later on forms the site of attachment of the discrete placenta, and a number of thin-walled sinuses pass through it, bringing blood to the intervillous spaces. It also serves as a barrier against the invasion of the muscle by the syncytio-trophoblast, and under normal conditions the chorionic tissue does not penetrate through the decidua into the muscle.

Decidua capsularis. This is the portion of the decidua which intervenes between the embryo and the uterine cavity, and it bounds the superficial half of the implantation cavity. As the ovum grows it bulges out into the cavity, and by the 12th week the growing embryo fills the cavity, so that the decidua capsularis becomes fused with the decidua vera.

Decidua vera. This is the portion of the decidua that is not related to the site of implantation, and lines the rest of the cavity of the uterus.

Two other terms need definition. The *decidual space* is the space bounded by the decidua vera and the decidua capsularis. It is obliterated by the 12th week of pregnancy. The *choriodecidual space* is the space between the chorionic villi and the decidua basalis. It contains maternal blood.

3

The placenta, cord and membranes

The previous chapter gave a general outline of the implantation and early development of the embryo, and we may now proceed to describe the growth and anatomy of the placenta in more detail.

In the primitive mammalian placenta the fetal chorion is merely applied to the surface of the maternal decidua, so that exchange of nutrients and excretory products between maternal and fetal blood must take place through these layers (epithelio-chorial placenta). In the human placenta the trophoblast erodes into the decidua, so that the endothelium of the maternal blood vessels is destroyed and maternal blood is in direct contact with the chorion, without the intervention of any decidual tissue (haemochorial placenta).

At first the syncytiotrophoblast forms an open reticulated mesh-work, whose lacunae are filled with maternal blood, and in part of the trophoblast replaces the maternal endothelium. At first the trophoblast is arranged in trabeculae which are covered by syncytiotrophoblast and have a core of cytotrophoblast. When the embryonic mesoderm appears it extends into each of these trabeculae, and finally the vascularization of the mesoderm completes the formation of chorionic villi by about the 16th day. At some points the trophoblast comes into direct contact with the decidua, thus anchoring the main villi to the maternal tissues at the junctional zone. Here can be seen, lying between the invading trophoblast and decidua, a wavy layer of fibrin—the layer of Nitabuch. The number of these anchoring villi is small, but by budding from them and from the chorion, true chorionic villi are formed, which differ from the former in that their outer ends protrude free into the intervillous space. The capillaries in the terminal parts of the villi are much convoluted, with an arrangement reminiscent of that in a renal glomerulus, but adjacent villi are not joined, i.e. the villi do not form a reticulum.

Structure of a chorionic villus. A villus has a core of mesoderm, or stroma, and an epithelial covering. Embedded in the stroma are numerous fetal blood vessels. In the main villous stems the arteries and veins have connective tissue walls, but in the terminal villi only capillaries are present. The arteries are branches of the umbilical arteries and end in the terminal villi as capillaries from which purified blood is collected into venous radicals to pass back into the veins of the main villous stems, and thence

Chorionic   Syncytio-trophoblast
villi   covering villus

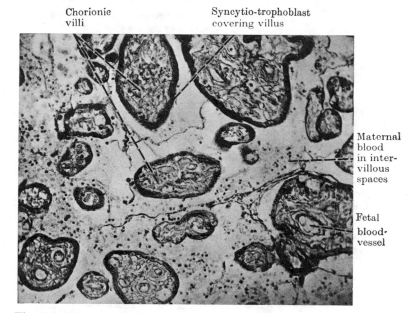

Maternal blood in inter-villous spaces

Fetal blood-vessel

Fig. 3.1 Microscopical section of placenta at term. × 170.

via the veins of the chorionic plate to the umbilical vein of the cord.

From the time of their formation in the 3rd week until the end of the 12th week, the epithelial covering consists of a single layer of cytotrophoblast and an outer layer of syncytiotrophoblast in immediate contact with the blood in the intervillous space. After the 20th week the cytotrophoblast begins to disappear until finally only a thin layer of syncytium remains.

Further development of the placenta. The chorionic villi are formed in immense number, and constitute the vast bulk of the villous system which covers the placental area. Thus comes about an arrangement whereby over a great surface, thin walled vessels carrying fetal blood are separated from the maternal blood only by the meagre connective tissue of the villi and a thin layer of trophoblast.

At first villi are formed all over the surface of the gestation sac, so that an ovum of 4 weeks' growth appears as a translucent thin walled sac covered by a spherical halo of soft villi (Fig. 3.3). As growth proceeds, the decidua capsularis becomes thinner and between the 12th and 16th weeks the villi on the capsular surface of the ovum rapidly degenerate, leaving this side of the chorion smooth (chorion laeve). In compensation, those on the surface opposed to the decidua basalis hypertrophy greatly (chorion frondosum) and become matted into a solid disc which is the fully developed discrete

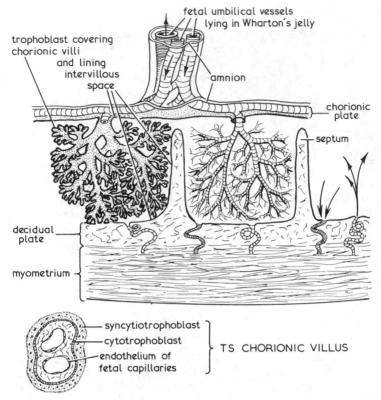

Fig. 3.2   Diagram to show structure of placenta. For clarity only the fetal arterioles are shown. The real villi are far more finely branched.

placenta. This is formed by the 12th week, though proportionately it then comprises a much larger part of the ovular surface than it does at term.

Increase in size of the placenta.   From the end of the 4th week, when the villi have penetrated towards the decidua basalis, there is no further invasion. Further growth in thickness of the placenta is now due to growth of the chorionic villi with an accompanying expansion of the intervillous sinuses. Until the end of the 16th week, the placenta grows both in thickness and circumference. Subsequently there is no increase in thickness, but the placenta continues to increase in size circumferentially until near term. The growth is proportionate with that of the fetus and of that part of the wall of the uterus to which the placenta is attached.

The placenta at term.   The placenta at term is circular in shape, forming a spongy disc 20 cm in diameter, and about 2.5 cm thick. It thins off towards its edge, which is abrupt. Its weight is about 500 g but there is some relationship with the fetal weight.

Placental wgt ≈ 1/6 Foetal weight

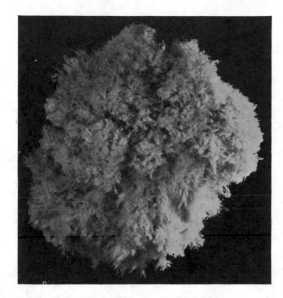

Fig. 3.3 Embryo, showing chorionic villi.

It has a fetal and a maternal surface. The fetal surface is covered by smooth amnion underneath which is the chorion. The blood vessels are visible beneath it as they radiate from the insertion of the umbilical cord. The maternal surface is rough and spongy, and presents a number of polygonal areas known as cotyledons, each being somewhat convex, and separated from those adjoining it by a shallow groove. Each cotyledon is formed by, and corresponds to, a main villous stem and its system of branch villi. The number of cotyledons, between 15 and 20, depends on the number of end arteries into which the umbilical artery divides, and this is determined by the number of the anchoring villi. The colour is a dull red, with a thin greyish and somewhat shaggy layer on the surface which is the remnant of that part of the decidua basalis which has come away with the placenta. Numerous small greyish spots are frequently seen on the maternal surface. They are due to the deposit of calcium in degenerate areas and are the result of normal senescence. They are more numerous in placentae at term. These deposits do not occur in the villi nor interfere with the maternal circulation in the intervillous spaces, and are of no importance.

The chorion spreads away from the edge of the placenta to form the outer layer of the two membranes which enclose the fetus and liquor amnii. Though the line of demarcation between the placental edge and the chorion is sharp, yet they are essentially one structure, for the placenta is a specialized part of the chorion.

The umbilical cord usually reaches the fetal surface of the placenta at about the middle of its disc, though sometimes at its edge (battledore placenta), and brings with it two umbilical arteries and one umbilical vein.

The area supplied by each artery varies but there is always a communication between the two arteries shortly after they have reached the placenta in order to equalize the pressure in the two systems. Except for this communication, the main trunks into which the arteries divide are terminal, and each ends in a tuft of capillary vessels. These tufts correspond to the cotyledons in which they are in free communication with the venules, which make up the corresponding tributaries of the umbilical vein.

The substance of the placenta is made up almost entirely of a multitude of chorionic villi, most of which protrude in an arborescent manner into the intervillous blood spaces. The placenta might be described as a space containing maternal blood, which is bounded on the maternal side by a decidual plate, and on the fetal side by a chorionic plate from which the chorionic villi branch into the maternal blood.

The intervillous space can be described as a lake of maternal blood which has left the maternal vessels to flow slowly round in a space bounded by fetal trophoblast. To supply this space arteries and large sinuses perforate the decidual plate. In the past some observers have maintained that the blood flows to the edge of the placenta to be collected in a 'marginal sinus' before leaving the intervillous space, but this is not now generally accepted, and vessels serving the arterial inflow and venous drainage appear to be scattered indiscriminately over the entire decidual plate.

Each cotyledon consists of between 10 and 20 lobules. Each lobule consists of a group of villi which are based on one large fetal artery which branches and rebranches to supply the villi. The lobule is like a sea-anemone floating in maternal blood. The maternal blood enters the intervillous space by about 200 arterioles which perforate the decidual (basal) plate. Each maternal arteriole spurts a jet of blood into the centre of a corresponding fetal lobule. The blood percolates through the branching villi of the lobule and then returns to the basal plate where it flows out through the decidual veins.

Functions of the placenta

The placenta has the following functions:
1. It enables the fetus to take oxygen and nutrients from the maternal blood.
2. It serves as the excretory organ of the fetus; carbon dioxide and other waste products pass from the fetal to the maternal blood.
3. It forms a barrier against the transfer of infection to the fetus, although a few organisms, such as the virus of rubella and the spirochaete of syphilis are able to pass.

4. The placenta secretes chorionic gonadotrophin, oestrogen and progesterone in large amounts, and also other hormones, which play an
essential part in the maintenance of the decidua and the growth of the
uterus and breasts.

Placental transport. In general the trophoblast and underlying
endothelium of the fetal vessels behave as a semi-permeable membrane,
allowing the free passage of water and soluble substances of relatively low
molecular weight according to the laws of osmotic equilibrium, but there
are several mechanisms of active transport, which allow more rapid diffusion of solutes, as well as transfer of larger molecules such as proteins and
lipids. The syncytium has a high degree of selectivity, permitting passage
of immune globulins, but excluding other potentially harmful large
molecules. The placenta not only transfers nutrients, but is also an important metabolic organ, with the ability to carry out metabolic processes of
which the immature fetus is incapable.

Substances with a molecular weight of less than 1000 are, in general, able
to pass the placental barrier, and most anaesthetic agents and drugs fall
into this class. The concentrations of water, sodium chloride, magnesium,
urea and uric acid are equal in maternal and fetal blood. A few substances,
including amino acids, nucleic acid, calcium and inorganic phosphorus,
are in higher concentration in fetal than in maternal blood, and there is no
doubt that the trophoblast has some power of selective transfer of these
substances, most of which are necessary for the building of fetal tissues.
Glucose is found in higher concentration in maternal than in fetal blood,
not because it does not pass the placenta freely, but probably because of its
continual utilization by the fetus.

Much of the fat in fetal tissues is synthesized from carbohydrate,
especially in late pregnancy. Although synthesis of fatty acids,
triglycerides, cholesterol and lipids takes place in fetal tissue, there is also a
contribution by direct transfer of maternal lipids.

The serum iron concentration in the fetus is higher than that in the
mother, but the mechanism of transfer is uncertain.

As regards hormones, oestrogens, androgens and thyroxine cross the
placenta, whereas insulin, parathyroid hormone and posterior pituitary
hormones do not. The vagina of the newborn female child shows evidence
of the oestrogenic action of maternal oestrogens in utero.

Despite the separation of the nucleated red cells in the vessels in the villi
from the maternal red cells in the intervillous space, on occasion a few fetal
red cells and fragments of villi may escape into the maternal circulation.
The entry of red cells from a fetus whose blood group differs from that of
its mother accounts for the development of haemolytic disease in certain
circumstances. See Chapter 41, p. 447.

Placental permeability increases as pregnancy progresses, probably
because the trophoblast becomes thinner, and also because the villi become
finer and more branched. The transfer of oxygen to the fetus is discussed
on p. 31.

The functional efficiency of the placenta. Placental transfer will depend upon the maternal blood flow through the intervillous space, the effective area of the surface of the chorionic villi, and the fetal blood flow through them.

The maternal blood flow is 500 – 700 ml per minute at term. The pressure in the intervillous space, which is of the order of 15 mm Hg, will be affected by uterine contractions. As the uterus contracts the veins in the myometrium are occluded first, so that the venous outflow ceases. The inflow of blood will continue until the uterine pressure equals the pressure of the arterial inflow. With a strong contraction the inflow also ceases, and the blood in the intervillous space is temporarily stagnant but the space does not empty because the veins are closed.

The volume of the intervillous space is about 140 ml. The blood in it is therefore exchanged about 4 times per minute. The area of the surface of the chorionic villi which is exposed to this 140 ml of blood has been estimated to be about 11 square metres. The blood therefore forms a very thin film over the surfaces. This large area, resulting from the fine branching of the villi, does not take into account microvilli on the trophoblast which can be seen with the electron microscope.

The volume of the fetal capillaries has been estimated to be about 60 ml and the fetal blood flow to be about 300 ml per minute, giving a total replacement of the fetal blood in the placenta about 5 times per minute. The pressure in the fetal capillaries in the villi is of the order of 30 mm Hg.

Placental hormones. The placenta secretes oestrogens, progesterone, chorionic gonadotrophin, lactogen, thyroid stimulating hormone, a hormone resembling adrenocorticotrophin, and possibly relaxin (a hormone which causes relaxation of pelvic ligaments in some species) into the maternal blood.

During pregnancy there is a progressive increase in the blood oestrogen and urinary oestrogen concentrations which reach their peak just before the onset of labour. The oestrogen found in the urine during pregnancy is chiefly oestradiol glucuronate. The placenta converts precursors which are formed in the fetal adrenal gland and liver to oestriol sulphate, which passes into the maternal blood before being conjugated with glucuronic acid by the maternal liver, finally to be excreted by the maternal kidney (see p. 34).

Until the end of the 8th week the corpus luteum continues to secrete progesterone. With the gradual cessation of function of this structure the placenta becomes responsible for the secretion of progesterone which, like oestrogen, reaches a peak just before labour. The excretion of progesterone in the urine in the form of pregnanediol is about 10 mg daily in the 8th week and reaches up to 80 mg daily by the end of pregnancy.

Chorionic gonadotrophin can be detected in the maternal plasma by raidoimmunoassay as early as 6 days after fertilization of the ovum, and is found in the urine soon after that. It reaches its peak concentration in urine at about 60 to 70 days, then the concentration falls to a low level at which it remains steady. The presence of this hormone in the urine forms the basis of the routine tests for pregnancy. It usually disappears from the urine if the fetus dies. It may persist for a time after delivery if placental tissue is retained.

Placental lactogen (HPL, formerly known as human chorionic somato-mammotrophin) closely resembles pituitary growth hormone in structure. Its secretion is first detectable about 35 days after fertilization, and it is produced in increasing amounts as pregnancy continues, maternal plasma levels reaching $6\,\mu g$ per ml. It is doubtful whether it has any somatotrophic or mammotrophic action in women, but it may have effects on carbohydrate and lipid metabolism.

The chorionic membrane

After the discrete placenta is formed the rest of the chorion atrophies and persists only as a thin, friable membrane intervening between the amnion and the decidua. On its outer surface vestiges of decidual cells and of the trophoblastic layer that formerly covered it can be distinguished micro-scopically, but the bulk of it is a fragile connective tissue, which is loosely attached to the amnion.

Sometimes vessels from the umbilical cord can be seen running across it, and occasionally the cord itself is attached to the chorion outside the placental margin, so that the umbilical arteries and veins run across it to reach the placenta (velamentous insertion).

The amnion

The first appearance of the amnion is a hollow space in the embryonic ectoderm. It is lined by cubical cells, which quickly become more columnar at the part which eventually forms the embryonic plate and the embryo. At first more or less spherical, the amniotic cavity soon becomes flattened down upon the embryo and closely applied to it. As the head and tail appear and the body walls fold round to enclose the embryonic coelom, the amnion attached at their margins is carried round also, so that the embryo is, as it were, pushed up and projects into the amniotic cavity. When the body cavity of the embryo is quite closed up, the amnion is attached all round the plate at which the ventral stalk emerges. (See Figs. 2.6(2) and 2.6(3).

At this period the embryo is relatively very small, and has the amnion closely applied to it, while the cavity of the blastocyst is relatively very large. Now a great change begins. The amniotic cavity enlarges out of proportion to the embryo, and becomes distended with fluid, and the embryo is gradually carried more and more into the amniotic cavity by elongation of the ventral stalk, which becomes the umbilical cord.

The enlargement of the amniotic cavity which brings about the complete investment of the umbilical cord likewise brings the amnion into close contact with the fetal surface of the placenta. This surface is, therefore, completely covered by the amnion. The amnion is attached to the placenta and chorion in a loose manner, and can be separated up to the insertion of the cord.

The amnion is lined by a single layer of cubical or flattened epithelial cells which is attached to a layer of connective tissue. The epithelium contains granules, fat droplets and vacuoles. The connective tissue upon the outer side of the amniotic membrane is closely applied to the similar connective tissue upon the inner side of the chorion; the two merely stick together, and are not organically united. They can easily be separated from one another at all periods of pregnancy. That portion of the amnion which covers the umbilical cord, however, is very closely incorporated with the connective tissue of the cord and cannot be stripped off.

Amniotic fluid.   The amniotic fluid is usually slightly turbid from the admixture of solid particles derived from the fetal skin and the amniotic epithelium. It may also be stained a greenish colour if any meconium has been passed into it. The solid matter is composed of lanugo hairs, epithelial cells and sebaceous material from the fetal skin, and cast-off amniotic epithelial cells.

The volume of the amniotic fluid at term is about 800 ml, but with a wide range of 400 to 1500 ml in normal cases. At 10 weeks the average volume is 30 ml, at 20 weeks 300 ml, and at 30 weeks 600 ml. The rate of increase is therefore about 30 ml per week, but the rate falls off at term. This is evident on clinical examination. On palpation at 30 weeks there seems to be a lot of liquor relative to the size of the fetus; nearer term there is less liquor, and when the expected date of delivery is passed the uterus seems to be 'full of baby'.

At term the liquor has a specific gravity of 1010. It contains 99 per cent of water, and its osmolality is less than that of maternal or fetal plasma. The liquor has organic, inorganic and cellular constituents. Concentrations of some of the important contents near term are as follows: Sodium, 130 mmol/l, urea 3 – 4 mmol/l, protein 3 g/l, lecithin 30 – 100 mg/l, α fetoprotein 0.5 – 5 mg/l. In addition traces of steroid and non-steroid hormones and of enzymes are present. It is mildly bacteriostatic.

The liquor is of both maternal and fetal origin, and the relative importance of the different mechanisms of production alters as pregnancy progresses. In very early pregnancy there is secretion from the amnion. Later, diffusion through the fetal skin accounts for much of the liquor, and there is increasing diffusion through the fetal membranes, including the part of the amnion that covers the fetal vessels in the cord and on the surface of the placenta. By the 20th week the skin loses its permeability, and from this time onwards the fetal kidneys play an increasing rôle in the production of liquor. By term about 500 ml per day is secreted as fetal urine, and tracheal fluid accounts for 200 ml. Studies with radio-isotopes have shown that near term 500 ml of water are exchanged hourly between the maternal plasma and the amniotic fluid. Disposal of the fluid is partly by absorption through the amnion into maternal plasma, and partly by fetal swallowing and absorption in the intestine to enter the fetal plasma.

In cases of renal agenesis (p. 175) there is oligohydramnios, and in conditions of defective swallowing such as anencephaly and oesophageal atresia there is polyhydramnios.

Functions of the liquor amnii. The liquor guards the fetus against mechanical shocks, equalizes the pressure exerted by uterine contractions, and allows it, at least in the early months, plenty of room for free movement. Since the temperature of the fluid is maintained by the mother the fetus is not subjected to loss of heat. Fetal metabolism is devoted entirely to growth and differentiation, and not dissipated in making good heat loss. Some of the fluid is swallowed, but it can hardly be regarded as a source of nutriment for the fetus as the content of protein and salts is so small. During labour the liquor contained in the bag of forewaters forms a fluid wedge which, with the uterine contractions, dilates the internal os uteri and cervical canal. When the membranes rupture during labour the liquor flushes the birth canal from downwards with fluid that is aseptic and bactericidal.

Investigation of the amniotic fluid. Samples of liquor can be obtained during pregnancy for various diagnostic purposes by abdominal amniocentesis. Not only can a variety of chemical estimations be made for normal and pathological constituents, but fetal amniotic cells can be obtained for tissue culture and chromosomal study. Details are given on p. 369.

The umbilical cord

The umbilical cord, or funis, forms the connection between the fetus and the placenta. It is derived from the ventral stalk and receives a close covering of amniotic epithelium. The constituents of the umbilical cord are as follows:

(1) The covering epithelium is a single layer of amnion. (2) Wharton's jelly is composed of cells with elongated anastomosing processes in a gelatinous fluid, and is part of the extra-embryonic mesoderm (see p. 13). (3) Blood vessels. These are at first four in number, two arteries and two veins. The embryonic umbilical veins fuse before the 3rd month leaving a single vessel. The two umbilical (hypogastric) arteries are derived from the internal iliac (hypogastric) arteries of the fetus, and carry reduced blood

from the fetus to the placenta. The umbilical vein carries oxygenated blood from the placenta to the fetus. (4) The umbilical vesicle and its vitelline duct, the shrivelled remnant of the yolk sac, may be found as a very small yellow body near the attachment of the cord to the placenta. (5) The allantois, which occasionally occurs as a blindly-ending tube just reaching into the cord, is continuous inside the fetus with the urachus and bladder.

The cord is commonly about 50 cm in length, but its length varies greatly, and may be as long as 180 cm, or as short as 7.5 cm. It is usually as thick as the little finger, but is not uniform since, as a rule, it presents nodes and swellings which are sometimes caused by dilatation of the umbilical vein, but more often by simple local increase in Wharton's jelly. At the earliest stage the cord is straight and somewhat flattened, but as early as the 12th week it shows a spiral twist. In addition to the nodes above mentioned, sometimes called false knots, the cord on rare occasions contains one or more true knots, due to the fetus passing through a loop in the cord. If such a true knot becomes drawn very tight the child will perish from obstruction to its circulation. The cord is often coiled round the child's body or neck, but this seldom gives rise to any serious trouble. Further reference will be made to anomalies of the cord in Chapter 15.

4

The fetus

Size of the fetus

The embryo at 4 weeks is about 2 cm in diameter, and at 6 to 8 weeks 5 cm. The length of the fetus is a more reliable index of its age than its weight. In the early weeks the measurement of the fetus is commonly taken from the vertex of the head to the coccyx (crown-rump length), but from the 20th week onwards the measurement is taken from the vertex to the heels. The table shows the approximate measurements:

Table 4.1

Gestation (weeks)	Length (cm)	Weight (g)
12	Crown-rump 7	14
16	Crown-rump 12	100
20	Vertex-heel 25	300
24	Vertex-heel 30	650
28	Vertex-heel 35	1100
32	Vertex-heel 40	1700
36	Vertex-heel 45	2500
40	Vertex-heel 50	3400

A rough guide to the length of the fetus after the 20th week is to multiply the number of lunar months by five.

Other characteristics of the growing fetus are useful in determining the age:

At 8 weeks the 2.5 cm fetus lies in a much enlarged amniotic cavity, the amnion is in contact with the chorion and the extra-embryonic coelom is obliterated. The ventral stalk and yolk sac have united to form the umbilical cord which is invested by amnion, and the primitive small intestine is contained in the dilated proximal part of the cord. The facial form has been completed by the formation of the nose and its separation from the mouth. The ears are completely formed externally, and the eyelids have appeared around the eyeball. The limbs are enlarging and show their jointed appearance, and the fingers and toes are formed. The flexion of the trunk has diminished, so that the vertex of the head now

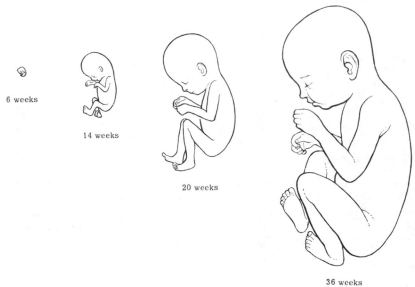

6 weeks

14 weeks

20 weeks

36 weeks

Fig. 4.1 Growth of the fetus.

forms the upper end of the embryo, rather than the back of the neck.

At 12 weeks the placenta is discoid. The amnion entirely fills the chorionic sac. The umbilical cord, still short and thick, shows a spiral twist. The primitive intestine is completely withdrawn into the body cavity. Nails have appeared on the fingers and toes, and the external sexual organs are differentiated. The crown-rump length is 7 cm, and the weight about 14 g.

At 28 weeks the fetus weighs about 1100 g. The subcutaneous fat is becoming more evident, so that the skin wrinkles begin to disappear. The testicles are in the inguinal canals. The eyelids open. At this period the fetus is said to be viable, and the law assumes that it can survive after birth, although the number of infants who survive such premature birth is small.

After this the weight of the fetus increases with comparative rapidity. The fetus becomes completely covered with vernix caseosa, a greasy substance composed of the secretion of sebaceous glands mixed with des-quamated epithelial cells. The scalp hair increases in length. Short colour-less hairs known as lanugo, which have previously appeared on the body and head, tend to disappear. The red colour of the skin changes to flesh colour owing to the thickness of subcutaneous fat. Just before the 36th week one testicle has usually descended into the scrotum. The nails reach the ends of the fingers but not of the toes.

At 40 weeks the fetus measures 50 cm and weighs as a rule between 2700 and 3600 g. The signs that the fetus has reached term are not always certain, but the length and weight are important. The nails usually project beyond the ends of the fingers and have reached the ends of the toes. The skin is pink and the lanugo has almost disappeared except over the shoulders. The whole of the intestine contains meconium. The umbilicus is almost at the centre of the body. Both testicles have descended into the scrotum. As a rule only one epiphysis has started to ossify, that at the lower end of the femur, but the centres of ossification of the upper epiphysis of the tibia and of the humerus may have appeared.

Babies weighing more than 4500 g at birth are very rare. If a baby weighs less than 2500 g at term it is probably dysmature and on this account may have a diminished chance of survival. It is different with twins; both may weigh less than 2500 g, and they tend to be born before term, and yet both are likely to survive. The heaviest children are likely to be born when the mother's age is between 25 and 35 years. The weight of the children tend to increase in successive pregnancies, provided that the mother's age is under 35. Very young mothers commonly have small babies. Male babies are heavier than females on average at birth.

Fetal circulation

The fetal circulation differs from that of the adult in several respects. Oxygen and nutriment is carried back from the placenta in the single large umbilical vein. Although there is free diffusion of oxygen across the thin barrier between the maternal and fetal circulations in the placenta, the oxygen saturation in the umbilical venous blood is already reduced from the 95 per cent level in maternal arterial blood to about 80 per cent because the active metabolism of the placenta has already used some of the oxygen. On entering the body of the fetus the vein communicates with the portal vein, so that some blood passes through the liver to the hepatic vein and inferior vena cava, but most of the oxygenated blood passes more directly through the ductus venosus to the vena cava (Fig. 4.2). In the inferior vena cava it mixes with the stream of desaturated blood returning from the lower limbs and abdominal organs, so that the oxygen saturation is reduced to less than 70 per cent by the time the blood enters the right atrium. By a remarkable anatomical arrangement most of the blood entering the right atrium from the inferior vena cava is directed through the foramen ovale into the left atrium, and from thence it passes into the left ventricle and out into the ascending aorta. By this arrangement the coronary arteries and the brain receive the most highly oxygenated blood.

Blood returning from the head and upper limbs through the superior vena cava streams towards the tricuspid valve to enter the right ventricle, taking with it a portion of the blood which has entered through the inferior vena cava. The unexpanded fetal lungs offer such high resistance to blood flow that the greater part of the right ventricular output passes from the main pulmonary artery through the widely patent ductus arteriosus into

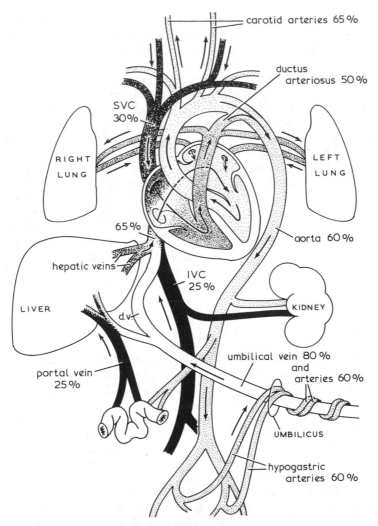

Fig. 4.2 Diagram of fetal circulation. SVC, superior vena cava; IVC, inferior vena cava; dv, ductus venosus.

the aorta to be distributed to the lower part of the body of the fetus and along the paired umbilical arteries to the placenta. The blood in the descending aorta has a saturation of about 60 per cent, which is lower than that in the ascending aorta because of the admixture of blood which has come from the ductus arteriosus.

In the fetus only 5 to 10 per cent of the total cardiac output goes directly to the lungs and returns to the left atrium via the pulmonary veins.

Although the left ventricle is pumping the most highly oxygenated blood to the brain and coronary arteries, the right ventricle is contributing more to the total cardiac output, and its wall is as thick as that of the left ventricle.

The greater part of the blood descending in the aorta leaves the body by the hypogastric (umbilical) arteries to be oxygenated in the placenta.

Changes in the circulation at birth

See p. 456.

Oxygen supply to the fetus

As the fetus grows it requires ever increasing amounts of oxygen. The placenta becomes more permeable as pregnancy proceeds, but in addition the fetal blood has the advantage of being able to take up more oxygen per unit volume than the maternal blood. This is possible because the fetal blood at term contains more haemoglobin per ml. Fetal haemoglobin, which has a different globin structure from adult haemoglobin, is formed in the liver and spleen rather than in the bone marrow. It does not itself have a higher affinity for oxygen than adult haemoglobin, although intact fetal blood does so because of the high haemoglobin concentration.

The fetal red cell count rises progressively from 1.5 million per cu mm at 10 weeks to 5.5 million at term. The cells are macrocytic, and the haemoglobin content at term is about 18 g per 100 ml. The maternal blood at term often contains less than 12 g per 100 ml.

The effect of these differences between maternal and fetal blood is that 100 ml of maternal blood can carry 16 ml of oxygen if it is fully saturated, but the same volume of fetal blood can carry 21 ml. In other words, the fetal blood can easily take up oxygen from the maternal blood. Maternal arterial blood is nearly fully saturated and carries about 15.7 ml of oxygen per 100 ml, whereas fetal blood in the ascending aorta is only about 60 per cent saturated and carries 13 ml of oxygen per 100 ml.

Nutrition of the fetus

Although the fetus is completely dependent on the maternal blood and the placenta for its nutritional requirements, it is a separate physiological entity, and it will take what it needs from the mother, even at the cost of reducing her reserves of some substances, for example calcium and iron. The details of fetal metabolism need not concern us here, except to point out that for nearly every substance the rate of fetal intake increases progressively, and is greatest in the late weeks of pregnancy.

Effect of teratogens on the fetus

A variety of agents will interfere with the development of the embryo, for example rubella virus (p. 227), drugs (p. 63) and radiation. The effect of a teratogen depends on the stage of development reached at the time of exposure. In early pregnancy abortion may occur, and major malformation may arise if the agent acts at the time of organogenesis. Minor malformations and functional defects are likely to be produced at a later stage of pregnancy.

5

Changes in maternal anatomy and physiology during pregnancy

Although the anatomical and physiological changes that occur during pregnancy chiefly involve the genital tract and the breasts, many other inter-related changes occur in other systems of the body. All these changes are initiated by hormones produced by the fetal chorionic tissue. The most important alterations in maternal physiology during pregnancy may be summarized thus:

1. *Hormonal changes.*   Placental hormones maintain the decidua, initiate the growth of the myometrium, increase the vascularity of the whole genital tract, and cause proliferation of the glandular tissue of the breasts. These hormones have other secondary effects, including the retention of water in the body, relaxation of smooth muscle especially in the urinary tract, and possibly relaxation of pelvic ligaments.

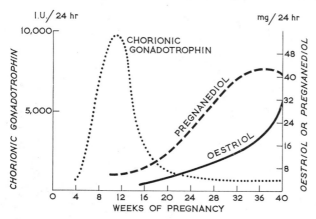

Fig. 5.1   Urinary excretion of hormones during pregnancy.

2. *Changes due to the uterine enlargement.*   The increased blood flow through the uterus, causes great changes in the maternal circulation, and the enlarged uterus alters the general posture and affects the mechanism of respiration.

3. *Metabolic changes.*   The fetal requirements of oxygen and food substances, and the growth of the uterus and preparation for lactation,

33

affect the mother's metabolism and dietary needs. We may now consider some of these changes in detail.

Endocrine system. (*a*) *Fetal hormones.* We have already described how the fetal trophoblast produces large amounts of chorionic gonadotrophin, especially in the first trimester of pregnancy (see p. 22). During pregnancy large quantities of this hormone are present in the blood and urine, and it is believed that high concentrations of this substance prolong the life span of the corpus luteum, which in turn continues to produce oestrogen and progesterone and so to maintain the uterine decidua until the output of oestrogen and progesterone from the placenta rises.

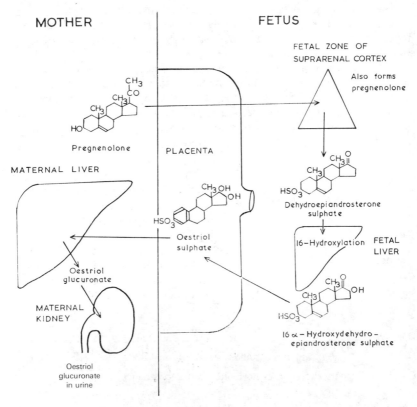

Fig. 5.2   Formation of oestriol during pregnancy.

Large amounts of oestrogens and progesterone are found in the blood and urine during pregnancy, at first secreted by the corpus luteum, but chiefly from the placenta after the 12th week. The oestrogen which appears in largest quantity in the maternal urine during pregnancy is oestriol. This is formed in the placenta from precursors which come from the fetal suprarenal cortex and liver (see Fig. 5.2), so that the urinary oestriol level is an index of both placental function and of fetal wellbeing.

The blood progesterone level rises during pregnancy, and therefore the urinary excretion of the metabolite pregnanediol increases. Even if the corpus luteum is removed in early pregnancy the hormone levels continue to rise, and it has been shown that the placenta contains large quantities of these hormones. Oestrogen and progesterone maintain the decidua of pregnancy, cause the growth and hyperaemia of the uterus and lower genital tract, and the hyperaemia and development of the breasts.

(*b*) *Other maternal endocrine changes.* During pregnancy the anterior lobe of the pituitary gland undergoes hypertrophy, with increase of both acidophil and basophil cells. No anatomical changes are evident in the posterior lobe of the pituitary gland.

The thyroid gland is slightly enlarged during pregnancy, and the basal metabolic rate is increased.

There is an increased concentration of adrenal glucocorticoid hormones in both the blood and the urine, and there is some evidence that the placenta secretes an adrenocorticotrophic substance, which may explain the eosinophilia which occurs during pregnancy. The observation that rheumatoid arthritis often undergoes a remission during pregnancy may be explained by the increased secretion of glucocorticoids. There is also some increase in the excretion of mineralocorticoids (aldosterone).

Uterus. During pregnancy the uterus is adapted to contain the growing fetus and placenta, and it also undergoes changes in preparation for its task of expelling the fetus during labour. The changes include development of the decidua, hypertrophy of the muscle coat, increased vascularity, formation of the lower segment and softening of the cervix.

At term the uterus is about 35 cm long and 23 cm in diameter. It weighs 1 kg, in contrast to the non-pregnant uterus which weighs 65 g. The pregnant uterus is usually slightly rotated on its long axis, so that the anterior surface faces a little to the right, and the fundus may also be inclined to one or other side, most often the right. At term the main axis of the cavity of the uterus is at a right angle to the plane of the pelvic brim. The enlargement of the uterus is greatest at the fundus, so that the points of entry of the Fallopian tubes appear to lie well below the top of the uterus.

The enormous growth of the myometrium during pregnancy is due to two factors—hormonal stimulation and distension. During early pregnancy the embryo does not fill the uterine cavity, and distension has no influence at this stage. An identical uterine enlargement occurs in cases of ectopic pregnancy when the embryo is outside the uterus. The growth is brought about by the action of oestrogen and progesterone. Later on, as the fetus and placenta become larger, the distension of the uterus provides a further stimulus to growth.

In early pregnancy active mitosis can be seen in the connective tissue and muscle cells, and the enlargement of the uterus is largely due to an increase in the number of cells. Later in pregnancy the enlargement is chiefly due to hypertrophy of the individual cells, and cell division is less active. At term each muscle cell is about ten times as long as it was before pregnancy. The blood supply to the uterus is greatly increased, and especially under the placental site the veins become converted to large sinuses, thicker than a pencil. Section of the nerve supply to the uterus has no effect on the growth of the uterus in pregnancy.

At the 12th week of pregnancy the body of the uterus is roughly spherical. Examination of the uterus at this stage will show that the lowest part of the body of the uterus, the part just above the internal os, forms a short narrow canal, sometimes termed the isthmus. At first the isthmus does not contain any part of the embryo, but as pregnancy proceeds the isthmus becomes stretched, and the embryo comes to occupy this part of the body of the uterus as well as the main cavity. The isthmus thus forms the *lower uterine segment,* and this is the part of the body of the uterus which will be stretched during labour by the more powerful contractions of the upper segment. In many cases the formation of the lower segment begins in late pregnancy and before labour starts, and at this stage the lower part of the uterine cavity has the form of a half sphere, with the internal os at its lowest point. During labour this half sphere will be converted into a cylinder which is continuous with the cervical canal. In most cases the lower segment is represented by that part of the uterus at term which is within a radius of 7.5 cm from the internal os, but it must be recognized that the distinction between the upper and lower uterine segments is physiological, rather than one that is capable of precise anatomical definition.

At term the wall of the uterus appears thin in relation to the enormous enlargement of the cavity, but in fact it is still about 1 cm thick. In late pregnancy it is possible to define three layers in the muscular wall of the uterus:

1. There is a thin outer layer of fibres that arch over the fundus. These are continuous laterally with the muscle of the round ligaments.
2. There is a thick intermediate layer, consisting of a meshwork of interlacing fibres, which pass around the blood vessels. The contraction of this layer will stop the blood flow in the vessels, and it is the strong contraction of this layer which prevents dangerous haemorrhage from the large placental sinuses in the third stage of labour.
3. The inner layer is thin, and arranged in a circular fashion, especially around the internal os and around the tubal openings.

During pregnancy the uterus contracts from time to time (Braxton Hicks contractions), and contractions can be stimulated by handling the uterus. The contractions are not so strong or so sustained as those of labour, and are painless.

The peritoneal coat grows to keep pace with the enlargement of the uterus. It preserves its usual relations to the uterus in front and behind, but at the sides the gradual distension of the lower segment has the effect of separating the layers of the lowest part of the broad ligament, so that its level is raised and a larger area at the side of the uterus is uncovered by peritoneum than in the non-pregnant organ.

The ovarian and uterine arteries and veins are greatly enlarged, and the latter become straighter in their course up the side of the uterus.

Cervix. Although the cervix hypertrophies to some extent during pregnancy, it does not do so to anything like the same extent as the body of the uterus. Three important changes occur in it, namely, hypertrophy of the glands of the cervical canal, softening of the cervix, and bluish colouration. Softening of the cervix begins in the early weeks, but its degree varies. It is due to increased vascularity and to a great increase in the gland spaces. The glands are distended with mucus, and the pattern of the glands becomes far more complex, so that the cervix seems to contain a honeycomb filled with mucus. This is sometimes described as a mucus plug, but the mucus is in the gland spaces, not free. The bluish colour is due to venous congestion, and appears earlier than the similar appearance in the vagina.

The cervical canal is normally still present at the end of pregnancy, although in many multiparae the external os is patulous. An intact and effective internal os is of importance in retaining the embryo safely; with an incompetent cervix there is a considerable risk of abortion, or of premature rupture of the membranes.

Because of the great activity of the columnar epithelium of the cervix, and the increased secretion of mucus, it is common for the stratified epithelium on the vaginal surface of the cervix to be replaced by an outward extension of the columnar epithelium—one type of cervical erosion. Such an appearance is not to be regarded as abnormal during pregnancy, and it will usually disappear in the puerperium.

Vagina and vulva. The increased vascularity already described in the cervix affects the vaginal walls a little later, and they eventually show the violet coloration right down to the vulva. The vaginal walls become softened and relaxed, and the same change occurs in the perineal body.

The watery transudation that normally occurs through the vaginal wall is increased during pregnancy. The hypertrophied cervical glands secrete more mucus, and this is added to the vaginal transudate and desquamated vaginal cells, so that the total discharge from the vagina is increased. The vaginal secretion is acid in reaction (pH 4.5 to 5) and is some protection against ascending infection.

Under the influence of placental hormones the vaginal epithelium is very active, and the desquamated cells often have their lateral edges rolled over, so that they appear boat-shaped (navicular cells), and these cells are usually clumped together. This normal epithelial activity should not be mistaken for carcinoma *in situ*.

As pregnancy advances the vulva shares in the increased vascularity, and shows some swelling in consequence. The violet colour is seen on the moist surfaces around the urethra and inner parts of the labia minora, and varicose veins may appear.

Breasts. During pregnancy the secretion of oestrogen in large amounts causes activity and thickening of the skin of the nipple, and active growth and branching of the underlying ducts. The added action of progesterone causes further hyperaemia, and proliferation of the glandular epithelium of the alveoli. Neither of these hormones causes the active secretion of milk, which only begins after delivery, when the level of oestrogen falls and prolactin from the anterior lobe of the pituitary gland causes secretion. (See p. 473.)

Slight changes in the breasts occur in the menstrual cycle, under the influence of oestrogen and progesterone, and the breasts may become tense and uncomfortable for a few days before the onset of the period. If pregnancy occurs these changes are more marked. The earliest change is a swelling of the breasts, especially at the periphery. The lobules of the gland can be felt easily and are harder than normal, these changes producing a knotty feeling in the breast. At the same time the breasts become a little tender, and the patient often describes a 'prickly' sensation in them. The increased blood-supply is shown by a very obvious network of veins under the skin. As a result of congestion, followed by actual growth of the glandular tissue, the breasts become more prominent. Plethysmographic studies have shown that each breast may increase in volume by about 200 ml, an increase of about one-third.

By about the 12th week of pregnancy the glands begin to secrete an almost clear fluid, which will appear in droplets if the breast is squeezed towards the nipple. Towards the end of pregnancy the secretion becomes more copious and is yellow in colour and creamy in consistence. It is then known as colostrum, and consists of water, fat, albumin, salts and colostrum corpuscles. The latter are cells shed whole from the gland acini, and filled with fat droplets. When the milk secretion is eventually established colostrum corpuscles are not found in it, because the fat is discharged from the secreting cells into the lumina of the acini, and the cells themselves are not detached.

Changes also occur in the nipple, which becomes larger and more readily erectile. The areolar skin is active and slightly raised above the surrounding skin. The areola becomes pigmented to a greater or lesser degree, the change being most marked in brunettes. Once the pigmentation has occurred it persists as a permanent change. The sebaceous glands on the areola are very active in pregnancy, and can be seen as a ring of about 12 to 20 small tubercles (Montgomery's tubercles).

At about the 20th week of pregnancy, in dark skinned women, further pigmentation may occur on the skin beyond the margin of the areola. This is termed the secondary areola, and is not a uniform pigmentation, but takes the form of patchy streaks. The secondary areola is not a permanent change, and it disappears after pregnancy.

The stretching of the skin over the breasts may produce striae like those which occur on the abdomen.

Sometimes outlying lobules of mammary tissue are found in the axillae; they enlarge during pregnancy and may form comparatively large swellings. Such breast tissue has inadequate drainage to the main duct system, and so may become tense and painful when lactation begins.

Abdominal wall. The muscles of the abdominal wall become stretched to accommodate the enlarging uterus, and although in perfect health subsequent recovery is complete, in not a few multiparae some loss of tone of these muscles persists. In late pregnancy the umbilicus may be flattened out, or even protrude.

Stretching of the abdominal skin may cause the formation of striae gravidarum. These are due to rupture of the elastic fibres of the skin, and they appear as curved lines, roughly concentric with the umbilicus, which may extend to the loins or thighs, and may sometimes occur on the breasts. At first the striae are pink or red, but after delivery they become silvery-white, and are then called lineae albicantes. After the first pregnancy the striae are apt to become pigmented in any subsequent pregnancy. Not all women develop striae; perhaps one-third do not. It is unusual to see striae in other conditions in which the abdominal wall is stretched, such as large ovarian cysts, ascites or gross obesity. The fact that they are frequently seen in Cushing's syndrome, when there is a high level of glucocorticoids in the blood, as there is in pregnancy, has led to the suggestion that the striae are partly due to the action of these hormones.

Pigmentation of the line from the pubes to the umbilicus (the linea nigra) may be seen in dark-skinned women during pregnancy, and tends to persist in part after the pregnancy.

Pelvic joints. The pelvic hyperaemia causes some softening and slight relaxation of the ligaments of the sacroiliac joints, and of the ligaments and fibrocartilage of the symphysis pubis, and the mobility at these joints is slightly increased in pregnancy. In some animals a specific hormone relaxin, derived from the ovary, or in some species from the placenta, causes relaxation of the pelvic joints, but it is uncertain whether such a hormone plays any part in human physiology.

The changes so far described have mostly been those directly related to the genital tract and the breasts. Numerous other changes occur in the rest of the body, and nearly every system is involved in some change. Yet pregnancy is a physiological and not a pathological process, and many women both feel and appear to be in better general health during pregnancy than at other times. Given good previous nutrition and sound emotional adjustment, the physiological changes of pregnancy are not to be regarded as a strain on the mother's health, but merely as a temporary adaptation to a normal activity.

Maternal metabolism during pregnancy. *Weight gain.* The body weight increases during pregnancy. The total gain varies between 7 and 17 kg in normal cases, with an average of 12 kg. After the 12th week the average normal gain is about 0.5 kg per week.

A fetus weighing 3.5 kg, a placenta of 0.5 kg, amniotic fluid weighing 0.5 kg, a uterus of 1 kg, and an increase in the weight of the breasts of about 1 kg would account for a total gain of 6.5 kg. The average additional gain of 5.5 kg represents the weight gained by the rest of the maternal tissues, and this is partly due to fluid retention (1.5 kg), and partly due to increase in the body fat and protein.

During pregnancy, apart from the fluid retained in the fetal tissues, there is some retention of fluid in the maternal tissues, chiefly in the extracellular components, including the blood plasma (see below). Corresponding quantities of sodium are retained, and at present it is believed that this retention of salt and water is due to the high concentrations of sex steroids during pregnancy, although the part played by mineralocorticoids has not yet been fully determined.

Metabolic changes. The basal metabolic rate during pregnancy is increased by between 10 and 25 per cent, but if allowance is made for the metabolism of the fetus and its supporting tissues the basal metabolic rate of the maternal tissues is probably unaltered.

The need for calories during pregnancy is increased, but not always to the degree that the patient's appetite may suggest. Apart from fluid retention in cases of pre-eclampsia, abnormal weight gain during pregnancy and the puerperium is often due to simple overeating, chiefly by an excessive intake of carbohydrate.

During pregnancy the renal threshold for the excretion of sugar from the blood is often lowered, so that glucose may appear in the urine although the blood sugar level is normal. This condition is of no importance but it must be distinguished from diabetes, by a blood-sugar curve if necessary (see p. 224). The escape of sugar is probably the result of increased glomerular filtration, which allows so much glucose to enter the tubules that they are unable to absorb it all. Lactose may appear in the urine during lactation, but is not found during pregnancy.

A high protein intake is required to supply the growing fetus, placenta, uterus and breasts. Yet during pregnancy, in spite of an increased excretion of amino acids, large quantities of nitrogen are retained, over and above the amounts required for these structures.

There are also changes in lipid metabolism during pregnancy. Plasma levels of triglycerides, cholesterol and free fatty acids rise, and there is a greater tendency to ketosis.

The maternal diet must not only supply the protein, carbohydrate and fat required, but also the essential minerals and vitamins. An ordinary diet provides adequate amounts of most of these substances, but in the case of iron and calcium there is some risk of a deficit, particularly during the last trimester when the fetal uptake is greatest. The fetal body at term contains about 25 g of calcium, but even with this large demand a mother taking a first class diet will increase her calcium reserve during pregnancy. However, with a less favourable diet there may be a deficiency in late pregnancy whch leads to decalcification of the maternal bones and dentine. Recalcification quickly occurs after lactation has been completed if the diet contains adequate calcium.

In the case of iron only about 1.2 mg is usually assimilated daily, an amount insufficient to meet the fetal needs, especially in late pregnancy. In addition the mother forms additional red cells during pregnancy. The blood volume is increased, and although the amount of haemoglobin per millilitre may be reduced, the increase in blood volume outweighs this, so that the total amount of haemoglobin in the maternal body is increased. Even in health, and with a normal diet, the maternal iron reserves in the liver, spleen and marrow may therefore be reduced during pregnancy. Not all the iron so used is lost; apart from the iron in the fetal tissues and blood, and the maternal blood lost at delivery, the iron built up into additional maternal red cells during pregnancy is later returned to her reserves.

Some figures may illustrate these facts. There are about 2400 mg of iron in the form of haemoglobin in the red cells, and there is also a reserve of 1000 mg in the form of transferrin and haemosiderin in the liver, spleen and bone marrow. The fetus and placenta require about 450 mg, and blood loss at delivery and in the milk during lactation accounts for about 300 mg. About 0.5 mg is excreted daily throughout pregnancy. The absorption of iron during pregnancy and lactation must therefore be about 890 mg, or 3 mg daily. As daily absorption is probably less than 1.5 mg even with an iron supplement to the diet, it is likely that the iron stores will be drawn upon, and iron should also be given for some weeks after delivery.

Changes in the blood during pregnancy. The total blood volume is increased during pregnancy by about 30 per cent. The uterus and the maternal blood spaces in the placenta contain a large volume of blood, perhaps 800 ml. The increase in blood volume is an adaptation to supply the needs of the new vascular bed. Although the total number and volume of red cells increase by about 20 per cent, the plasma volume increases by about 50 per cent, with the result that the blood becomes more dilute and the red cell count and the haemoglobin concentration fall. A red cell count of 4 million per cu. mm and a haemoglobin concentration of 11 g per 100 ml are usually accepted as normal during pregnancy. Although such levels are commonly observed in completely healthy women in pregnancy, if supplemental iron is given in a form that is well absorbed then in many of these women the red cell count and haemoglobin concentration remain higher. The question which is still by no means decided is whether this gives any additional benefit. However, many women have poor iron reserves and inadequate diets, and for them iron supplements are essential (see pp. 212–3).

A very high leucocytosis is often observed during labour and the early puerperium, but not during normal pregnancy, when the count does not exceed 11,000 per cubic millimetre. The platelet count is normal. The erythrocyte sedimentation rate is much increased during normal pregnancy. Readings of up to 100 mm per hour are not unusual without any detectable abnormality.

Changes in the circulation during pregnancy. The cardiac output rises considerably during pregnancy, usually rising by about 30 per cent by the 34th week, and it remains at or above this level until after delivery. It was previously believed that the cardiac output fell at the 36th week, and if observations are made on patients lying in the dorsal position this may appear to be the case, because the large uterus obstructs the venous return. If the same patients are turned over onto their sides the cardiac output will be found to remain elevated in late pregnancy. Because of this interference with the venous return a few women complain of faintness when they lie on their backs in late pregnancy (supine hypotensive syndrome).

The blood pressure does not rise during normal pregnancy—indeed it falls slightly during the second trimester—and the pulse rate rises only slightly, so that the greatly increased cardiac output must be achieved by the expulsion of an increased volume of blood from the heart at each beat. This extra cardiac work is well within the reserve of the normal heart. The heart is displaced upward in late pregnancy and the apex is rotated outward, so that the apex beat is displaced outward and the electrical axis is altered. There may be slight left axis deviation and inversion of the T-wave in an electrocardiograph, but there is little evidence of muscular hypertrophy.

The large blood flow through the uterus may be regarded as an arteriovenous shunt across the main circulation, and the increase in cardiac output and in the blood volume may be related to this. In addition there is increased renal blood flow and some dilatation of peripheral vessels. The hands and feet are often noticeably warm during pregnancy, and the skin capillaries are dilated.

The enlarged uterus interferes with the venous return from the legs, so that there is stasis in the large veins and slight oedema of the ankles may occur, even in normal cases. Haemorrhoids or varicose veins may appear for the first time or become worse during pregnancy.

Changes in the respiratory system during pregnancy. Pulmonary ventilation is increased by about 40 per cent, as a result of increased tidal volume. This is probably an effect of progesterone on the respiratory system. Oxygen requirements only increase by 20 per cent, and this over-breathing leads to a fall in PCO_2. The low PCO_2 gives rise to a sensation of dyspnoea, which may be accentuated by elevation of the diaphragm. When the fetal head engages in the pelvis in late pregnancy the breathlessness diminishes.

Changes in the alimentary tract during pregnancy. The most striking change in the digestive function in pregnancy is nausea or morning sickness, which occurs in greater or less degree in about a third of pregnancies. As a rule it begins at the 6th week and stops spontaneously before the 14th week. Although it is generally limited to the early morning it may occur at other times of the day. Usually the symptoms are slight; excessive or prolonged vomiting is certainly pathological. The cause is uncertain. The most acceptable of the many theories that have been brought forward is that it is related to the high levels of chorionic gonadotrophin in the blood during early pregnancy. The fact that morning sickness, or at least nausea, occurs in so many pregnant women, and only troubles them in the morning, are obvious objections to the view that it is entirely of psychological origin. On the other hand, cases of excessive vomiting are often neurotic. See also p. 61 for further discussion and description of the treatment.

As a rule the appetite is good during pregnancy, but minor digestive upsets are common, probably due to the relaxant effect of progesterone on smooth muscle. Sometimes gastric or intestinal distension occurs, and especially in early pregnancy this causes a feeling of abdominal enlargement. Heartburn is a common complaint, and is caused by relaxation of the cardiac sphincter of the stomach. In a few of the more severe cases this symptom is caused by a hiatus hernia (p. 230). The emptying time of the stomach is prolonged during pregnancy, and even more so during labour (a fact of considerable importance in relation to the risk of vomiting during anaesthesia). The gastric acidity is often reduced, and peptic ulcers almost invariably become quiescent during pregnancy.

Constipation is not uncommon, and this, together with the pelvic hyperaemia and pressure of the enlarged uterus, may lead to the formation or increase in size of haemorrhoids.

Changes in the urinary tract during pregnancy. Frequency of micturition occurs during the first 12 weeks, when the enlarging uterus is still in the pelvic cavity and rests on the bladder. It may also occur in the last month of pregnancy when the presenting part of the fetus is engaging in the pelvis.

From about the 16th week of pregnancy onwards there is considerable and progressive dilatation of the renal pelvis and of the ureters down as far as the level of the pelvic brim. Direct measurement of the intra-ureteric pressure shows that it is lowered rather than raised, and the dilatation is chiefly caused by loss of muscle tone, although pressure from the uterus may explain the greater degree of change which is usually seen on the right side. These changes are important in relation to pyelonephritis during pregnancy (see p. 205). The dilatation disappears during the puerperium, so long as there is no infection of the tract. They are thought to be caused by progesterone.

Changes in the skin during pregnancy.   The striae gravidarum and linea nigra of the abdomen, and the primary and secondary areolae of the breast have already been mentioned. Pigmentation also occurs on the face, mainly as irregularly shaped brown patches on the forehead or cheeks, known as the chloasma or mask of pregnancy. These patches completely disappear after pregnancy. The cause of these changes is unknown, but may be related to adrenal hormones or an increase in melanocyte stimulating hormone.

Emotional changes during pregnancy.   See Chapter 40, p. 438.

Changes in immune reactivity.   The fetus carries antigens derived from the father, and is therefore an allograft which is foreign to the mother. It might be expected that the mother's immune system would reject the fetus. The protection of the fetus from immunological rejection is far from fully understood, but it seems likely that immune tolerance develops because of depression of maternal T-lymphocyte formation. It may be that some abortions and congenital defects are caused by a breakdown of this system, with consequent rejection. It is of interest that many diseases which are thought to have an auto-immune basis tend to remission during pregnancy.

6

Clinical signs and diagnosis of pregnancy

The duration of pregnancy. In cases in which pregnancy has followed a single coitus the average duration of pregnancy from the date of intercourse is 266 days. If the calculation is made from the first day of the last menstrual period the average duration is 280 days, and these observations support the belief that ovulation most frequently occurs on the 14th day of a 28 day menstrual cycle. However, there is considerable variation in the duration of normal pregnancy, even in cases in which the menstrual cycles were previously regular and of normal length, and also in cases in which the date of a single coitus is known. The method of estimating the most likely day of delivery is discussed on p. 52.

Symptoms of pregnancy

Amenorrhoea. Amenorrhoea is the earliest symptom of pregnancy. In a healthy woman whose menstrual periods were previously regular, if there is a sudden cessation of the periods the presumption must always be that she is pregnant unless some other cause for the amenorrhoea can be found. Amenorrhoea has not the same significance in the case of a woman whose periods were previously irregular, nor may it have any significance in a woman of menopausal age. Pregnancy has been known to occur in a young girl before a menstrual period has been observed, and it may arise during a period of amenorrhoea, for example during lactation or following discontinuation of oral contraception.

Difficulty may also arise if there is bleeding during early pregnancy. Such bleeding may come from the cavity of the uterus before the decidua capsularis fuses with the decidua vera, but it is not to be regarded as menstrual bleeding. Although a pregnancy with slight bleeding in the early weeks may prove to be completely normal, such bleeding should always be viewed as a threat to miscarry.

Morning sickness. This may start as early as the first missed period. See p. 61.

Breast symptoms. In the early weeks of pregnancy some tenderness and fullness of the breasts may be noticed.

Frequency of micturition. During the first 12 weeks, when the

45

uterus is still a pelvic organ, there is often some frequency of micturition, because the enlarging uterus presses on the bladder slightly, particularly in the daytime when the woman is standing.

Abdominal enlargement.   Many women notice some abdominal fullness in early pregnancy at a time when the uterus is not much enlarged. This can only be the result of slight intestinal distention. Later on the uterine enlargement becomes evident, and sometimes it is this that first brings the patient to the doctor, especially in a case in which the menstrual periods were previously irregular. On the other hand, a woman sometimes thinks that she is pregnant because of abdominal swelling from some other cause, such as fat or an ovarian cyst.

Quickening.   A primigravida usually first feels fetal movements between the 18th and 20th weeks of pregnancy, but multiparae may recognize the movements about 2 weeks earlier. At first the movements are slight, and may be confused with movement of wind in the intestine. This very subjective symptom is not of much value in the diagnosis of pregnancy, as a woman who believes that she is pregnant will commonly declare that she feels movements.

Signs of pregnancy

It will be seen that it is not possible to make a certain diagnosis of pregnancy from any of the symptoms given above, although a combination of them may be highly suggestive. The clinical diagnosis of pregnancy, especially in the first half, depends on a combination of symptoms and signs, and in every case an examination to seek confirmatory physical signs is required. Only when the pregnancy has advanced far enough for the parts of the fetus to be recognized clearly, for fetal movements to be palpable, or the fetal heart sounds to be heard, can the physical signs be said to be absolute.

Although radiological demonstration of the fetal skeleton is also an absolute sign of pregnancy this method is no longer used if the fetus is possibly alive because of the hazard of radiation to the fetus. Ultrasonic examination, either to show fetal parts or fetal heart movements, has taken its place (p. 111).

Signs due to changes in the uterus.   The earliest alteration in the uterus that can be detected is slight *enlargement of the body of the uterus*, but it is difficult to be certain of this if the patient has had a previous pregnancy. On bimanual examination the body is felt to be globular, and as progressive enlargement occurs the diagnosis becomes more evident.

Softening of the uterus due to its increased vascularity is a useful sign, for although there are many other causes for uterine enlargement they do not as a rule cause softening. The lowest part of the body of the uterus softens first, and because of this on bimanual examination the globular fundus may feel distinct from the still unsoftened cervix until about the 9th week of pregnancy (Hegar's sign). Deliberate attempts to elicit this sign should not be made, as they may well cause bleeding and even miscarriage.

Softening and blue discolouration of the cervix soon follow, and are usually complete by the 16th week. When these changes are marked they are reliable signs of pregnancy, but in a few cases the cervix remains firm during pregnancy.

By the 12th week the fundus of the uterus is palpable in the abdomen just above the symphysis pubis, and *progressive enlargement of the uterus* follows. (Fig. 6.1.) The fundus reaches the level of the umbilicus at about the 22nd week, and is just below the ensiform cartilage at the 36th week. If the presenting part of the fetus then sinks into the pelvis the fundus descends slightly, so that at term it is again at the level it occupied at the 34th week. The level of the fundus may be higher than expected from the duration of the pregnancy in cases of multiple pregnancy or hydramnios; and at a lower level than expected with an abnormal, growth-retarded or dead fetus.

The pregnant uterus varies in consistency on palpation because it has intermittent *painless contractions*. If the patient is easy to examine these may be felt even when the uterus is still in the pelvis. When the uterus rises up into the abdomen the contractions are more easily felt, and are reliable evidence that any swelling under examination is in fact the uterus.

Because the blood flow through the vessels in the broad ligament is greatly increased during pregnancy, on auscultation with a stethoscope pressed firmly against the side of the uterus the *uterine souffle* may be heard at any time after the 20th week. It is a blowing murmur, synchronous with the maternal pulse. It is not diagnostic of pregnancy, as it may also be heard with some large uterine fibromyomata.

Signs due to the presence of the fetus. From the 16th week until about the 30th week the sign known as *ballottement* may occasionally be observed. It depends upon the fact that at this stage of pregnancy the fetus is floating in a relatively large amount of liquor amnii. Internal ballottement is felt on vaginal examination. A finger is placed in the anterior fornix with the patient lying on her back. If the fetus can be felt it is pushed upward when it will be felt to float away and then fall back on the finger. External ballottement is elicited on abdominal examination of a breech presentation, when the head may be felt to move between the two hands placed on either side of the fundus of the uterus.

Abdominal *palpation of fetal parts* is usually possible from the 24th week onwards, and at a later stage the definite recognition of the head, back and limbs of the fetus is an absolute sign of pregnancy. During palpation *fetal movements* may be felt, and this is also an absolute sign. In a thin patient the movements can often be seen as well.

On auscultation of the abdomen with the fetal stethoscope the *fetal heart sounds* may be heard after the 24th week. The fetal heart rate varies be-

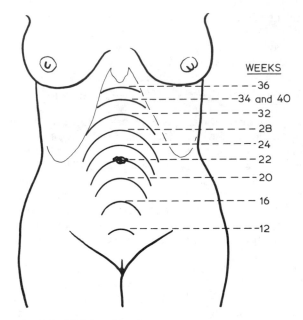

Fig. 6.1   Height of fundus.

tween 120 and 160 beats per minute, and is therefore at roughly double the rate of the maternal pulse. The sounds are described as resembling the ticking of a watch under a pillow; there is a double sound to each beat, but more equal than the maternal double beat, and at a different pitch.

Fetal heart movements can be detected at a much earlier stage of pregnancy, even from the 10th week, with *ultrasound* (see p. 50), and this is now part of routine clinical examination, using a small portable apparatus.

The *funic souffle* is occasionally heard if the fetal stethoscope happens to lie directly over the umbilical cord as a soft blowing murmur synchronous with the fetal heart sounds.

Signs due to changes in the breasts and the skin.   Some of these have already been described (pp. 38 – 9) but they may be summarized here. The earliest sign is due to proliferation of the peripheral lobules of the breast, which may give rise to a knotty feeling at the edge of the gland. Pigmentation of the areola of the nipple occurs as early as the 8th week, but may be very slight in fair women. This *primary areola* persists after the first pregnancy, so that the sign is useless in the diagnosis of any subsequent pregnancy. The sebaceous glands around the areola become enlarged to form a ring of small tubercles (*Montgomery's tubercles*) and the subcutaneous veins over the breast become more evident.

By the 12th week a clear secretion can be expressed from the nipple, but this sign too is only of value in a first pregnancy, as secretion can often be expressed from the breast of any patient who has once been pregnant, even when she is not again pregnant.

In a second or subsequent pregnancy only one change in the breast is absolutely diagnostic, and that is the *secondary areola*, which is patchy pigmentation of the skin outside the primary areola. This only occurs in dark skinned women, and after the 20th week. It fades during the puerperium.

The appearance of *striae on the abdomen* and the *linea nigra* (p. 39) are also only helpful in the diagnosis of a first pregnancy, as they tend to persist afterwards. In a subsequent pregnancy striae may become freshly pigmented.

Diagnosis by detection of chorionic gonadotrophin

Various tests depend on the fact that during pregnancy the trophoblast of the embryo secretes large quantities of gonadotrophic hormone, which is found in maternal serum and excreted in maternal urine.

Tests performed on maternal urine. The most certain results are obtained if the urine is concentrated, and for that reason it is best to test the first morning specimen.

Immunological tests. Essentially these tests consist of two steps: (1) the addition of antibody against chorionic gonadotrophin (anti-HCG) to the urine to be tested and (2) the use of an indicator to see whether a reaction has occurred. If the patient is pregnant her urine will contain HCG. When anti-HCG is added to the urine it combines with the HCG and is neutralized. The mixture is now tested for anti-HCG and if none is found the test is positive for pregnancy.

If the patient is not pregnant, the urine does not contain HCG and the anti-HCG remains unfixed and will react with the indicator. A change in the indicator shows that the patient is *not* pregnant.

The anti-HCG is obtained from rabbits or sheep which have been immunized against HCG. Various indicators have been used, including HCG-coated latex particles or HCG-coated red blood cells. If the patient is not pregnant the latex particles are precipitated or the red cells are agglutinated. The following Table 6.1 illustrates this:

Table 6.1

Pregnant	*Not pregnant*
Urine contains HCG	Urine contains no HCG
Add antiserum containing HCG antibodies	
HCG antibodies neutralized	HCG antibodies not neutralized
Add latex particles coated with HCG	
No flocculation	Flocculation

Radioimmunoassay for HCG can now be performed on urine as well as blood (see below).

The urinary output of gonadotrophin during pregnancy rises rapidly to reach a peak at about 12 weeks and then falls again to a much lower level (Fig. 5.1). Tests for urinary gonadotrophins are unlikely to be positive for 7 to 10 days after the missed period, and the tests may give weak or even negative results after the 16th week, but by then clinical diagnosis is easier.

Tests performed on maternal serum.   *Radioimmunoassay* may be used to detect HCG or its β subunit. Pregnancy may be diagnosed 9 to 12 days after conception and before a period has been missed, but these tests require expensive reagents and laboratory equipment and are not used routinely. The β subunit assay is more accurate because HCG may cross-react with luteinizing hormone to give a false positive result.

Laboratory tests for pregnancy are used when it is important to make an early diagnosis of pregnancy for either medical or social reasons. In addition to the risk of false positive reactions from cross-reactions with LH, error may also arise in the climacteric when the tests may reflect the rising levels of pituitary gonadotrophin which may occur at that time. In the diagnosis of vesicular mole or choriocarcinoma urine tests can be used quantitatively by performing them in serial dilutions of urine and noting the dilution (e.g. 1:200) at which the test becomes negative, but the more accurate methods of radioimmunoassay of serum are now preferred for these cases. High titres will also be obtained in cases of multiple pregnancy. The test is sometimes of assistance in the diagnosis of ectopic pregnancy, but if the embryo has been killed by the haemorrhage the result may be negative. The test is weakly positive in some cases of missed abortion.

Ultrasonic diagnosis of pregnancy

By the use of B scan (p. 111) to demonstrate the gestation sac pregnancy can often be diagnosed as early as 6 weeks from the first day of the last menstrual period, and by 7 or 8 weeks echoes representing the fetus within the sac can be obtained. With combined A and B scan pulsation of the fetal heart may be detected at this time. While ultrasound apparatus used for these observations may cost thousands of pounds much simpler, cheaper and easily portable machines (e.g. Sonicaid, Doptone) are available which employ a different principle. Ultrasonic waves are emitted by the head of the machine, which is placed against the skin of the abdomen. If the waves strike a moving surface, such as flowing blood, the reflected waves have an altered wave-length according to the Doppler principle. The alteration is detected by the apparatus, and in the case of the fetal heart the rhythmic changes in wave-length are converted into audible signals, which are surprisingly similar to the fetal heart sounds. Blood flowing in any large maternal vessel will give the same effect, but the characteristic rate of the fetal heart makes the source of the signals clear. With these machines the fetal heart beat can be recognized at the 10th week and occasionally earlier.

Differential diagnosis of pregnancy

The pregnant uterus has to be distinguished from other abdomino-pelvic swellings, of which the commonest are fibromyomata, ovarian cysts and a distended bladder. Pregnancy may also be associated with these.

Ovarian cysts. In many cases on bimanual palpation the unenlarged uterus can be felt separately from the ovarian cyst. Ovarian neoplasms will not cause amenorrhoea except in the unlikely event of their being bilateral and totally destroying both ovaries. A thrill or fluctuation is common with ovarian cysts, but is only felt in the pregnant uterus in cases of hydramnios. There is no clinical evidence of the presence of a fetus, and the pregnancy test is negative. Ultrasonic examination will show the cyst wall and absence of fetal parts.

Uterine fibromyomata. When these tumours are deeply placed in the uterus they may enlarge it symetrically, and they are sometimes soft enough to stimulate the consistency of the pregnant uterus. However they do not cause amenorrhoea and pregnancy tests are negative.

Distended bladder. The bladder may become distended and then mistaken for the uterus if there is retention of urine from incarceration of a retroverted gravid uterus (p. 240). The direction of the cervix and the passage of a catheter disclose the diagnosis.

Pregnancy associated with an ovarian cyst. Two swellings are usually evident, the pregnant uterus presenting its usual characters in accordance with the duration of the pregnancy and the cyst, but in some cases they are in such close juxtaposition that it is not easy to distinguish two swellings. The combined swelling will then be larger than expected for the duration of pregnancy. Ultrasonic scan will reveal the fetus within the uterus and the cyst as a separate cavity.

Pregnancy associated with fibromyomata. It can sometimes be difficult to diagnose pregnancy in a uterus with multiple fibromyomata. Pregnancy tests and ultrasonic examination will be of value in early pregnancy. Later on small tumours can easily be mistaken for fetal parts. A fibromyoma in the uterine wall is immobile, unlike a fetal limb which alters its position from time to time. When the uterus contracts fetal parts become more difficult to feel, whereas a fibromyoma may become more evident. A fibromyoma in the pelvis may even be mistaken for the fetal head.

Pseudocyesis

Pseudocyesis is a psychological disorder in which the patient has a false but fixed idea that she is pregnant. The term does not include the uncommon instances of wilful and conscious deception; the patient honestly believes that she is pregnant. Pregnancy fantasies may occur with other delusions in psychoses, but most patients with pseudocyesis do not have serious mental illness.

It is frequently, but not always, seen near or after the menopause, and not invariably in patients without children. There may be amenorrhoea, and the patient may declare that she has morning sickness and breast enlargement, and that she can feel fetal movements. The abdomen may appear distended, either by air collected in the stomach by aerophagy, by intestinal distention, by persistent contraction of the diaphragm with exaggerated lumbar lordosis, or sometimes just by fat. The shape of the swelling is not that of the pregnant uterus, and fetal parts cannot be felt nor the fetal heart heard. If the patient is fat a pregnancy test, ultrasonic scan or even an x-ray examination may be justified. The difficulty is to convince the patient that she is not pregnant.

Estimation of the expected date of delivery and assessment of maturity

Since there is no exact means of knowing the time at which conception occurred, it is usual and convenient to calculate the date on which delivery is to be expected from the first day of the last menstrual cycle, with the assumption that ovulation took place about 14 days after that. A simple practical method is to count forward 9 calendar months (or backward 3 months) from the first day of the last period, and to add 7 days. This gives an average of 280 days, with a little variation as the lengths of the calendar months are not uniform. If the previous menstrual cycles were irregular or prolonged no reliance can be put on this method. Even if the previous cycles were regular, in as many as 40 per cent of cases labour begins more than 7 days before or after the calculated date.

An attempt has often to be made to estimate the probable date of delivery or the maturity of the gestation when the date of the last menstrual period has been forgotten, or when conception occurred during a phase of amenorrhoea, for example during lactation or when conception took place soon after discontinuation of oral contraception. When decisions have to be made towards the end of pregnancy about the optimum moment for delivery it will be found extremely useful to have an accurate record of observations made in early pregnancy; these sometimes prove to be more reliable than those made later on.

Clinical observations. The date at which the patient first felt fetal movements gives a rough indication of maturity. Primigravidae usually feel fetal movements between 18 and 20 weeks, and multiparae may recognize the movements a little sooner, but a patient who cannot remember the date of her last period is seldom able to give an accurate report of the date of quickening.

Bimanual examination by an experienced clinician performed between 6 and 12 weeks gives a fairly accurate assessment of uterine size. Subsequent repeated measurements of the height of the uterine fundus give only approximate estimates, with an error of perhaps ± 4 weeks, and measurements of the abdominal girth are also an imprecise guide.

Ultrasonic scan. This is the most accurate method available. The crown-rump length of the fetus can be measured between 7 and 14 weeks, and the biparietal diameter of the fetal head after this time. The measurements are compared with standard curves showing normal increments of growth, and there is a straight-line relationship between the size of the fetal head and the duration of pregnancy before the 30th week; subsequently there is more variation.

Radiological examination. This shows the presence or absence of fetal centres of ossification. Those most easily seen are the lower femoral and upper tibial epiphyses which appear between the 36th and 40th weeks, and the cuboid centre which is present near term. There is considerable variation in times of appearance, and because of radiation hazard this method cannot be used until the last few weeks. It is now seldom employed.

Cytological examination of liquor amnii. Liquor may be obtained by amniocentesis and centrifuged to give a smear of epithelial cells. The cells are stained with Nile blue sulphate. After 36 weeks mature cells containing orange-coloured fat are seen against a background of blue-stained cells. If there are more than 10 per cent of orange cells the maturity is likely to be more than 36 weeks, and if there are more than 50 per cent the maturity is likely to be 38 weeks or more. The test is not often used now.

Chemical examination of liquor amnii. Creatinine levels in liquor rise as pregnancy progresses and levels higher than 2 mg/100 ml are seldom found before 37 weeks. The difference between the urea concentration in liquor and in maternal serum also gives some indication of maturity because of the increasing activity of the fetal kidneys. It has been suggested that a combination of cytological and chemical examination of liquor in a scoring system will give an accuracy of ± 2 weeks in 90 per cent of cases, but this is hardly more than can be achieved by clinical judgement.

The surfactant activity of liquor can also be determined by measurement of its lecithin content (see p. 369). This gives a good indication of the functional maturity of the fetal lung, but does not necessarily equate with gestational age.

7

Antenatal care

Antenatal care and investigation is an important part of preventive medicine, its object being to maintain the mother in health of body and mind, to anticipate difficulties and complications of labour, to ensure the birth of a healthy infant, and to help the mother rear the child.

The number of times a patient needs to be seen during her pregnancy must vary, but in an uncomplicated case the following care is desirable. The first visit, when the patient comes to make arrangements, should be as early in pregnancy as possible. Thereafter the patient should be seen every 4 weeks until the 28th week, fortnightly until the 36th week, and then every week until the onset of labour. If complications arise more frequent visits may be necessary.

Today hospital delivery is advocated for the majority of patients, but not all antenatal care has necessarily to be in hospital clinics. Shared care between the hospital and the patient's general practitioner may be preferred in many normal cases, as this may save the patient travelling, promote better doctor-patient relationships, and allow more individual care by reducing the numbers of patients attending hospital clinics. Patients having shared care should attend at the hospital to see the obstetrician for the booking visit. Thereafter, if all is well, hospital visits are usually at 28 and 36 weeks, and weekly from the 39th week until the onset of labour, all other visits being to the general practitioner.

Antenatal care

Booking visit

At the first visit the following procedure is followed:

General medical history. It is important to know whether the patient has had any serious illness, including cardiac disease, renal disease, diabetes, rubella or a blood transfusion. Previous surgical treatment, particularly gynaecological operations, may be relevant.

Family history. Any disease with a hereditary tendency, including hypertension and diabetes, is recorded. A family history of twins may be significant.

Past obstetric history. If the patient has been pregnant before she is questioned about previous pregnancies and labours. For example, a history of repeated abortion or premature labour might suggest cervical incompetence, and intrauterine fetal death might suggest the possibility of hypertension, diabetes or rhesus incompatibility. A history of raised blood pressure might suggest pre-eclampsia, with the possibility of recurrence.

The history of previous labours is a guide to what may be expected in the coming labour. For example, if the patient has had a long labour ending in instrumental delivery, resulting perhaps in the birth of a dead or injured child, it is possible that she has pelvic contraction. A history of postpartum haemorrhage would be a warning of potential recurrence. It is essential to know the birth-weights of any previous children. The cause of any stillbirth or neonatal death should be ascertained whenever possible, sometimes by writing to the doctor who was then in charge of the patient.

It is important to know whether the children were breast fed, and of any feeding difficulties which may possibly be overcome by special advice.

History of the present pregnancy. This should then be taken. The date of the first day of the last menstrual period must be carefully recorded, with a note of her normal cycle and of any irregularities. If the patient was using oral contraception this may be relevant.

The doctor will then proceed to examine the patient:

General examination. The patient is weighed, and her height and development are noted, including any abnormal gait or deformity. The heart and lungs are examined. Routine radiological examination of the chest is not performed, but it may be wise in the case of immigrants from countries in which tuberculosis is still common. The blood pressure is recorded, and the urine is examined for protein and sugar. It is now routine practice to examine a midstream specimen of urine for bacteriuria (see p. 203).

A sample of blood is taken for determination of the blood group, and if the patient is rhesus negative an antibody test is made. The haemoglobin concentration is estimated, and for negro patients and those of Mediterranean origin plasmapheresis is performed to screen for haemoglobinopathy (p. 215). Serological tests for syphilis are carried out. Rubella antibody titres are investigated, and if the result indicates that the patient is not immune a note is made to offer vaccination in the puerperium. In many clinics the serum is examined for α-fetoprotein as a screening test for neural tube defects (p. 370). This test is most reliable between the 16th and 18th weeks. The presence in the blood of hepatitis B antigen may also be detected, so that precautions can be taken to avoid infection of attendants during blood-letting or delivery.

The teeth should be inspected and, if necessary, overhauled. Septic teeth or gums may be the origin of infection, and progression of caries may be prevented.

Obstetric examination. After examining the breasts an examination of the abdomen is made, including auscultation of the fetal heart sounds if the pregnancy has reached 24 weeks. Before this time fetal blood flow may be detected with the portable ultrasound apparatus. Details of the method of abdominal examination are given on p. 100.

In most clinics a vaginal examination is made at the patient's first visit. By this the position of the uterus (anteverted or retroverted) and particularly its size in relation to the menstrual history are determined, and any extrauterine abnormality such as an ovarian cyst or a fibromyoma may be discovered. A cervical smear is taken for cytological examination. Some idea of the general shape of the pelvis may be gained, but efforts to estimate pelvic capacity are usually better postponed until the 36th week, when the tissues are more relaxed. For details see pp. 105 and 304.

Subsequent visits

At every subsequent visit the blood pressure is recorded and the urine is tested. A careful check is kept on the patient's weight. Provided that it is within normal limits at the outset, the increase should not exceed 12 kg during the pregnancy. There is little, if any, increase during the first 12 weeks. From the 16th to the 28th week the average gain is about 6 kg, and thereafter weight is gained at about 2 kg every 4 weeks. Excessive weight gain should raise suspicion that the patient is developing pre-eclampsia, or that she has an excessive intake of carbohydrate which needs to be checked.

The haemoglobin concentration will be estimated again at the 30th and 36th weeks.

At every visit the height of the fundus is recorded, and from the 32nd week onwards the presentation of the fetus. After the 36th week it is important to determine whether the widest diameter of the fetal head has entered the brim of the pelvis, or if it has not done so, whether it can be made to engage (see p. 101). Any suspicion that fetal growth is impaired calls for full investigation of the case, usually by ultrasonic measurement of the fetus. In a few well-equipped units a routine ultrasonic examination of the fetus is made during early pregnancy.

What has been described is routine antenatal care. Any abnormality will demand further investigation and treatment, with more frequent visits to the clinic or admission to hospital for observation. Some special tests are described in the next section.

Antenatal monitoring of the fetus and placental function tests

A variety of tests are now in use for assessment of the state of the fetus during pregnancy. Reference to these will be made in later chapters, but it may be helpful to summarize them here.

Indications of progesterone production in early pregnancy. It is possible that some miscarriages are caused by progesterone deficiency, and the production of this hormone can best be measured by assay of maternal blood. Indirect indications of progestogenic activity may be obtained by examination of vaginal smears or cervical mucus, but these tests are not very reliable. During normal pregnancy vaginal epithelial cells are clumped together and have rolled edges, and if cervical mucus is dried on a slide it does *not* show fern-like salt crystals. Lack of clumping of the cells or ferning of the mucus may be an indication of progesterone deficiency.

Assay of hormones and enzymes to assess feto-placental function. Many tests have been proposed; three are in common use:

1. The placenta produces lactogen (HPL. See p. 23) and measurement of this hormone in maternal blood by radioimmunoassay is used as an index of placental function.

2. The placenta produces many enzymes, including heat-stable alkaline phosphatase. Assay of this in maternal serum is used as an index of placental function.

3. During pregnancy the fetal adrenal cortex produces large amounts of dehydroepiandrosterone sulphate which is converted in the fetal liver and the placenta to oestriol sulphate, and then excreted in the maternal urine as oestriol glycosuronidate (see p. 34). Estimation of the level of oestrogens in maternal blood or urine is therefore an index of both fetal and placental activity. If all is well the excretion of oestrogens rises progressively during pregnancy, but with wide daily variation. Repeated estimations are made and compared with the normal curve of excretion.

Measurements of fetal growth. Repeated ultrasonic measurement of the biparietal diameter of the fetal head, especially after the 30th week, will show whether normal fetal growth is occurring.

Investigation of circulatory and other fetal responses. Apart from asking the mother to keep records of the fetal movements ('kick counts') ultrasonic examination may permit observation of fetal respiratory movements and will allow accurate recording of the fetal heart rate over a period of several minutes or hours. Signals from the fetal electrocardiograph can also be recorded with a ratemeter from an abdominal electrode.

A normal fetus has periods of inactivity during which the heart rate shows little variation, and episodes of active movement, during which the heart rate shows much beat-to-beat variation. Uterine contractions of pregnancy may cause temporary slowing of the rate, and the effect of giving a small dose of oxytocin by intravenous injection is sometimes used as a stress test. A fetus that shows none of the normal variations in heart rate, or one that shows prolonged slowing of the heart rate with a uterine contraction, may be at risk.

Amnioscopy. In late pregnancy an amnioscope can be passed through the cervix to inspect the colour of the liquor through the intact membranes. If meconium staining is seen the fetus may be at risk, but since clear liquor does not exclude risk this test is now seldom used.

Tests for fetal maturity.   See p. 52.

Investigations to exclude fetal abnormalities.   Ultrasonic screening will 'visualize' the fetal sac and the fetus from very early in pregnancy. In late pregnancy radiological examination is occasionally used if fetal abnormality or fetal death is suspected.

Liquor amnii may be obtained by abdominal paracentesis so that fetal cells found in it can be grown in tissue culture for chromosomal analysis, for example in cases of Down's syndrome (p. 502). In some other inherited diseases biochemical study of the liquor is also helpful.

In cases of open neural tube defects α-fetoprotein may be found in excess in maternal serum, and amniocentesis is then performed so that estimation of fetoprotein in the liquor can be done for confirmation.

Estimations of rhesus antibody titres in maternal blood and of bilirubin concentrations in liquor amnii are frequently used in the management of cases of haemolytic disease (p. 450).

Fetoscopy, performed by passing a fine cannula and fibreoptic system into the uterus through the abdominal wall, will allow inspection of the fetus, and aspiration of a blood sample for electrophoresis and other tests.

Advice to the patient during pregnancy

During pregnancy the patient should be advised to attend the education classes which are now generally available at antenatal clinics. It is also convenient to give each patient a booklet which she can read at leisure, giving explanations of events in pregnancy and labour, advice about the care of her health, and information about services available. With the advent of so many special investigations such as blood tests and ultrasound many clinics also have leaflets to explain these. The patient will also need information about financial grants and social services.

Diet.   A number of investigations on the effect of diet on the outcome of pregnancy have been made. It has been shown that a poor quality diet predisposes to premature labour and increased perinatal mortality, but claims that pre-eclampsia can be prevented by modification of the diet during pregnancy have not been substantiated.

There is no need for a large increase in calorie value of the diet; 2400 calories is recommended but the distribution of its constituents requires consideration. Protein should be increased, and at least two-thirds of the protein should be of animal origin, i.e. meat, milk, eggs, cheese and fish. The intake of fats will be adequate if these are taken. Carbohydrates can be reduced slightly to compensate for the increased calorie value of the protein, and more severely restricted if weight reduction is necessary.

In the latter half of pregnancy there is need for a considerable increase in the intake of calcium, phosphorus and iron, and probably of other trace elements, to supply the needs of the growing fetus and to prepare for lactation. Milk, cheese, eggs, meat and fresh green vegetables are foods rich in mineral salts, and a well balanced diet will contain sufficient minerals except perhaps for calcium and iron.

Calcium. The amount of calcium required daily by an adult is 0.5 g; during pregnancy the amount is increased to 1.5 g. It is contained in milk, cheese, some vegetables and bread. It is difficult to be sure that all the calcium taken is absorbed; for example, the phytic acid of bread flour produces an insoluble salt of calcium.

Iron. Many women have poor iron reserves at the beginning of pregnancy, so it is necessary to check the haemoglobin level throughout pregnancy. The daily absorption of iron from an ordinary diet is about 1.2 mg, while the requirement during pregnancy averages 3 mg (see p. 212). An iron supplement is therefore often given. The preparation often used is ferrous sulphate 200 mg 3 times daily. This may cause gastric irritation in some patients and constipation in others, when ferrous fumarate 300 mg daily may be used or a slow-release preparation. During pregnancy anaemia from deficiency of folic acid may occur, and in many clinics combined pills are used, containing iron with a daily dose of 0.5 mg of folic acid.

Rest and exercise. Although violent exercise is imprudent during pregnancy, the patient should be encouraged to continue all ordinary activities. Adequate sleep must be secured, with a sufficient number of hours in bed. Sleeplessness is occasionally troublesome towards the end of pregnancy. It may be treated, if it is severe enough, with sedatives such as promezathine hydrochloride 10 mg, benzodiazepines such as flurazepam (Dalmane) 15 mg, or the chloral preparation dichloralphenazone (Welldorm) 1300 mg. Barbiturates are best avoided because they may be habit forming.

Regulation of the bowels. Constipation is a troublesome complication in many pregnant women. Strong purgatives are to be avoided as they may cause premature labour. With a diet containing plenty of fruit and vegetables a daily action of the bowel can usually be ensured; otherwise mild aperients such as senna and cascara may be prescribed. Liquid paraffin is unsuitable as it impairs absorption from the gut.

Coitus. Patients can be reassured that coitus is not harmful during pregnancy except when there is a threat to miscarry or a previous history of abortion. It should be avoided if there has been antepartum haemorrhage, and near term because of the possible introduction of infection.

Preparation for lactation. The best preparation for lactation is to ensure that the expectant mother is aware of the normal course of events following delivery and is mentally prepared for breast feeding.

Attention must be given during antenatal examination to the nipples. A poorly developed, retracted or inverted nipple cannot be drawn into the infant's mouth, and may be traumatized because the baby cannot fix onto the nipple properly. The nipples should be examined to see whether they are retracted or inverted, and to ascertain whether they will protract. The external appearance of the nipple is not a certain guide and the base of the nipple should be gently pinched to make it protrude. If the nipples are retracted the mother should wear glass nipple shields during the day, and at night during the later part of pregnancy, and this will in some cases correct the abnormality.

There should be no attempt to harden the nipples with spirit; only ordinary washing is necessary. Dry skin on the nipples may be treated with an occasional application of lanoline. Expression of the breasts during the last few weeks of pregnancy has been advocated as a way in which congestion may be prevented, but this requires special instruction to the mothers, and not all of them find it easy.

Corsets.   During pregnancy no more abdominal support is usually needed than is customarily worn. A few parous patients with very relaxed abdominal muscles may require more support, but this should be as simple as possible. The breasts should be supported by a well-fitting brassiere which does not press upon the nipples.

Education of the expectant mother.   It is obvious that the young mother will benefit from some instruction, and in most clinics classes are arranged for this purpose. There are many subjects on which instruction will be useful, such as the preparation of the baby's clothes, the advantages of breast feeding and its method. It is important to allay any anxiety about labour. A simple explanation of the stages of labour should be given to the patient so that she will know what to expect. This is a convenient time to discuss analgesia and to demonstrate the use of the gas and air or trilene apparatus. It is helpful if the labour ward sister can meet the patient so that when she arrives in labour she does not find herself among complete strangers. If the husband is to be present during labour he should also be given preparatory instruction.

In many clinics patients are given instruction in antenatal exercises. These are directed more to the patients' posture and general physique than to the muscles especially concerned with childbirth. Many patients benefit from instruction in muscular relaxation, so that they may be able to relax voluntarily during the uterine contractions of the first stage of labour. Relaxation may also be achieved by deep breathing during pains. This is the basis of the method of so-called psychoprophylaxis.

Disorders of pregnancy

The more serious disorders of pregnancy, such as abortion, antepartum haemorrhage, hypertensive conditions and hydramnios are described separately in later chapters. The complications mentioned here are of less consequence.

Vomiting of pregnancy (morning sickness). From about the 6th to the 12th week of pregnancy nausea or vomiting in the early morning is so common that it is accepted as a symptom of normal pregnancy. It usually occurs soon after waking, and is often retching rather than vomiting. It nearly always stops before the 14th week and does not disturb the patient's health or her pregnancy.

Since these symptoms can sometimes occur when the woman does not know that she is pregnant they appear to be caused by something other than a psychological reaction to pregnancy, and the increased incidence of vomiting in cases of twins and vesicular mole led to the theory that it was the result of higher production of chorionic gonadotrophin or of sensitivity to it. The vomiting occurs at the time of peak output of this hormone in normal pregnancy, but studies comparing hormone levels and sensitivities in cases of excessive vomiting with those of normal controls have not consistently supported this theory.

If the vomiting is persistent and disturbs the patient's health it is termed *hyperemesis gravidarum*. In these severe cases the only biochemical abnormalities which have been found are those which are secondary to vomiting, starvation and dehydration, namely ketosis, electrolyte imbalance and vitamin deficiency. In the years before the management of electrolyte imbalance was understood hyperemesis was a significant cause of maternal mortality, and in fatal cases severe weight loss, tachycardia and hypotension, oliguria, neurological disorders from vitamin B deficiency, and jaundice from hepatic necrosis were seen. In the last 20 years the incidence of hyperemesis in the United Kingdom has greatly diminished, and maternal deaths or cases requiring termination of pregnancy are now virtually unknown.

In some of the severe cases there may be psychological factors. Mere removal to hospital without any other treatment often leads to dramatic and immediate improvement. It has been stated that the incidence of hyperemesis decreases during times of national stress, such as wartime, when other problems outweigh any anxieties about pregnancy. Hyperemesis is almost unknown in so-called underdeveloped countries.

Management. In any case of severe or persistent vomiting it is essential to exclude any other possible cause for it such as pyelonephritis, intestinal obstruction, infective hepatitis or cerebral tumour.

Ordinary morning sickness can be simply treated by reassurance and sometimes by giving one of the anti-emetics which have been proven to be non-teratogenic such as meclozine 25 mg, cyclizine 50 mg or promezathine 25 mg, all three times daily.

If the vomiting is severe the patient is admitted to hospital. if the vomiting continues her dehydration, ketosis and electrolyte imbalance require treatment by intravenous infusion of 4 per cent glucose solution with $\frac{1}{5}$ N saline, with sedatives and sometimes with vitamin supplements. The treatment is regulated by twice daily studies of the blood chemistry; and cessation of vomiting, normal urinary output and weight gain are indications of recovery. Oral feeding is begun as soon as possible, starting with fluids and progressing to semi-solids and eventually to a full diet. The possible need for psychotherapy must be considered.

Ptyalism.   An apparent increase in the amount of saliva occasionally occurs during early pregnancy. The patient spits out her saliva instead of swallowing it and lives in an aura of wet handkerchiefs. Treatment is unsatisfactory. Psychological factors should be borne in mind.

Varicose veins.   Varicose veins of the legs may cause considerable discomfort during pregnancy, and may be associated with oedema, eczema or ulceration, and thrombosis. Fortunately pulmonary embolism from such thrombi is extremely rare. Support by elastic stockings may give some relief. Surgical treatment is not advised during pregnancy because the condition often improves considerably after delivery. The residual lesion should be assessed about three months after delivery before deciding on surgical treatment.

Vulval varices may be uncomfortable during pregnancy, and are an occasional cause of a vulval haematoma during labour.

Haemorrhoids.   Haemorrhoids may first appear or be made worse during pregnancy. Surgical treatment is not advised during pregnancy except to evacuate a painful perianal haematoma under local anaesthesia. Aperients should be prescribed; the anal region should be carefully washed and dried after defaecation, and analgesic ointment applied.

Pruritus vulvae and vaginal discharge.   An excess of vaginal discharge from any cause may lead to vulval pruritus. The commonest cause during pregnancy is infection with *Candida albicans* (monilia) which may be associated with the lowered renal threshold for sugar which occurs in many pregnant women. In all cases of pruritus the urine should be tested for glucose, and if there is any reason to suspect the possibility of diabetes a glucose tolerance test will be required. In candidiasis there may be vulvitis with redness of the skin, or vaginitis with masses or plaques of white cheesy material lightly adherent to the epithelium. Microscopical examination of a little of the discharge in a drop of normal saline will show mycelial threads, and *Candida* will be grown on culture. A variety of fungicides may be used for treatment, including nystatin pessaries 100 000 units to be inserted for 14 successive nights with nystatin cream to the vulva, or clotrimazole (Canesten) pessaries and cream for 6 nights.

Vaginitis during pregnancy may be caused by *Trichomonas vaginalis*, which causes a profuse offensive purulent discharge, in which the organisms can be found on microscopical examination. Metronidazole tablets 200 mg 3 times daily by mouth for 10 days may be used during pregnancy. No adverse effect on the fetus has ever been shown with this drug, but it may be wiser to rely on local treatment before the 12th week, using acetarsol pessaries, 1 or 2 inserted nightly for 21 days.

Cramps in the legs.   Transient nocturnal painful spasms of the small muscles of the feet or of the muscles of the legs sometimes occur during pregnancy. Such cramps have been attributed to calcium deficiency, but there is no satisfactory evidence to support this. It is more likely that they are due to temporary circulatory insufficiency. The cramp tends to improve spontaneously in late pregnancy, but can be troublesome during labour.

Acroparaesthesia. This is not uncommon during pregnancy. There is a sensation of pins and needles in the hands with some sensory loss, and sometimes weakness of the small muscles. The patient finds it difficult to use her hands for fine work. Acroparaesthesia has been attributed to oedema in the carpal tunnel involving the median nerve, and this will explain the cases in which the signs have the appropriate distribution, but in many cases the ulnar border of the hand is chiefly involved, and sometimes even the forearm, and in these cases pressure on the lowest part of the brachial plexus near the first rib must be considered. There may be sagging of the shoulder girdle in pregnancy.

Some, but not all, patients obtain relief from diuretics such as chlorothiazide. Splinting the wrists at night is sometimes helpful. Recovery after delivery is the rule.

Meralgia paraesthetica. Pain, numbness and tingling may occur on the lateral side of the thigh from compression of the lateral cutaneous nerve as it passes under the inguinal ligament. The symptoms resolve after delivery.

Harmful effects of drugs on the fetus

After the discovery that the drug thalidomide given to pregnant women could cause gross fetal deformities, all drugs used during pregnancy have come under close scrutiny. Thalidomide was used as a sedative and anti-emetic but was withdrawn in 1962 after it was found to cause gross limb deformities (phocomelia) and other fetal abnormalities if given to the mother between the 30th and 70th days of pregnancy. Yet care is necessary before attributing any solitary case of deformity to a particular drug. In every 1000 viable births there will be about 5 perinatal deaths from congenital malformation, and more than 10 other infants with malformations of clinical significance. The great majority of these malformations occur as a result of genetic disturbance or pathological events entirely unrelated to any drugs which the mothers may have taken during pregnancy. Properly controlled statistical study is always necessary in studying such relationships.

There are few drugs which do not pass the placental barrier, and possible effects on the fetus must always be considered when drugs are prescribed during pregnancy. It is an important principle of teratology that it is not so much the nature of any harmful agent as the time in embryonic development at which it acts that chiefly determines the abnormality produced. In general, the earlier in pregnancy that a teratogenic agent acts the more severe will be the malformation. Furthermore, there is a short critical period during which each developing structure is particularly vulnerable. If a drug is so harmful that it immediately kills the fetus, there will be no malformation. In addition there seem to be many maternal factors which affect the outcome, such as the standard of nutrition and hormone levels. It should be a general principle to avoid the administration of any drug during the early weeks of pregnancy unless it is clearly necessary for the treatment of a maternal condition.

There is now in Great Britain an expert Committee on the Safety of Drugs which insists that adequate tests are carried out on pregnant animals before a drug is used for women. There is a scheme for the voluntary notification by doctors to the General Register Office through regional medical officers of all malformations present at birth, whether the baby is born alive or is stillborn. A central register is kept, and it is hoped that any national or regional incidence of malformations will be noticed and can be investigated.

A brief account of possible teratogenic and other adverse effects of drugs during pregnancy follow.

Sedatives and analgesics.   *Morphine* or *pethidine* given within 2 or 3 hours of delivery will depress the fetal respiratory centre. (This effect can be antagonized by an injection of naloxone, (p. 464). If the mother is a *heroin* addict the baby may show withdrawal symptoms after delivery, with restlessness and failure to feed, and consequent loss of weight. *Diazepam* (Valium) administered in large doses before delivery will depress the fetal medullary centres and cause loss of the normal base-line variation of the heart rate, and there is hypotonia after delivery. *Phenytoin* (Epanutin) given to control epilepsy is a folic acid antagonist, and if it is used during pregnancy additional folic acid must also be given.

Drugs affecting the cardiovascular system.   Digitalis has no harmful effect on the fetus. *Hexamethonium* may cause ileus in the newborn child, and *reserpine* will cause a transitory non-infective nasal discharge in the infant, but neither of these drugs is now often used. With *propanolol* there may be neonatal circulatory depression. Methyldopa, bethanidine, guanethidine and hydrallazine seem to have no harmful effect on the fetus. Both atropine and scopolamine accelerate the fetal heart rate, but the effect is transitory and not harmful.

Anticoagulant drugs.   Heparin does not cross the placenta. *Oral anticoagulants* reach the fetus, and there have been a few cases of retroplacental haemorrhage or bleeding into fetal tissues, with intrauterine death, and these drugs should only be used during pregnancy when they are essential because of some real risk to the mother.

Antibacterial drugs.   *Sulphonamides* compete with bilirubin for binding sites on serum albumin, and therefore increase any possible risk of kernicterus after birth, and *salicylates* may act in a similar way, so that it is wise to discontinue these drugs before birth if there is any probability of premature birth or if there is rhesus incompatibility. The children of mothers taking *tetracyclines* during pregnancy may have greenish-yellow staining of their milk teeth, and there may be interference with their bone growth. With *streptomycin* there is a theoretical risk of damage to the 8th nerve of the fetus, but with ordinary doses this seems to be very rare. *Chloramphenicol* may cause postnatal collapse and hypothermia. The penicillins, erythromycin and most other antibiotics pass into fetal blood and the amniotic fluid, but seem to have no harmful effect.

Hormones. *Androgens* such as testosterone should not be given to the mother during pregnancy as they may cause virilization of a female fetus. However, *synthetic progestogens* whose structure is related to that of testosterone given in cases of threatened or habitual abortion have also caused virilization. Norethynodrel and dydrogesterone are safer than ethisterone or norethisterone, and 17α-hydroxyprogesterone caproate seems to be without risk (although it is of doubtful value for this purpose. See p. 140). *Diethyl stilboestrol* should not be given to pregnant women as it may cause vaginal septal defects in female fetuses, or vaginal adenosis which may proceed to vaginal carcinoma 15 to 20 years later.

Adrenal steroids may be given in physiological doses to pregnant women with Addison's disease without risk to the fetus. In a few uncommon diseases such as lupus erythematosus, polyarteritis nodosa, status asthmaticus and thrombocytopenic purpura steroids are used in larger pharmacological doses. Animal experiments have suggested that there may be some risk of fetal cleft palate, but human evidence is doubtful, and it is justifiable to use these drugs for severe maternal illness.

Radioactive substances. Radioactive isotopes of iodine, strontium and phosphorus cross the placenta and become localized in fetal tissus. Neither these substances nor any others which emit gamma rays, should be used during pregnancy.

Antithyroid drugs. Drugs such as *thiouracil* or large doses of *iodine* may cause fetal goitre of hypothyroidism.

Cytotoxic and alkylating drugs. All of these, including methotrexate, busulphan, cyclophosphamide, chlorambucil and many others may harm the fetus. They are unlikely to be called for during pregnancy, but if there is a disease such as leukaemia in the mother it may be necessary to give such drugs in spite of the fetal risk.

Smoking during pregnancy

Smoking during pregnancy is harmful to the fetus and will cause reduction in birth weight with an increase in perinatal mortality. It is uncertain whether this is entirely caused by nicotine, which causes vasoconstriction of maternal vessels in the placental bed, or because raised maternal carbon monoxide levels interfere with oxygen transport.

Alcoholism during pregnancy

Children born to mothers who are severely addicted to alcohol have a low birth weight and a few will have a characteristic facial appearance, with a broad base to the nose, epicanthic folds, a long upper lip and a small lower jaw, with mental retardation. This syndrome must raise the whole question of alcohol intake by pregnant women. All that can be said is that no harmful effect can be demonstrated from small doses of alcohol, but on general principles it must be undesirable in the early weeks.

8

The stages of normal labour

The causes of the onset of labour

The uterus normally contracts strongly to expel any foreign body or solid tumour from its cavity. In discussing the cause of the onset of labour the problem is not to discover why the uterus starts to contract at term, but to find out why it remains quiescent during pregnancy. The uterus clearly has the power of expelling its contents before term, as in cases of miscarriage and of premature labour, and also in cases in which labour is induced before term.

It has been suggested that the uterine muscle is inhibited during pregnancy by progesterone. In rabbits the onset of labour can be postponed by giving large doses of progesterone, but this is not the case in women. Nor has it been shown that the concentration of progesterone falls in the blood or urine before term.

It has also been suggested that the rising levels of oestrogen during pregnancy sensitize the uterine muscle, so that it eventually responds more easily to stimuli or to oxytocin. There is no increase in secretion of oxytocin at term, and labour starts normally in hypophysectomized animals.

There is some evidence that the fetal adrenal gland plays a part in initiating labour. Anencephalic fetuses may have defective adrenal cortices and with some of these fetuses pregnancy is greatly prolonged unless labour is induced artificially.

The possible part played by prostaglandins in the onset of labour has yet to be fully investigated. It has been shown that mechanical stimulation of the cervix by the insertion of a finger and separation of the membranes leads to local secretion of prostaglandins. Prostaglandins are present in the decidua of late pregnancy. A prostaglandin pessary placed in the vaginal vault near term induces labour.

During normal pregnancy the growth of the uterus keeps pace with that of its contents and the limit of stretch is probably not reached even at term; the intrauterine pressure does not rise. However, in cases of hydramnios or of twins premature labour is common, so that in abnormal cases overstretching of the uterus may play some part in the onset of labour.

Quite apart from the natural mechanism of onset, in some instances labour may be started artificially by stimulation of the uterus by rupture of the membranes, by oxytocin infusions and by the local or systemic administration of prostaglandins.

Labour follows intrauterine death of the fetus, but there is usually an interval of several days or even weeks before its onset.

During normal pregnancy the uterus contracts intermittently, but these contractions are not strong enough to overcome the resistance of the normal cervix. However, if the internal os of the cervix is damaged or incompetent even these weak contractions may dilate the cervix and labour will follow.

The uterine segments

In describing the phenomena of labour the uterus may be divided into two functional segments. The upper part of the uterus, known as the *upper segment*, contracts strongly, and with each successive contraction becomes shorter and thicker. The powerful upper segment draws up the weaker,

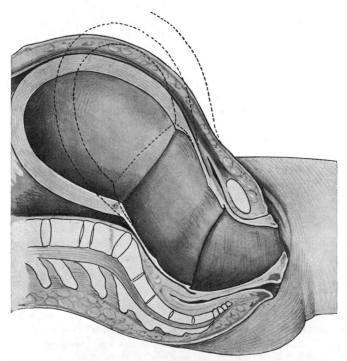

Fig. 8.1 Diagram to show the thickened upper uterine segment and the thin lower uterine segment. The dotted line shows the position assumed by the uterus during contraction.

thinner and more passive lower part of the uterus over its contents, and in so doing 'takes up' and then dilates the cervix. The *lower segment*, consisting of the lower part of the body of the uterus and the cervix, can contract (as is evident if ergometrine is given) but is relatively passive as compared to the upper segment.

Late in labour these two distinct segments can be clearly seen and the transition between them is quite abrupt (Fig. 8.1). In the non-pregnant uterus and during early pregnancy it is not possible to define the limits of the eventual lower segment, but at the end of pregnancy the lower segment is recognizable, and in front it corresponds fairly well with the lower limit of firm peritoneal attachment to the uterus. Below this point the uterovesical peritoneum is loosely attached.

During labour, as the cervix dilates and the lower segment is drawn up its shape changes from a hemisphere to a cylinder. If there is obstruction to delivery the retraction of the upper segment is even more pronounced, and the junction between the two segments forms a distinct ring known as the *retraction ring of Bandl*. In extreme cases this may be palpable and visible per abdomen.

In labour the lower uterine segment, cervix, vagina, pelvic floor and vulval outlet are dilated until there is one continuous birth canal (see Fig. 8.1). The forces which bring about this dilatation and expel the fetus are supplied by the contraction and retraction of the muscle of the upper uterine segment, with assistance in the second stage from the abdominal muscles, including the diaphragm.

The muscle fibres of the upper segment of the uterus not only contract but *retract*. When contracting the fibres become shorter and thicker. When the active contraction passes off the fibres lengthen again, but not to their original length. If contraction was followed by complete relaxation no progress would be made. In retraction some of the shortening of the fibres is maintained. Each successive contraction starts at the point which its predecessor attained, so that the uterine cavity becomes progressively smaller with each contraction. Retraction is a property which, though not peculiar to uterine muscle, is more marked in the uterus than any other organ. Later in labour when the placenta is expelled retraction enables the uterine walls to come together so that there is hardly more than a potential cavity.

The stages of labour

Labour is divided into three stages:
1. The first stage, or stage of dilatation, lasts from the onset of true labour until the cervix is fully dilated.
2. The second stage, or stage of expulsion of the fetus, lasts from full dilatation of the cervix until the fetus is born.
3. The third stage lasts from the birth of the child until the placenta and

membranes are delivered and the uterus has retracted firmly to compress the uterine blood sinuses.

Premonitory symptoms.   In most primigravidae the presenting part sinks into the pelvis during the last 3 or 4 weeks of pregnancy, and in lay terms this is spoken of as 'lightening' because the descent of the fundus of the uterus, together with the reduction in the amount of liquor in late pregnancy, reduces the upper abdominal distension, making the patient more comfortable.

In many multiparae the presenting part does not engage in the pelvis until labour begins. Multiparae not infrequently have uterine contractions which are strong enough to be painful for some days before real labour starts. Such 'false pains' only differ from 'labour pains' in that they are less regular and are ineffective in dilating the lower segment and cervix.

Symptoms and signs of the onset of labour.   These are (1) painful contractions, (2) the show, (3) shortening and dilatation of the cervix and (4) sometimes rupture of the membranes.

1. *The contractions.*   The uterus contracts irregularly and painlessly throughout pregnancy (Braxton Hicks contractions). Labour is recognized by the changes in the contractions, in that they become regular and painful enough to distract the patient from her usual activities. The uterus can be felt to harden during each contraction which begins gradually, works up to a period of maximal intensity and then dies away, the whole lasting about 45 seconds. At the onset of labour the interval between contractions is variable and may be as long as 20 minutes, but then the contractions increase in frequency, strength and their painful quality, until at the end of the first stage they are coming every 2 or 3 minutes and lasting as long as 1 minute.

The contractions are not within the control of the patient's will and occur even when she is unconscious, although they may be lessened in frequency or temporarily abolished by emotional disturbance or by distension of the bladder or rectum. They may be increased in strength and frequency by such stimuli as a purgative or enema, stretching of the cervix or pelvic floor by the presenting part, or by injection of oxytocin.

The pain of labour has the same character as that of spasmodic dysmenorrhoea and probably has the same cause—ischaemia of the uterine muscle from compression of the blood vessels in the wall of the uterus. It is analogous to myocardial pain which occurs when the blood flow in the coronary arteries is restricted. The fact that the contractions are intermittent and not continuous is of great importance to both the fetus and the mother. During a contraction the circulation through the uterine wall is stopped, and if the uterus contracted continuously the fetus would die from lack of oxygen. The intervals between the pains allow the placental circulation to be re-established, and give the mother time to recover from the fatiguing effect of the contraction. The uterus is a very large muscle, and contractions use up much of the patient's energy; if continued too long this would produce maternal exhaustion.

Electrical records of the pattern of uterine contractions show that in normal labour each contraction wave starts near one or other uterine cornu. The contraction spreads as a wave in the myometrium, taking 10 to 30 seconds to spread over the whole uterus. As each point is reached by the wave, contraction starts and takes about another 30 seconds to reach its peak.

The upper part of the uterus contracts more strongly than the lower part, and the duration of the contraction is longer in the upper than in the lower segment. This dominance of the upper segment leads to the stretching and thinning of the lower segment and to dilatation of the cervix.

If the wave pattern is abnormal, with the lower part of the uterus contracting first or as strongly as the upper part, no progress in labour will be made. In other cases the wave spreads erratically in the myometrium and the contractions are incoordinate (see p. 309 et seq.).

The duration and strength of each contraction are relevant both to their efficiency and to the pain felt by the patient. The resting tone between contractions in early labour is about 10 mm Hg; the intrauterine pressure at which a contraction can be felt by the hand of an observer is about 20 mm Hg; and the pressure at which the patient feels pain is about 25 mm Hg. Efficient first stage contractions reach 50 mm Hg, and they may reach 75 mm Hg in the second stage. The pain threshold of patients varies, and may vary in one woman during labour. It is the anxious worried patient, long in labour, who may feel pain at a pressure as low as 15 mm Hg.

2. *The show.*   This is a mucous discharge from the cervix, mixed with a little blood. As the internal os is pulled open the membranes are separated from the lower uterine segment, and a variable amount of oozing of blood results.

3. *Shortening and dilatation of the cervix.*   At the beginning of labour the cervix of a nulliparous woman is often a thick-walled canal at least 2 cm long. In other cases the cervix may be found to be completely 'taken up' and partly dilated in the later weeks of pregnancy.

When labour begins the contraction and retraction of the upper uterine segment stretches the lower segment and the upper part of the cervix, while the lower part of the cervical canal remains at first unaltered. As the internal os is pulled open, the cervix is dilated from above downwards, becoming shorter until at length no projection into the vagina is felt, but only a more-or-less thick rim at the external os, the whole cervix being 'taken up' and its cavity made one with that of the body of the uterus. Without true shortening of the cervix it is unwise to diagnose that a primigravida is in labour (Fig. 8.2).

In women who have borne children the external os will often admit a finger before labour has begun, and the finger-tip can sometimes be passed through the internal os. Very often the cervix has been taken up. In this case the projection of a small bag of membranes during a pain will show that labour has begun.

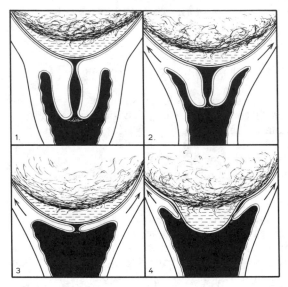

Fig. 8.2 Diagrams to show how the cervix is taken up and then dilated during labour.

4. *Rupture of the membranes.*   The membranes may rupture at any time during labour. When the membranes rupture spontaneously near term it is probable that labour will begin within a short time, although in a few instances the onset is still delayed. Early rupture of the membranes is more likely to occur if the presenting part is not engaged, but it also occurs in many normal cases.

The first stage of labour

The contractions of the uterus dilate the cervix. The dilatation of the internal os causes separation of the chorion from the decidua in its immediate neighbourhood. Thus a small bag of membranes is formed and is forced into the internal os by the intrauterine pressure. At the beginning of each contraction a little more liquor is forced into the bag of membranes, the head then comes down like a ball valve and separates the liquor amnii which is above it from that in the bag, called respectively the hind and forewaters. The bag of membranes may remain intact until nearly the end of the first stage, but even if the membranes rupture early the cervix will normally still become dilated as it is drawn up over the presenting part by the retraction of the upper segment.

During the first stage the fetus is moved downwards very little. When a certain amount of liquor has left the uterus after the membranes have ruptured a new form of pressure comes into play, namely the *fetal axis pressure*. The upper pole of the fetus, normally the breech, is pressed on by the fundus of the uterus, while the lower pole is pressed down onto the lower segment and cervix. When the membranes rupture early the fetal axis pressure will operate at an early stage, and in modern practice the membranes are often deliberately ruptured during labour.

The normal first stage should not exceed 12 hours in a primigravida, and should be even shorter in a multipara. During the early part of the first stage the pains may not be very severe, but towards the end of this stage they are often very distressing. They recur frequently, and as progress in dilatation of the cervix is not apparent to the patient she thinks that they are doing no good. Vomiting is not uncommon at this time. This is often the most painful part of labour.

In the past much has been written about the disadvantage of early rupture of the membranes, but today it is agreed that in normal vertex presentations early rupture is of no consequence. So long as the bag of membranes is intact the intrauterine pressure is distributed equally over all parts of the fetus. This is still true in a normal case after the membranes have ruptured except for the small part of the fetus which is related to the cervix, because the well-fitting presenting part prevents much liquor from draining away. If, however, there is a malpresentation or disproportion, early rupture of the membranes may be followed by loss of nearly all the liquor and the uterus becomes closely applied to the fetus. If labour is prolonged the placenta and cord may be unduly compressed by the retraction of the uterus, and in extreme cases the fetus may die.

If the membranes remain unruptured when the cervix is fully dilated the onset of the expulsive stage is delayed, the cervix not receiving the pressure of the head which should stimulate the uterus to increased activity. If the membranes remain intact after full dilatation they should be ruptured with toothed forceps during a contraction.

The second stage of labour

There is very little descent of the fetus during the first stage. In the second stage the resistance offered by the lower uterine segment and the cervix has been overcome, and the presenting part can be pushed down onto the pelvic floor, the resistance of which has then to be overcome by the uterine contractions aided by the action of the voluntary muscles of the abdominal wall and the diaphragm.

The normal second stage should not be much more than an hour in a primigravida, and may be very much shorter in a multipara. The pain felt during the second stage is often less than that at the end of the first stage, partly because cervical dilatation is now complete. The patient realizes that some progress is being made and that she can help herself. As the head passes through the pelvis she may complain of cramp in the legs from pressure on the sacral nerves. Especially in first labours there is again sharp discomfort during the stretching of the vulval outlet.

The character of the pains is different from that of first stage pains. As the contraction comes on the patient takes a deep breath, then holds her breath and bears down with all the force of her abdominal muscles. During the height of the pain there may be expiratory groans. These expulsive efforts are partly voluntary but largely reflex.

During a contraction the fetal heart rate is often slowed, but it regains its normal rate as soon as the contraction has passed. Such transient brady-cardia is of little significance, but if bradycardia is prolonged after each contraction this is often a sign of fetal distress (see p. 354 et seq.).

With each contraction the presenting part is forced down onto the pelvic floor. During the intervals between the contractions, however, the pelvic floor at first pushes the presenting part up again. Retraction now plays an important part, so that the progress made by each contraction is not com-pletely lost during the succeeding interval. Eventually, after being pushed down many times by the contractions and slipping back in the intervals between them a time comes when the presenting part is stationary at the end of a contraction. The uterus and abdominal muscles press the head downwards, while the muscles of the pelvic floor push upwards and for-wards. The resultant of these two forces is mainly forwards. The axis of the outlet of the bony pelvis is downwards and forwards and that of the soft parts below the bones is almost directly forwards. In a primigravida the head may be visible for some time at the vulva before it can emerge. When the widest diameter of the head distends the vulva it is said to be crowned.

As the head passes through the vulva of a primigravida the stretching pain may be very severe, and will probably cause the patient to cry out, and so to cease from bearing down. To some extent this saves the perineum from damage, as it is likely to be torn if the patient bears down hard while the head is passing through the vulval orifice. It is at this stage that episiotomy is frequently necessary (see p. 375).

The body of the child is generally born by the next contraction if not by the contraction which expelled the head, and is followed by a gush of liquor.

The caput succedaneum. That part of the head which is most in advance is free from pressure during labour while all the rest of the head is pressed upon by the cervix and lower segment. As a result of venous con-gestion serum is exuded and an oedematous swelling forms on the scalp, superficial to the periosteum of the cranial bones and not limited by them. This is known as the caput succedaneum. It gradually disappears in the course of a few hours or days.

If some other part presents, e.g. the face or breech, a comparable oedematous swelling will be formed over the part most in advance.

Moulding. The change in the shape of the head by which the diameters of the skull most pressed upon become diminished is called moulding.

The bones of the base of the skull are incompressible, and are joined to each other in such a way that movement is not possible between them, but the bones of the vault of the skull are compressible, and the sutures allow some movement between the individual bones. The parietal bones and the tabular portions of the occipital and frontal bones can be shaped by pressure, and when much compressed the parietal bones can override the occipital and frontal bones, and one parietal bone can override its fellow. By moulding and overlap the biparietal diameter can be reduced by as much as 1 cm, but excessive moulding may result in intracranial damage.

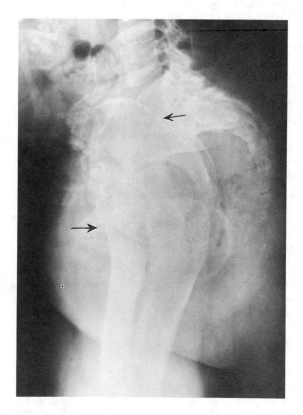

Fig. 8.3 Lateral view of the pelvis, showing moulding of the fetal head during labour. The arrows point, respectively, to the sacral promontory and to the lower border of the symphysis pubis.

The third stage of labour

The uterus follows down the body of the child, and after its expulsion the fundus lies about 5 cm below the level of the umbilicus. As a rule, unless oxytocic drugs are given, contractions are absent for a few minutes after the expulsion of the child but the uterus remains retracted on the placenta. After a variable interval rhythmical contractions, which are not usually felt by the patient, begin again. As the uterine walls become thicker and the cavity of the uterus becomes smaller the placental site shrinks until it reaches a stage when detachment of the placenta must occur unless it is abnormally adherent. Separation of the placenta occurs in two ways: (1) A part of the placenta near its centre separates and bleeding occurs at this point. With further contractions and bleeding the placenta is gradually pushed down through the cervix with its fetal surface presenting. The placenta is delivered first, dragging the membranes behind it (Schultze mechanism). (2) In other patients separation begins at the lower pole of the placenta which gradually slides into the cervical canal, the upper pole of the placenta being the last part to leave the uterine cavity. Either the edge or the uterine surface of the placenta presents (Matthews Duncan mechanism).

The separation of the placenta and membranes from the uterine wall takes place through the decidual layer, part of which comes away covering the uterine surface of the placenta and membranes, while the rest remains in the uterus.

There is generally a gush of blood, not amounting to more than 200 ml as the placenta is expelled. If the uterus does not retract well there is further bleeding, but in the great majority of cases the strong retraction of the uterine muscle fibres compresses the uterine sinuses so effectively that there is little further loss. The uterus is then felt as a hard, round ball about the size of a fetal head, with the top of the uterus just below the umbilicus.

When the placenta is expelled into the vagina the patient may be able to deliver it by voluntary use of her abdominal muscles, but in practice the accoucheur often assists its delivery by Brandt-Andrews' method (see p. 125).

Duration of labour

Labour in primiparae usually lasts 8 to 16 hours; the precise time of onset is often uncertain. In multiparae 4 to 8 hours might be usual. The first stage in primiparae usually lasts 7 to 14 hours, the cervix taking much longer to dilate than in multiparae. In the second stage the perineum and vaginal orifice also offer greater resistance in primiparae. In some multiparae labour may last only 2 or 3 hours and in them the child may be born with only two or three contractions after full dilatation of the cervix.

9

Anatomy of the normal female pelvis and the fetal skull

Knowledge of the shape and dimensions of the normal female pelvis and of the fetal skull is essential for proper understanding of the mechanism of labour and its abnormalities.

The pelvis

Although some sexual differences may be recognizable at birth the female pelvic characteristics are chiefly developed between that time and puberty. Radiological surveys have shown that variations in the shape of the pelvis are very common. What is described as the normal female pelvis, the rounded *gynaecoid pelvis*, occurs in only 40 per cent of white women. Some of the others have pelves with male characteristics (*android pelvis*), in others there is a slight increase in the antero-posterior diameter of the pelvis (*anthropoid pelvis*), while in the remainder the pelvis is slightly flattened (*platypelloid pelvis*). (See also p. 297.) Only the typical gynaecoid pelvis will be described here.

The part of the pelvis above the brim is described as the false pelvis and that below the brim as the true pelvis. The obstetrician is only concerned with the latter. The true pelvis may be described in terms of the brim, the cavity and the outlet.

The pelvic brim lies almost exactly in one plane bounded in front by the symphysis pubis, on each side by the upper margin of the pubic bone, the ilio-pectineal line and the ala of the sacrum, and posteriorly by the promontory of the sacrum. In the gynaecoid pelvis the brim is rounded except for the slight projection of the promontory.

The pelvic cavity is sometimes described in terms of an imaginary plane bounded in front by the middle of the symphysis pubis, on each side by the pubic bone, the obturator fascia, the inner aspect of the ischial bone, and posteriorly by the junction of the 2nd and 3rd pieces of the sacrum. The ischial spines lie slightly below this plane. In the gynaecoid pelvis the cavity is roomy because the sacrum is inclined backwards and well curved, and the sacro-sciatic notches are wide.

The pelvic outlet is roughly diamond shaped and is bounded in front by the lower margin of the symphysis pubis, on each side by the descend-

77

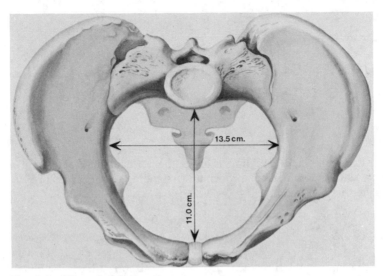

Fig. 9.1   The pelvic brim.

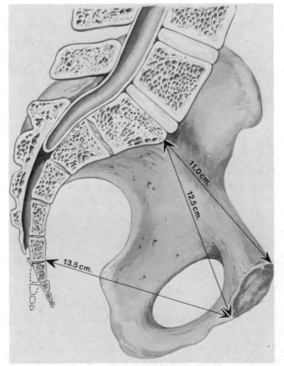

Fig. 9.2   Sagittal section of pelvis. The true and diagonal conjugate diameter.

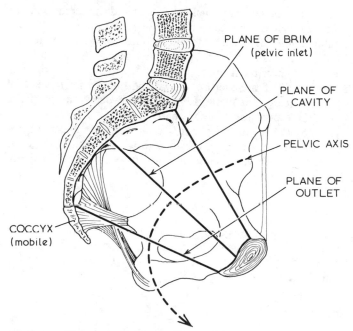

Fig. 9.3 The planes and axes of the pelvis.

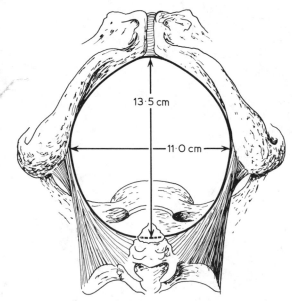

Fig. 9.4 The pelvic outlet.

ing ramus of the pubic bone, the ischial tuberosity and the sacro-tuberous ligament, and posteriorly by the last piece of the sacrum (*not* the coccyx, which is mobile). Unlike the brim the outlet does not have boundaries which lie in a single plane, but an imaginary plane of the outlet is sometimes described, passing from the lower margin of the symphysis pubis to the last piece of the sacrum. It will be noted that the ischial tuberosities lie well below this plane. In a gynaecoid pelvis the subpubic arch is wide and the tuberosities are far apart.

During pregnancy the ligaments of the sacro-iliac joints and the symphysis pubis become softened and there is slightly increased mobility at these joints. The sacro-coccygeal joint allows the coccyx to move freely backwards during delivery.

The pelvic axis

The axis of the pelvis is an imaginary curved line which shows the path which the centre of the fetal head follows during its passage through the pelvis. It is obtained by taking several antero-posterior diameters of the pelvis and joining their centres (Fig. 9.3).

Pelvic inclination

By this is meant the angle that any pelvic plane makes with the horizontal. In the erect position the brim is normally inclined at 60 degrees. In negro

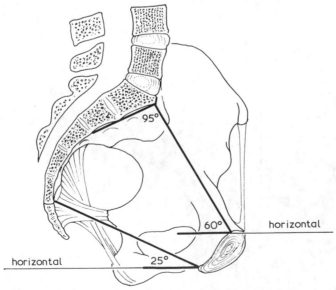

Fig. 9.5 Angles of inclination of the pelvic brim and pelvic outlet.

women this angle may approach 90 degrees and because of this the head may be slow to engage during labour.

The pelvic outlet is inclined at about 25 degrees to the horizontal.

The inclination of the sacrum is measured differently. It is the angle between the front of the first piece of the sacrum and the plane of the pelvic brim. It may affect the available space in the upper part of the pelvic cavity (Fig. 9.5).

Average dimensions of the normal pelvis

It must be clearly understood that the pelvic diameters vary just as much as women's heights vary, and that the diameters will also be affected by the pelvic shape. What matters during delivery is not the absolute size of the pelvis but the size relative to that of the fetal head. However, in a woman of average height with a normal pelvis the following measurements are to be expected.

Diameters of the brim. The antero-posterior diameter of the brim (or true conjugate) is measured from the back of the upper part of the symphysis pubis to the promontory of the sacrum and is 11 cm. The transverse diameter of the brim measures 13.5 cm.

Diameters of the pelvic cavity. The plane of the cavity has already been defined. The antero-posterior and transverse diameters both measure 12 cm.

Diameters of the pelvic outlet. The outlet does not lie in a simple plane like the brim. The antero-posterior diameter of the outlet is measured from the lower part of the symphysis pubis to the end of the sacrum (*not* the coccyx) and is 13.5 cm. The transverse diameter is measured between the inner surfaces of the ischial tuberosities and is 11 cm. However, the fetal head cannot occupy all the space under the subpubic arch so the simple antero-posterior measurement of the outlet is of less significance than the sum of the transverse distance between the ischial tuberosities and the posterior sagittal diameter. The latter is measured from the centre of the transverse intertuberous diameter backwards to the end of the sacrum. The sum of these two measurements normally exceeds 15 cm (Fig. 9.6).

The average normal measurements are summarized in Table 9.1:

Table 9.1

	Anterior-posterior	Transverse
Brim	11 cm	13.5 cm
Cavity	12 cm	12 cm
Outlet	13.5 cm	11 cm

The brim is a transverse oval, the cavity is round and the outlet is an antero-posterior oval.

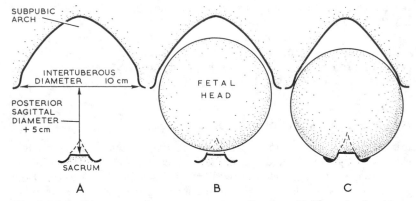

Fig. 9.6   A. Diagram to show measurements of outlet.   B. Normal subpubic arch.   C. The head cannot enter a narrow subpubic arch, and the effective size of the outlet is reduced.

Clinical examination of the pelvis

A pelvic examination is usually made early in pregnancy to confirm the diagnosis of pregnancy and its duration, to exclude abnormalities of the pelvic organs and to assess the capacity of the pelvis. If the patient has miscarried or threatened to miscarry previously it is wise to postpone any internal examination until later, and in any case a further pelvic examination is usually performed at about the 36th week. At this time the pelvic floor is more relaxed, and also the size of the fetal head can be related to that of the pelvic brim.

External measurements cannot give an accurate picture of the size or shape of the pelvic brim or cavity, and they are no longer used for this purpose.

Vaginal assessment of the pelvis.   (1) *The brim.*   The sacral promontory cannot be reached with an examining finger in a normal pelvis unless the patient is anaesthetized. If it can be felt it is likely that the true conjugate is considerably reduced, and in such a case it may be possible to estimate the diagonal conjugate with the exploring finger. This is the distance between the promontory and the lower margin of the symphysis pubis. The true conjugate may be derived by subtracting 1.5 cm from the diagonal conjugate. (See Fig. 9.2.)

(2) *The pelvic cavity.*   On vaginal examination a general idea of the capacity of the pelvic cavity can be gained. The anterior surface of the sacrum is palpated from above downwards, noting whether it is straight or concave. The position of the ischial spines may be assessed by palpation of the sacro-spinous ligaments, which should be of a length that will accommodate three finger-breadths. The spines are sometimes unduly promi-

nent, but it is the distance between them rather than their prominence that matters.

(3) *The pelvic outlet.* The intertuberous diameter and the posterior sagittal diameter (see above) can be determined by external palpation, but vaginal examination gives the best assessment of the width of the subpubic arch and of the position of the sacrum.

Radiological pelvimetry. The internal diameters of the pelvis can be measured by radiological methods. These are described on p. 305.

The pelvic floor. Although this is not part of the bony pelvis it is mentioned here because it forms part of the birth canal and plays an important part in the mechanism of labour. The two levator ani muscles, with their fascia, form a musculo-fascial gutter during the second stage of labour, with the opening of the vagina looking forward between the sides of the gutter. (Fig. 9.7.) The pelvic floor directs the most salient portion of the presenting part forwards under the subpubic arch.

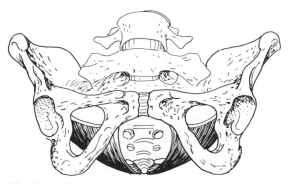

Fig. 9.7   The levator sling.

The fetal skull

The fetal skull may be divided into the vault, face and base. By the time of birth the bones of the face and base are all firmly united, but the bones of the vault are not so well ossified and are only joined by unossified membranes at the sutures. During labour the bones of the vault can undergo *moulding*, by which the shape of the skull can be altered with reduction of some of its diameters.

The bones which form the vault are the two parietal bones, and parts of the occipital, frontal and temporal bones (Fig. 9.8). At birth the frontal bone is divided into two parts. Three sutures are of obstetric importance:
1. The sagittal suture lies between the superior borders of the parietal bones.

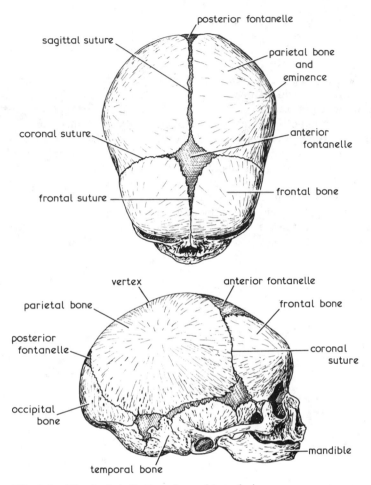

Fig. 9.8   The fetal skull. Superior and lateral views.

2. The frontal suture, which is a forward continuation of the sagittal suture, lies between the two parts of the frontal bone.
3. The coronal suture lies between the anterior borders of the parietal bones and the posterior borders of the frontal bones.

   Fontanelles.   The points of junction of the various sutures are termed fontanelles; the anterior and posterior fontanelles are important in obstetrics. The anterior fontanelle lies where the sagittal, frontal and coronal sutures meet. The posterior fontanelle lies at the posterior end of the sagittal suture, between the two parietal bones and the occipital bone. The position of these two fontanelles, when felt on vaginal examination, indicates in which direction the occiput is pointing and the degree of flexion or extension of the head.

The anterior fontanelle (or bregma) is much the larger of the two, is roughly kite shaped, has four sutures running into it, is always patent at birth, and takes about 20 months to close. The posterior fontanelle is triangular in shape, has three sutures running into it, in most cases cannot be felt as a space during labour, and closes soon afterwards.

The area of the fetal skull bounded by the two parietal eminences and the anterior and posterior fontanelles is termed the *vertex*. It is the part of the head which presents in normal labour.

Diameters of the fetal skull

The diameters of the fetal skull which are important in the mechanism of labour may be divided into vertical, longitudinal, and transverse.

Vertical and longitudinal diameters. The fetal head is ovoid in shape. In normal labour the head is well flexed so that the least diameters of the ovoid, namely the suboccipito-bregmatic and biparietal (transverse) diameters are those which engage. The *suboccipito-bregmatic diameter* is measured from the suboccipital region to the centre of the anterior fontanelle (bregma) and is 9.5 cm. (Figs. 9.9, 9.10.)

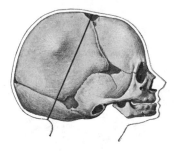

Fig. 9.9   Suboccipito-bregmatic diameter, 9.5 cm.

If the head is less well flexed the *suboccipito-frontal diameter* is involved. This is taken from the suboccipital region to the prominence of the forehead and measures 10 cm. This is the diameter of the head which passes through the vulval orifice at the moment of delivery of the head (Fig. 9.11).

With further extension of the head the *occipito-frontal diameter* engages. This is measured from the root of the nose (glabella) to the posterior fontanelle and is 11.5 cm (Fig. 9.12). This diameter meets the pelvis with a persistent occipito-posterior position (Fig. 9.13).

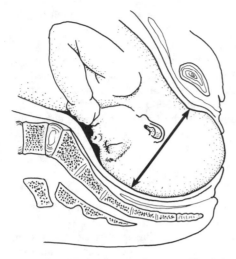

Fig. 9.10 To show the diameter, Fig. 9.9, engaged in the pelvis when the head is fully flexed.

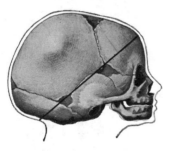

Fig. 9.11 Suboccipito-frontal diameter, 10 cm.

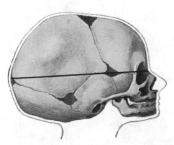

Fig. 9.12 Occipito-frontal diameter, 11.5 cm.

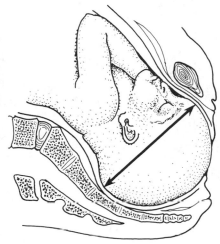

Fig. 9.13 To show the diameter, Fig. 9.12, engaged in the pelvis in an occipito-posterior position.

The greatest longitudinal diameter is the *mento-vertical*, which is taken from the chin to the furthest point of the vertex and measures 13 cm. This is the diameter which is thrown across the pelvis in a brow presentation (Figs. 9.14, 9.15) and is too large to pass through a normal pelvis.

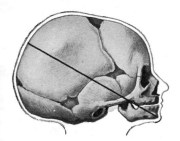

Fig. 9.14 Mento-vertical diameter, 13 cm.

Beyond this point further extension of the head so that the face presents results in a smaller vertical diameter, i.e. the other end of the ovoid presents. The *submento-bregmatic diameter* is taken from below the chin to the anterior fontanelle and measures 9.5 cm. (Figs. 9.16, 9.17.)

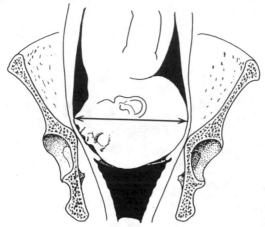

Fig. 9.15   To show the diameter meeting the pelvis in a brow presentation.

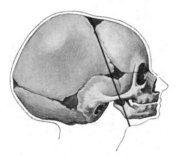

Fig. 9.16   Submento-bregmatic diameter, 9.5 cm.

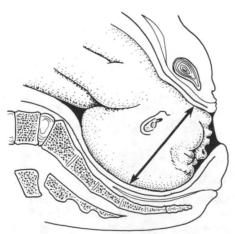

Fig. 9.17   To show the diameter, Fig. 9.16, engaged in the pelvis in a face presentation with the head completely extended.

Transverse diameter. The biparietal diameter, measured from one parietal eminence to the other, is 9.5 cm.

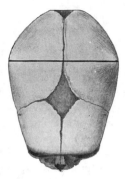

Fig. 9.18 Bi-parietal diameter, 9.5 cm.

Circumference of the fetal head

The smallest circumference of the fetal head is in the plane of the suboccipito-bregmatic diameter and measures 29 cm. A somewhat larger circumference is in the plane of the suboccipito-frontal diameter, and this distends the vulval orifice in normal labour. The largest circumference is in the plane of the mento-vertical diameter and measures 38 cm.

Processes of the dura mater

The great folds of the dura mater, the falx cerebri and the tentorium cerebelli, act in some degree as internal liagments, resisting too great deformation of the fetal head both in the longitudinal and the transverse directions. If moulding is excessive, or if the fetal head is subjected to severe and sudden stresses, these parts of the dura mater are liable to be torn. Some of the great venous sinuses are then in danger of rupture as well. These are the inferior longitudinal sinus, running in the free edge of the falx cerebri and receiving the great cerebral veins of Galen from the brain, and the straight sinus running between the falx cerebi and the tentorium cerebelli.

Diameters of the fetal trunk

The *bis-acromial diameter* is taken between the parts furthest apart on the shoulders and is 12 cm. The *bitrochanteric* diameter measures 10 cm.

10

The fetal position and the mechanism of normal labour

Certain terms used to describe the position of the fetus in relation to the uterus and the pelvis must be explained.

Lie. By the lie of the fetus is meant the relation which the long axis of the fetus bears to that of the uterus. The lie may be longitudinal, oblique or transverse.

Presentation. The presenting part of the fetus is that part which is in or over the pelvic brim and in relation to the cervix. When the head occupies the lower segment of the uterus the presentation is termed cephalic. If the head is flexed on the spine the vertex presents and the presentation is so designated. If the head is fully extended in the spine there is a face presentation, and if it is partly extended a brow presentation.

If the breech occupies the lower segment the presentation is termed podalic.

If the fetus lies obliquely the shoulder generally lies over the cervix and this is called a shoulder presentation.

Any presentation other than a vertex presentation is described as a malpresentation.

Position. By this term is meant the relation which some selected part of the fetus bears to the maternal pelvis. The indicator is a point on the presenting part, chosen according to the presentation which is being described. With a vertex presentation the indicator is the occiput, with a face presentation the chin (mentum) is the indicator, and with a breech presentation the sacrum.

It is conventional to describe four positions. For example with a vertex presentation the occiput could be related to:
1. The left ilio-pectineal eminence—left occipito-anterior position (LOA).
2. The right ilio-pectineal eminence—right occipito-anterior position (ROA).
3. The right sacro-iliac joint—right occipito-posterior position (ROP).
4. The left sacro-iliac joint—left occipito-posterior position (LOP).

However, the occiput most commonly lies in the transverse diameter of the pelvic brim, and the terms left occipito-transverse position (LOT) and right occipito-transverse position (ROT) are useful. It is extremely rare for the occiput to lie directly anteriorly or posteriorly in the brim, although it will do so at the outlet later in labour.

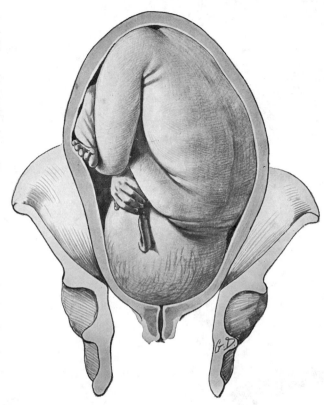

Fig. 10.1 Left occipito-anterior position.

Attitude. This term refers to the relation of the different parts of the fetus to one another. Normally the head, back and limbs of the fetus are flexed. In some abnormal presentations, which will be described in later chapters, the head or limbs may be extended.

In 96 per cent of cases at term the fetus lies longitudinally, with the head presenting. The reason for this is that the fetus adapts itself by its movements to the shape of the uterus. In the early months of pregnancy the liquor amnii is comparatively more abundant, and the fetus can float freely; but as pregnancy advances the fetus rapidly increases in size and the volume of liquor becomes comparatively less, so that the fetus is constrained to fit the shape of the uterus. When the attitude is one of complete flexion the buttocks, together with the adjacent parts of the thighs and the feet, constitute a mass which is larger than the head. The cavity of the uterus at term is pear-shaped, with the wider end uppermost; therefore the

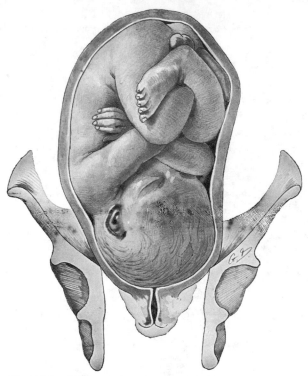

Fig. 10.2 Right occipito-posterior position.

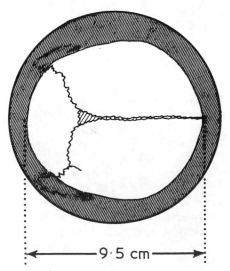

Fig. 10.3 Vaginal palpation of head in right occipito-lateral position. The circle represents the pelvic cavity with a diameter of 11 cm. The head is well flexed and only the posterior fontanelle is felt.

fetus fits into it best when the breech lies in the upper part of the uterus and the head in the lower part.

In premature labours presentations other than those of the head are more common than in labour at term because the liquor before term is comparatively more abundant, and because the head is comparatively larger in premature fetuses.

If the head cannot readily enter the brim of the pelvis a malpresentation may occur, for instance when the pelvic brim is severely contracted, or when a low-lying placenta or a pelvic tumour reduces the available space in the lower segment.

If the tone of the uterine and abdominal muscles is poor, as may be the case in a woman who has had many children, the factors which normally constrain the fetus to lie longitudinally are absent, and there may be a transverse or oblique lie. If the fetus is dead it may lie abnormally because it does not move and lacks muscular tone.

Mechanism of labour with vertex presentations

The term mechanism refers to the series of changes in position and attitude which the fetus undergoes during its passage through the birth canal. These should be studied with the help of a fetal model and a pelvis, as well as by observation of patients in labour.

The head is a more or less oval body and it fits fairly tightly into the birth canal through which it is pushed. The longest diameter of the pelvis is transverse at the inlet and antero-posterior at the outlet. At the outlet the pelvic floor offers resistance to the head on both sides and behind, while it leaves a free space in front (see Fig. 9.7). Consequently the head, which enters the brim in the transverse or one of the oblique diameters, does not maintain the same position throughout its passage, but undergoes some rotation and also some change in its attitude as it passes through the pelvic cavity. If the head and pelvis are both of normal size the mechanism of labour is determined by the soft parts rather than the bony pelvis.

Although four oblique positions of the occiput are conventionally described, in most cases the fetal head enters the brim in the transverse diameter (LOT or ROT). In less than 15 per cent of cases the occiput lies in relation to one of the sacro-iliac joints (ROP or LOP); it is never in direct relation to the promontory of the sacrum.

The degree of flexion or extension of the head is a most important factor in determining the mechanism of labour and therefore its outcome.

Mechanism with the occiput in the transverse or anterior position

For convenience of description the mechanism will be described in this section for the LOT or LOA positions. (For the ROT or ROA positions the same description applies, but with substitution of 'right' for 'left' throughout, and vice versa).

While the head is descending it makes five movements:

1. Flexion
2. Internal rotation
3. Extension
4. Restitution
5. External rotation

Flexion.   With LOT and LOA positions the head is usually flexed before labour begins. If flexion is incomplete it becomes complete as the head is pressed down onto the lower segment and cervix. This complete flexion, which brings the occiput to a lower level than the forehead (sinciput), occurs because of (1) the shape of the birth canal, (2) the shape of the head, and (3) the 'head lever'.

The shape of the birth canal.   There is more space in the front of the canal than at the back; whichever part of the head is in front will descend more readily.

The shape of the head.   Any ovoid body being pushed through a tube will tend to adapt its long diameter to the long axis of the tube. When the head is completely flexed its longest diameter, the mento-vertical, lies in the long axis of the canal.

The slope of the posterior end of the head is much steeper than that of the anterior end; consequently the occiput can descend more easily, with less friction, than can the forehead.

The head lever.   When the breech is pressed on by the fundus of the uterus and the fetus is subjected to fetal axis pressure the so-called head

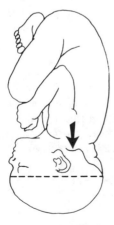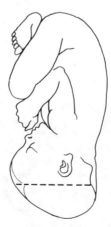

Fig. 10.4   Flexion of the head during labour. The arrow shows the direction of fetal axis pressure, and the dotted line indicates the reduction in diameter of the flexed head.

lever comes into play. The occipito-spinal joint is nearer to the occiput than to the forehead, so the head can be regarded as a lever with a short posterior and a long anterior arm (Fig. 10.4). As the fetus is pushed downwards the long anterior arm meets with more resistance than the short posterior arm, and so the forehead does not descend so deeply as the occiput.

The effect of complete flexion is to bring the posterior fontanelle, which lies in front and to the left, to a lower level than the anterior fontanelle, which lies to the right and behind.

Internal rotation. In the second stage of labour the head is pressed further downwards. As the occiput is furthest down the birth canal it meets the resistance of the pelvic floor first. The floor is a sloping gutter formed by the levatores ani muscles which leads to a free space under the pubic arch (Fig. 9.7). As the occiput is pushed down it rotates away from the resistance of the pelvic floor, sliding forwards along the left side of the pelvis towards the free space under the pubic arch. As it descends the long axis of the head rotates from the transverse or oblique diameter into the antero-posterior diameter of the pelvis. The head thus comes to lie with the sagittal suture in this diameter, with the occiput and posterior fontanelle in front under the pubic arch, with the forehead and anterior fontanelle behind in the hollow of the sacrum, and with the nape of the neck against the symphysis pubis. (Fig. 10.5.)

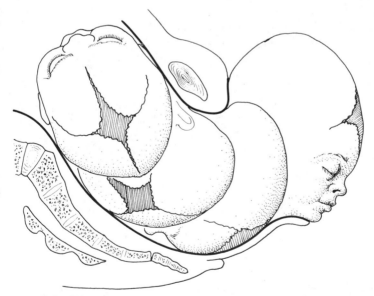

Fig. 10.5 Diagram to show descent and flexion of head, followed by internal rotation and ending in birth of the head by extension.

Extension.   The uterus and abdominal muscles now press the head downwards, while the pelvic floor presses it upwards and forwards. The resultant of these two forces directs the head forwards. It cannot move forward as a whole because the nape of the neck is pressed against the symphysis pubis; the only way in which the head can go forwards is by a movement of extension, the chin leaving the chest, and the occiput escaping under the pubic arch. The occiput is free already, and the vertex stretches the vaginal outlet until the head is crowned and can emerge, the vertex, forehead, face and chin successively gliding forward from under the perineum. (Fig. 10.5.)

Restitution.   As the head descends with its suboccipito-frontal diameter in the transverse or right oblique diameter of the pelvis the shoulders enter the pelvic brim in the antero-posterior or the left oblique diameter. When internal rotation of the head takes place the head is twisted a little on the shoulders. As soon as it is completely born it resumes its natural position with regard to the shoulders, the occiput turning towards the mother's left thigh. This movement, which sometimes occurs almost with a jerk, is called restitution, because by it the neck becomes untwisted and the head is restored to its natural relation to the shoulders.

External rotation.   As the shoulders descend the right and anterior shoulder is the lower and it meets the resistance of the pelvic floor before

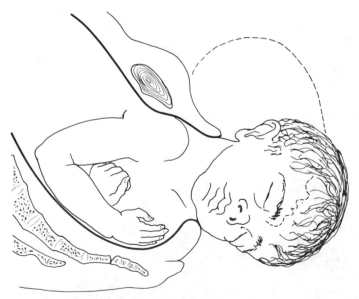

Fig. 10.6   To show external rotation of the head after delivery as the anterior shoulder rotates forward to pass under the subpelvic arch.

the left shoulder. The right shoulder rotates to the space in front, as did the occiput, and the shoulders now occupy the antero-posterior diameter of the pelvis. As they rotate the head, which has already been born, rotates with them and may make a further movement towards the mother's left thigh. The head now lies with the face to the right and the occiput to the left (Fig. 10.6).

Delivery of the body. The shoulders then emerge, the right one escaping under the pubic arch, while the left slides over the perineum. The rest of the body is usually born without any difficulty as its diameters are less than those of the head or the shoulders. The arms are usually folded on the chest, with the hands under the chin.

Mechanism with the occiput in the posterior position

The mechanism in the occipito-posterior positions depends on whether the head is well flexed or incompletely flexed.

The well-flexed head. If the head is well flexed the occiput is in advance when the head meets the resistance of the pelvic floor. The occiput slides down the gutter formed by the levator muscles, undergoing long rotation through three-eighths of a circle, to reach the free space under the pubic arch.

When the occiput lies behind and to the right (ROP) it rotates along the right side of the pelvis to reach the front, the shoulders rotating with the head from the left oblique diameter into the antero-posterior diameter. From this point the mechanism is the same as that of the ROA position, with birth of the head by extension.

(Similarly in the less common LOP position the occiput makes a long rotation along the left side of the pelvis).

Delay which occurs in some cases of occipito-posterior position is not because of this additional long rotation. If the head is fully flexed, as it must be for long rotation to occur, there is no delay in the labour and no difficulty. The cause of delay, if it occurs, is incomplete flexion, so that normal long rotation does not occur.

The incompletely flexed head. When the occiput occupies the posterior part of one of the oblique diameters of the pelvis the biparietal diameter lies in the sacro-cotyloid region of the pelvic brim. (This is the bay to one side of the promontory). When the head is pushed down into the pelvis in this position the biparietal diameter is hindered in descending if the pelvis is small or the head is large, and so the forepart of the head descends more easily than the occiput, and the head enters the pelvis incompletely flexed.

If the head is incompletely flexed the larger occipito-frontal diameter of the head, which measures 11.5 cm, has to pass through the pelvis, instead of the suboccipito-bregmatic diameter, which measures 9.5 cm. It is this, and the fact that sometimes neither the occiput or the sinciput is suffi-

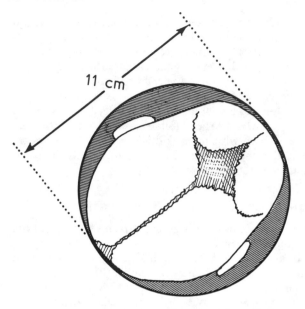

Fig. 10.7   Vaginal palpation of head in right occipito-posterior position. The circle represents the pelvic cavity with a diameter of 11 cm. The head is poorly flexed, so that the anterior fontanelle presents.

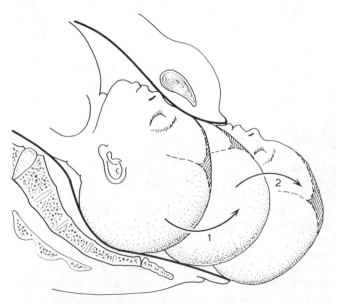

Fig. 10.8   Delivery of head in face-to-pubes position.

ciently in advance of the other to influence rotation, that explain why some cases of occipito-posterior positions cause difficult and prolonged labour. However, in some cases in which long rotation of the occiput does not occur spontaneous delivery takes place by an alternative mechanism, as follows.

If the head is incompletely flexed with an occipito-posterior position the forehead is as low as the occiput, and being at the anterior end of the oblique diameter of the pelvis it meets the resistance of the pelvic floor before the occiput. The forehead rotates to the front to the free space under the pubic arch, turning through one-eighth of a circle, while the occiput rotates backwards into the hollow of the sacrum. The head may now be born with the face towards the posterior surface of the symphysis pubis. The root of the nose is pressed against the bone, and the head flexes about this fixed point. The vertex is born by *flexion* and followed by the occiput. As soon as the occiput is born the head extends, the face and chin emerging from under the pubic arch. The vulval orifice is stretched by the occipito-frontal instead of the suboccipito-frontal diameter, with a difference in size of 2 cm, and a severe perineal tear may result. (Fig. 10.8.)

Deep transverse arrest of the head

In some cases the head becomes arrested with its long axis in the transverse diameter of the pelvis, the degree of extension being such that neither the occiput nor the forehead is sufficiently in advance to influence rotation.

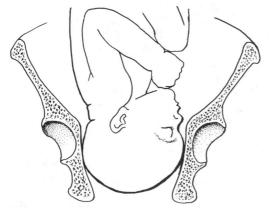

Fig. 10.9 Deep transverse arrest of head.

This is described as deep transverse arrest of the head and calls for interference (See p. 267). Some of these cases are the result of incomplete forward rotation from an occipito-posterior position; others, perhaps the majority, are the result of the descent of a head which originally lay in the occipito-transverse position and which has failed to rotate anteriorly.

11

Obstetrical examination

Reference should be made to the previous chapter for the definition of terms used here. Any obstetrical examination should be preceded by consideration of the history, including the past medical record, the past obstetric history and the record of the present pregnancy.

Abdominal examination

Abdominal examination is most important, and should always precede vaginal examination. By abdominal examination it is possible to ascertain:
1. The size of the uterus and to note whether it corresponds with the period of amenorrhoea.
2. The size of the fetus.
3. The lie, presentation and attitude of the fetus.
4. Whether the presenting part has entered the pelvis or not, and so to form an idea as to the relative sizes of the brim of the pelvis and the presenting part.
5. Whether the fetus is alive.
6. The presence of abnormal conditions, such as excess of liquor amnii, twin pregnancy or abdominal tumours.

Inspection. The examination should begin with inspection. An impression of the height of the fundus and the general shape and size of the uterus can be gained, and fetal parts and movements may be seen. In primigravidae with the head engaged in the pelvis, if the occiput is anterior and the back of the fetus is to the front the abdomen will appear smoothly convex; if the occiput is posterior a flattening of the abdomen may be seen above the symphysis pubis. If the lie is transverse the uterus will be wider than usual, and the height of the fundus may be a little lower than with a longitudinal lie. If twins are present the uterus also appears wide but the height of the fundus will be higher than normal.

Fetal movements may be observed.

Palpation. The fingers of both hands are used, and laid flat on the abdomen. The hands must be warm, and if the patient is nervous she should be reassured. The obstetrician stands on the patient's right side. A regular routine is followed:

(1) The level of the fundus is accurately determined by using the ulnar

border of the hand and moving it downwards from the xiphisternum (Fig. 11.1A).

(2) As the majority of fetuses present by the vertex, the lower part of the uterus should be palpated next to establish whether there is a cephalic presentation. This is done by placing both hands on the lower abdomen above the pelvic brim (Fig. 11.1B). The head is recognized because it is rounder and harder than the breech. Its mobility will depend upon its relation to the pelvic brim. If it is completely above the brim it is freely

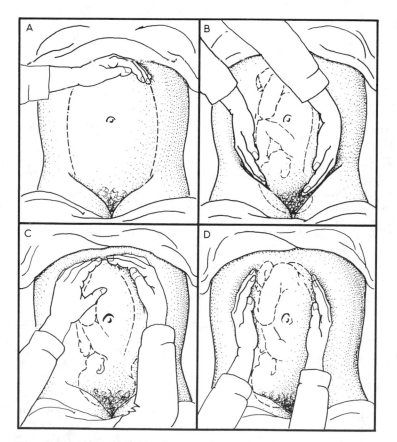

Fig. 11.1 Abdominal palpation. **A.** Determination of the level of the fundus of the uterus. **B.** Palpation of the lower pole of the uterus. In this case the head is well flexed and the occiput is deeply in the pelvis. The sinciput is felt at a higher level with the right hand. **C.** Palpation of the upper pole of the uterus. The breech is felt. **D.** Palpation of the sides of the uterus. The back is felt on the right and the limbs on the left.

movable and is spoken of as a 'floating head', and the fingers of both hands can be made to meet below it; if the widest diameter has entered or passed through the brim the head is usually fixed and is said to be engaged in the brim; if the head is deeply sunk in the pelvic cavity it may be difficult to feel it except with the finger tips.

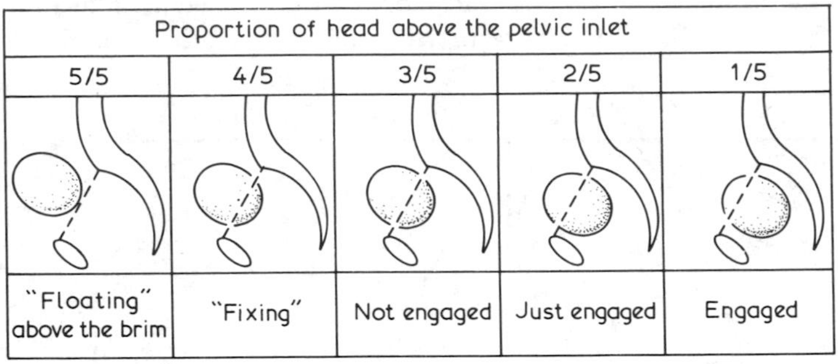

Proportion of head above the pelvic inlet				
5/5	4/5	3/5	2/5	1/5
"Floating" above the brim	"Fixing"	Not engaged	Just engaged	Engaged

Fig. 11.2 Diagram to explain the description of the position of the head in 'fifths'.

In many clinics the relationship between the head and the pelvis is now described in 'fifths'. A head that is completely free is described as 5/5; one that is beginning to enter the brim as 4/5, and one that has a major part in the brim as 3/5. Once the widest diameter has passed the brim the notation 2/5 is used, and for a head deeply engaged in the pelvis 1/5. The 'fifths' refer to the proportion of the head still palpable above the brim.

The degree of flexion of the head can often be made out by abdominal palpation. For example with a LOT position of the occiput the well-defined forehead (sinciput) will be felt on the right, but the occiput is less easily felt on the left as it is at a lower level, indicating that the head is well flexed. In such a case the anterior shoulder may be palpable near the midline.

If the head is above the brim of the pelvis it may be felt more easily by the single-handed grip shown in Fig. 11.3, but this method is of no use if the head is lower down.

(3) The fundus should then be palpated with both hands (Fig. 11.1C). If the breech occupies the fundus a broad mass will be felt, not so round or hard as the head. The breech is continuous with the fetal back, and a foot or knee can often be felt near it, and may move under the hand. If the head occupies the fundus it is felt as a harder, rounder, smoother and more mobile mass than the breech. The head can be moved independently of the body, and it can sometimes be balloted between the two hands. The fundus of the uterus is usually narrower when it contains the head than when it contains the breech.

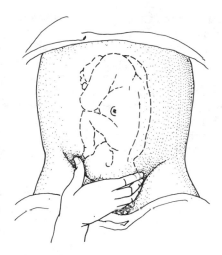

Fig. 11.3   Palpation of lower pole of uterus. Pawlik's grip of the head is only possible when the head is not engaged.

(4) The sides of the abdomen are then palpated to discover on which side the back lies. If the back is directed more to the front than behind a broad smooth surface will be felt on one side of the abdomen, and on the other side a number of small knobs, which are the limbs (Fig. 11.1D). If these small parts are felt all over the abdomen the back must be directed posteriorly and to the side, and deeper palpation may be necessary to feel it.

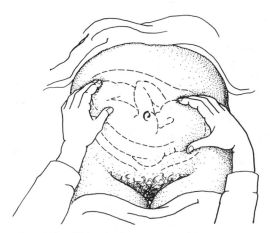

Fig. 11.4   Abdominal palpation of fetus lying transversely.

If the fetus is lying obliquely the head is often felt in one iliac fossa, and the breech higher up on the opposite side (Fig. 11.4).

(5) In the last 4 weeks of pregnancy if the head is presenting but is above the brim an attempt is made to discover if it will engage, and thus to exclude brim disproportion. This may be done by moderate pressure on the head in a backwards and downwards direction. Another method is to raise the patient's head and shoulders asking her to take the weight of her trunk on her hands or elbows, when the head will often enter the brim (Fig. 11.5). Perhaps the best method of all to test whether the head will engage is to examine the patient when she is standing.

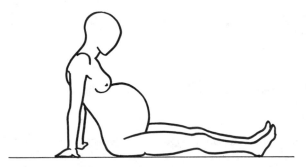

Fig. 11.5   Abdominal palpation. The patient is asked to sit up (or to lean on her elbows) to test whether the head will engage.

At each visit the level of the fundus and the size of the fetus must be carefully noted. If the duration of pregnancy is uncertain repeated observations are most useful, and any suggestion that the fetus is small-for-dates or is not growing normally calls for full investigation (see p. 250). If the uterus is larger than expected there may be an excess of liquor amnii or a multiple pregnancy. Twins may be diagnosed by palpation of more than two fetal poles, and often two heads are clearly recognized.

Auscultation.   The fetal heart sounds are next listened for. They are best heard over the back of the fetus in vertex and breech presentations; only in face presentations are they usually heard over the heart. In occipito-posterior positions, in which the back is directed to one side and posteriorly, the sounds may be heard either in the flank or near the midline.

In breech presentations the heart sounds will often be heard at a point higher up than in vertex presentations, at the level of or a little above the umbilicus.

Vaginal examination

A vaginal examination is usually made at the patient's first attendance at the antenatal clinic to confirm the pregnancy and its duration, to determine the position of the uterus, and to exclude other abnormalities such as ovarian cysts. The bony pelvis may also be examined, but the best time to assess the size and shape of the pelvis is at about the 36th week, by which time the soft tissues will be more relaxed and examination is easier. Further details of pelvic assessment are given on p. 304.

After the 36th week, and for any patient who may be in labour, full aseptic precautions are required for any pelvic examination. During labour the most important observations will be the degree of dilatation of the cervix, whether the membranes are ruptured or not, the recognition of the presenting part, and the determination of its position and level in the pelvis.

Some obstetricians use the *Bishop score* to record the state of the cervix (Table 11.1). It enables different observers to relate their findings accurately. A score of less than 5 suggests that labour is unlikely to start without ripening of the cervix; a score of 7 indicates that labour has begun or is imminent.

Table 11.1 Modified Bishop score

Score	0	1	2	3
Dilatation of cervix (cm)	0	1 or 2	3 or 4	5 or more
Consistency of cervix	Firm	Medium	Soft	—
Length of cervical canal (cm)	>2	2 − 1	1 − 0.5	<0.5
Position of cervix	Posterior	Central	Anterior	
Station of presenting part (cm above ischial spines)	3	2	1 or 0	Below

The ischial spines are useful landmarks in determining the level of the presenting part during labour, and the degree of flexion or extension of the head can be found by palpation of the fontanelles.

Radiological examination

The place of radiological examination in obstetrics is diminishing. While it will often give useful information, irradiation of the fetus, particularly in the early weeks, may produce fetal abnormalities or cause abnormal mutations in the genes of the sex cells. It has also been suggested that even moderate exposure to irradiation in utero may increase the incidence of leukaemia in childhood, although this has not been universally accepted. It is therefore wise to avoid radiological examination as far as possible during pregnancy, and whenever the required information can be obtained by ultrasonic examination that is to be preferred. However, if ultrasound is not available or is not applicable to the problem and there is a serious maternal or fetal diagnostic problem, X-ray examination is still sometimes justified.

X-rays are no longer used for the diagnosis of pregnancy. Ultrasonic examination can show the presence of a fetus (or the gestation sac) in early weeks, and the fetal heart movements by the Doppler effect.

Attempts to estimate fetal maturity by radiological examination of the ossific centres have not proved to be reliable (p. 53). It is possible to measure the fetal skull in utero by radiological cephalometry, but ultrasonic techniques are much better.

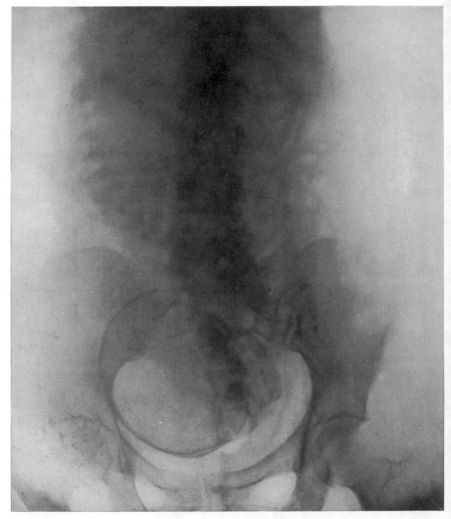

Fig. 11.6   Pregnancy of 36 weeks. Brow presentation.

Although the presentation and attitude of the fetus can always be determined by radiological examination in late pregnancy this should seldom be necessary, except perhaps in cases of gross obesity or of hydramnios.

Multiple pregnancy, including the rare higher multiples, can be diagnosed with certainty with x-rays, but such examination is unwise before the 30th week of pregnancy. Conjoined twins may be recognized.

When a *fetal abnormality* is suspected, and in all cases of hydramnios, radiological examination is justified. Anencephaly and gross hydrocephaly

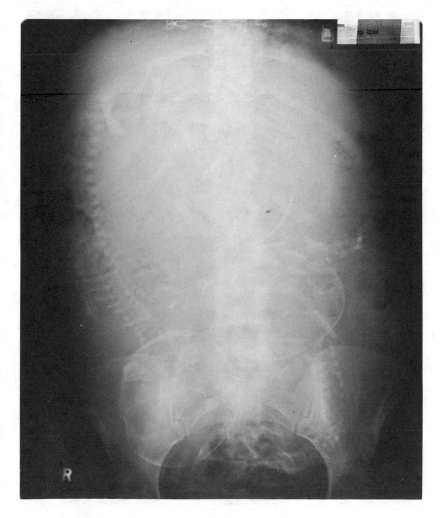

Fig. 11.7 Radiograph showing triplets.

are easily recognized, but lesser degrees of hydrocephaly should be diagnosed with caution as the position of the head relative to the film may give a false appearance of enlargement, especially in an antero-posterior view of a breech presentation. Spina bifida may occasionally be seen, and fetal ascites and hydrops can be recognized.

Intra-uterine death of the fetus. The most reliable radiological sign of fetal death in utero is over-riding of the bones of the vault of the skull

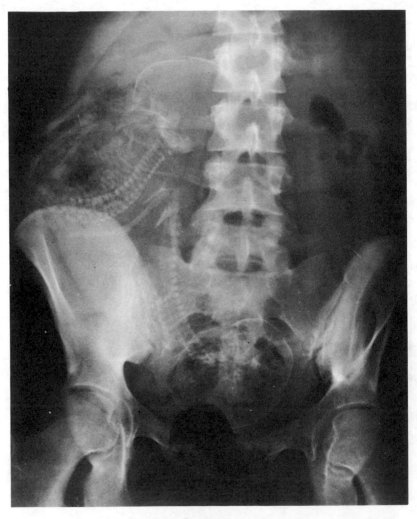

Fig. 11.8 Twin pregnancy. The smaller fetus is dead. The skull bones overlap (Spalding's sign) and the limbs and trunk are compressed together.

(Spalding's sign). This may be demonstrable 2 days after fetal death, but is often delayed for more than a week. Some overlapping of the skull bones may occur during labour from moulding, but with this exception over-riding can be taken as definite evidence of fetal death. Minor degrees of overlapping should be interpreted with caution, and of course its absence does not prove that the fetus is alive. Hyperflexion of the fetus or contortionist attitudes of its limbs give supporting evidence of fetal death. Nitrogen gas is sometimes seen in the large blood vessels of the fetus when it has been dead for about 4 days (Roberts' sign).

Placenta praevia. Radiological methods of localization of the placental site have been superseded by utlrasonic techniques (p. 169).

Pelvimetry. This still has a place in obstetrics, and is discussed on p. 305.

Ultrasonic examination

Ultrasonic waves are sound waves of high frequency, above the range of hearing. For clinical work very low power is used, and no tissue damage has ever been shown to occur. For diagnostic purposes a beam of ultrasonic waves is directed through the tissues. Whenever the beam encounters an interface between tissues of different physical properties partial reflection occurs. The echoes return to a piezo-electric crystal and the electrical signals produced are amplified and analysed by cathode-ray oscillography, finally appearing on a visual screen.

In the original A-scan method a dot of light on a screen was deflected to a degree which corresponded to the strength of the echo i.e. to the depth at which it originated. This allowed the relative distances of two interfaces such as the two sides of the fetal skull to be measured.

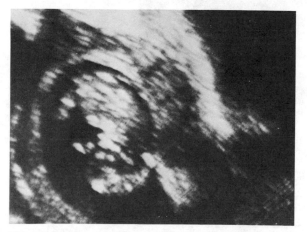

Fig. 11.9 Ultrasonic scan. Pregnancy of 11 weeks.

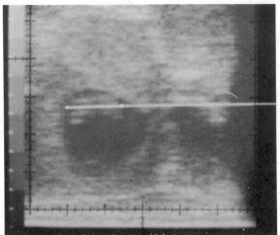

Fig. 11.10 Real-time ultrasonic scan. Fetal crown-rump length is marked for measurement.

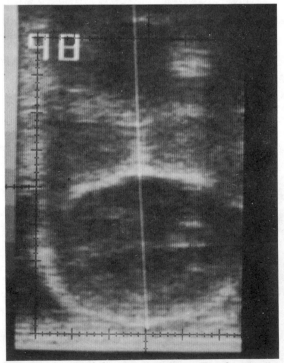

Fig. 11.11 Real-time ultrasonic scan. The fetal head is shown with the falx cerebri and ventricles. The biparietal diameter is marked for measurement.

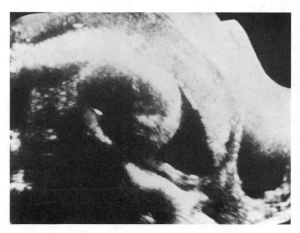

Fig. 11.12 Ultrasonic scan. The placenta is seen extending in front of the head on to the lower uterus segment above the bladder.

In B-scan, which has superseded A-scan, the brightness of a dot of light is made to vary according to the strength of the signal, and a composite two-dimensional section (tomograph) is built up on the screen as the beam is swung to and fro across the subject, not unlike the image on a radar screen. The B-scan has allowed the development of precise measurement, but the machine is relatively cumbersome and expensive, and it requires a skilled operator to get good results.

'Real time' ultrasound machines are currently under evaluation. Their advantage is that they are more portable and easier to use. Image resolution is less good, so that measurements are less accurate, but soft tissue outlines, fetal movements and some fetal abnormalities are well demonstrated. They can be operated by staff with minimal training, and may become part of the equipment of antenatal clinics, leaving the B-scan machines for the relatively few patients for whom accurate measurement is of importance.

With ultrasound the biparietal diameter of the fetal skull can be measured with an error of less than 1 mm. Repeated examinations can safely be made in order to follow the growth of the fetal head, and also to assist in the estimation of maturity in cases of doubt. When the fetus is small-for-dates, and in cases of maternal disease complicating pregnancy such as hypertension, renal disease or diabetes, weekly observations can be made for comparison with normal curves. (Fig. 11.13.)

Ultrasound can be used for the diagnosis of early pregnancy. The gestation sac can be recognized as early as the 6th week. The crown-rump length of the fetus will give an accurate assessment of fetal age at a very early stage, and after 12 weeks the fetal head can be independently demonstrated.

Twins can be diagnosed early in pregnancy when radiological examination is undesirable. Vesicular mole can be distinguished from a normal

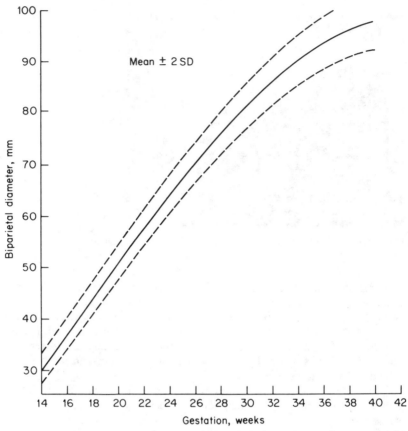

Fig. 11.13   Ultrasonic measurement of biparietal diameter at various stages of pregnancy. (Campbell and Newman, 1971.)

pregnancy, and an expert can determine whether an abortion is complete. Ultrasound can be used for the diagnosis of the presentation of the fetus.

A most useful application is for localization of the placental site in cases of suspected placenta praevia. Results should be interpreted cautiously before the 30th week, because a placenta which then appears to be low-lying may not be found to be attached to the lower segment when that is fully formed in late pregnancy. Localization of the placenta is also per-formed before amniocentesis.

Another application of ultrasound in obstetrics makes use of the Doppler principle. When the ultrasound waves are reflected from a moving surface their frequency is altered. By electronic means the alteration in frequency is recognized, and translated into audible signals which are curiously similar to the heart sounds heard through a stethoscope. The pulsation of the fetal heart or the blood flow in the fetal vessels or in the placenta will

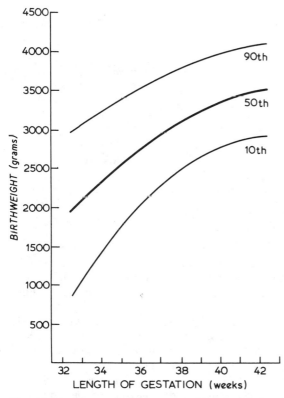

Fig. 11.14 Curves to show average birth weight according to length of gestation, with percentiles.

give signals whose rate is clearly different from the rate of those obtained from maternal vessels. Such machines as Sonicaid or Doptone are small and portable, and allow recognition of the fetal circulation as early as the 12th week. The presence, or absence, of signs of fetal life is often helpful to the clinician in cases of threatened abortion, suspected fetal death or vesicular mole.

Other obstetric diagnostic procedures

Some of these are discussed in other chapters:

Immunological test for pregnancy, p. 49.
Amniocentesis, p. 369.
Estimation of α fetoprotein in serum and liquor amnii, p. 370
Fetoscopy, pp. 58, 213.
Placental function tests, p. 251.
Fetal monitoring and fetal blood sampling, pp. 352, 359.

12

Management of normal labour

Today the majority of patients are confined in hospital. As soon as the patient is admitted her antenatal record is reviewed to discover whether there have been abnormal features of the pregnancy, and she is examined to confirm that the presentation remains satisfactory. In a few cases the patient will not have had any antenatal supervision; in that case complete examination will be necessary.

If the patient is to be delivered in her own home the doctor should go to see her as soon as labour begins. In domiciliary cases the midwife should previously have visited the house and arranged a supply of sterile towels, dressings, antiseptic etc., but the doctor should check that everything necessary is present.

In the routine management of normal labour the obstetrician's duty is (1) to maintain constant observation of the general condition of the mother, the progress of the labour and the state of the fetus, (2) to supervise nursing care, (3) to alleviate pain, and (4) to prevent infection.

No labour is certainly normal until the third stage is safely concluded. Danger, especially to the fetus, can arise suddenly and unexpectedly, and to secure the greatest safety of the mother and baby labour is best managed by 'intensive care' techniques. There is no reason why modern methods of monitoring during labour should be psychologically harmful or lead to interference with normal labour; indeed there is some evidence that they can sometimes prevent unnecessary intervention. If their purpose is explained to the patient they are also reassuring to her.

Although the dangers of infection have been much reduced by the use of antibiotics, it is still very important to minimize the risk of introducing infection into the genital tract during labour. Full sterile precautions must be taken by those delivering the patient and by any other persons present in the labour room. Vaginal examinations should be limited as far as possible.

The first stage of labour is proceeding normally if the cervix is progressively dilating and the fetal condition is satisfactory. The second stage is normal when there is progressive descent of the head and the fetus is in good condition. These statements may seem very obvious, but they are the basis on which most of the observations made during labour rest.

Management of the first stage

On admission the general condition of the patient is assessed, her pulse rate and blood pressure are recorded, and her urine is tested for protein. By abdominal examination the presentation and position of the fetus, and the relation of the presenting part to the brim of the pelvis, are determined. Abdominal examination will also show the frequency and strength of the uterine contractions. The fetal heart rate is counted for a full minute, and any abnormality of rate or rhythm is noted. A vaginal examination will show the degree of dilatation of the cervix, whether the membranes are intact or ruptured, and the level and position of the presenting part.

Although it is common practice to give an enema and to clip or shave the vulval hair, there is little to show that either of these practices is necessary, and many women dislike them. The patient may have a bath or a shower.

If each patient is told in simple language what to expect in each stage much of the apprehension from which so many women suffer can be removed before labour begins. If it is explained that the first stage of labour is the long one, during which she herself is not likely to appreciate much progress, it will be much more easy to reassure her and maintain her patience. She should always be kept informed of progress, although it is unwise to forecast the probable further duration of the labour. The patient should never be left alone, for it is then that fears and misunderstandings arise, and the midwife or the husband should be with the patient for as much of the first stage as possible. The purpose of any intervention or the reason for the use of any monitoring device should always be explained.

If the head is engaged there is no need for the patient to remain in bed during early labour. If she is up and about the weight of the liquor and the fetus helps to dilate the cervix, and pressure on the lower segment stimulates the uterus to contract. If the presenting part is not engaged the patient is kept in bed to diminish the likelihood of prolapse of the cord when the membranes rupture.

The pain during the early part of the first stage may not be very severe, although in primiparae it may cause distress. Towards the end of the first stage the pains become much more severe, and the patient may vomit at this time. If epidural analgesia (see p. 364) is not employed, drugs such as pethidine 100 mg intramuscularly may be given when labour is established and the patient is distressed, but a patient who has been intelligently prepared for labour should be allowed to decide for herself whether she wants the drug and when she needs the first dose. The knowledge that this help is available gives her confidence and she may prefer to defer its use for a time. As pethidine sometimes causes nausea metoclopramide (Maxolon) 10 mg may also be injected intramuscularly.

There may be a frequent desire to pass water during the first stage. If the bladder becomes full and the patient cannot empty it a soft catheter should be passed, as a full bladder has an inhibiting effect on the uterine contractions.

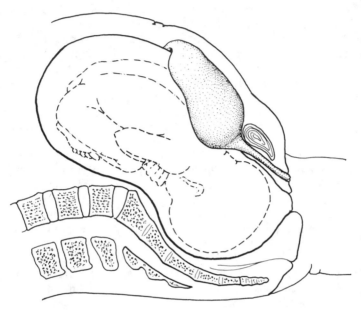

Fig. 12.1　Full bladder during labour.

During labour a patient must only be given fluid or sieved foods, as there is always the possibility that she may need a general anaesthetic for delivery. Once labour is established solid food is withheld so as to reduce the risk of vomiting during induction of anaesthesia and the risk of inhalation of vomit. If there is any evidence of dehydration or of ketosis appropriate fluid is given intravenously.

If epidural analgesia is not used, administration of nitrous oxide and oxygen, or of trilene and air, with the onset of each contraction may be started towards the end of the first stage (see p. 365).

Partogram.　Once labour has become established or the membranes have ruptured all events during labour are noted on a partogram—a most useful graphical record of the course of labour. Routine observations of the mother's pulse rate and blood pressure, with an assessment of the strength of the uterine contractions are entered on it. Records of the findings at successive vaginal examinations are plotted on a graph, showing the dilatation of the cervix in centimetres against the time in hours. The curve obtained

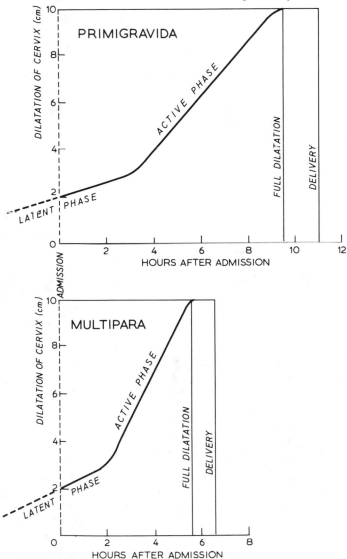

Fig. 12.2 Friedman curves based on observations made on the patients of a particular hospital, showing average normal progress during labour in that population. The time of admission will vary from patient to patient, and therefore the starting point of the observations will also vary. In general, the active phase of labour begins when the cervix is about 3 cm dilated. For practical use in the labour ward it is possible to prepare a series of stencils which can be superimposed on the partogram according to the parity of the patient and the degree of dilatation when she is first seen.

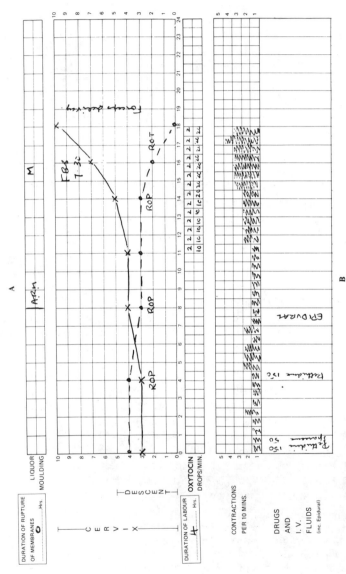

Fig. 12.3   Example of partogram. Only the middle section is shown. At A (above) there is a chart of the fetal heart rate, and at B (below) there is a chart of the maternal blood pressure and pulse rate. In the illustrative case shown there was a prolonged latent phase. With intravenous oxytocin (2 units/500 ml) at 20 drops per minute the uterine contractions improved and the active phase soon followed. At the point marked M meconium was seen in the liquor and there were some decelerations in the fetal heart rate, but a fetal blood sample showed a pH of 7.3 and labour was allowed to continue, ending in an easy forceps delivery. (The partograph shown is part of that devised by Mr J. Studd and used at Kings College Hospital.)

is compared with an average normal curve for primigravidae or multigravidae as may be appropriate. If the patient's progress is normal her curve will correspond with the normal curve, or 'lie to the left' of it.

Friedman has described two phases of labour: (1) The *latent phase*, from the onset of labour until the cervix is about 3 cm dilated, may last 5 to 8 hours in a primigravida. (2) This is followed by the *active phase*, during which dilatation up to 10 cm is more rapid, taking 2 to 5 hours, so that the slope of the partogram curve will be steeper in this phase. (Fig. 12.2.)

If for any reason labour is not progressing normally dilatation of the cervix will become slower or may cease, and the patient's partogram will be 'to the right' of the normal curve. A vaginal examination should be made every 2 or 3 hours, and if there is delay the membranes should be ruptured if they are intact, and augmentation of the uterine action by administration of an oxytocic infusion is to be considered (see p. 411).

The other important observations which must be made during labour relate to the fetus. If simple clinical observations are all that are possible these must be made and recorded regularly. The fetal heart rate is counted with a stethoscope at half-hourly intervals in early labour, and at 10 minute intervals in the active phase of labour. The normal rate is between 120 and 160 beats per minute, and there is no change in rate, or only a very transient slowing, with the uterine contractions. The signs of fetal distress are discussed on p. 351.

Fetal monitoring.   Many hospitals now employ fetal monitoring during labour. Where resources are limited this may only be possible for high-risk cases and those in which clinical signs suggesting fetal distress appear, but the ideal may be to monitor all cases because 50 per cent of instances of fetal hypoxia occur without evident preceding high-risk factors.

The uterine contractions can be recorded with a strain gauge strapped to the mother's abdomen, and the fetal heart rate can be monitored from an ultrasonic device attached in the same way. A better method is to attach a clip to the fetal scalp (through the cervix) from which a lead passes to a machine which calculates the heart rate continuously by measuring the intervals between R waves in the fetal electrocardiographic cycles. In normal labour the basal heart rate between contractions is between 120 and 160 beats per minute, with a continuous slight 'beat-to-beat' variation of the order of 5 beats per minute. In a normal case the heart rate may slow with each uterine contraction, but the slowing is neither profound nor prolonged. Prolonged deceleration or loss of beat-to-beat variation may be sinister signs. Details of these and other abnormalities which may be observed in the trace are discussed on p. 352.

If the ratemeter or clinical observations suggest that there may be fetal distress a sample of fetal blood is taken from the fetal scalp to determine its pH and thus indirectly whether there is fetal hypoxia or not. (See p. 359.)

All this information about the strength and frequency of the uterine contractions, the dilatation of the cervix and (later in labour) descent of the head, and the state of the mother and fetus can be shown graphically on the partogram. Drugs that are given can also be recorded there. These rather technical methods of checking that all is well with mother and baby must never be allowed to take the place of close clinical contact between doctors and midwives and the patient, and clinical assessment of well-being must not be omitted or disregarded. The disadvantage that some monitoring methods restrict the patient's mobility may perhaps be overcome in the future with apparatus that sends radio signals to the recording machine.

Management of the second stage

During the second stage the patient should be in bed, and the midwife or doctor should stay with her. In most cases it does not matter what position the patient adopts. Some women seem to use their voluntary muscles better in the dorsal position with their knees drawn up, but sometimes slowing or other changes in the fetal heart rate occur with the patient in this position because of supine hypotension (see p. 42). If such changes occur the patient is turned onto her side.

When the head begins to appear at the vulva it must be decided whether the patient is to be delivered on her back or on her side. In domiciliary practice with little help available the left lateral position is probably better, and it may be easier to control the birth of the head in this position. In hospital where assistance is usually available most patients are delivered in the dorsal position, in which it is easier to maintain good aseptic technique.

As each uterine contraction pushes the head down onto the pelvic floor the expulsive reflex comes into play and the patient will generally take a deep breath, hold it, and strain down. In a first labour the patient needs to be encouraged to relax the muscles of the pelvic floor at the time of the contraction. The progress of the descent of the head can be judged by watching the perineum. At first there is a slight general bulge as the patient strains. When the head stretches the perineum the anus will begin to open, and soon after this the caput will be seen at the vulva at the height of each contraction. Between contractions the elastic tone of the perineal muscles will push the head back to the cavity of the pelvis. The perineal body and vulval outlet become more and more stretched until eventually the head is low enough to pass forwards under the subpubic arch. When the head no longer recedes between contractions this indicates that it has passed through the pelvic floor and that delivery is imminent.

If delivery is left entirely to nature laceration of the perineum often occurs during birth of the head. By the time that the head begins to appear at the vulva some form of analgesia is usually desirable. A pudenal block may be used (see p. 366) but alternatively inhalation of a mixture of nitrous oxide and oxygen, or of trilene and air, is often effective.

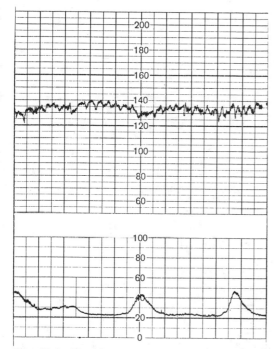

Fig. 12.4 Fetal heart rate. Normal trace. The lower trace records the uterine contractions.

At this stage the accoucheur must control the head to prevent its being born suddenly, and it must be kept flexed until the largest diameter has passed the vulval outlet. Once the head is 'crowned' the patient should be discouraged from bearing down by telling her to take rapid shallow breaths. The head may now be delivered carefully by pressure through the perineum onto the fore part of the head by means of a finger and thumb placed on either side of the anus, pushing the head forwards slowly before it is allowed to extend and complete its delivery. (See Fig. 12.5.)

If extension of the head begins before the biparietal diameter has passed through the vulval orifice a larger diameter than the suboccipito-frontal will distend the vulva and a tear may result. Even if the head has become crowned gradually, perineal rupture may occur if the head is then expelled suddenly and rapidly; it is important that the head should be born slowly and in the interval between pains.

Episiotomy, or incision of the perineal body, is necessary in some cases (see p. 375) and a clean incision is always preferable to an irregular laceration, or even to a grossly overstretched perineal body.

Directly the head is born a finger is inserted to feel whether a loop of cord is round the neck. Such a loop should be slipped over the head; if this

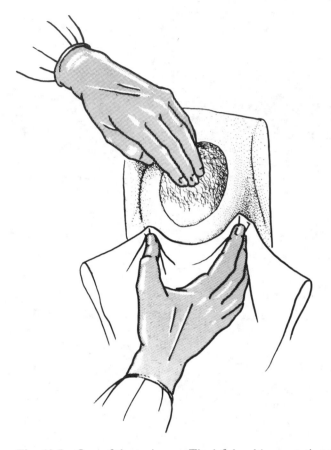

Fig. 12.5 Care of the perineum. The left hand is preventing sudden expulsion of the head, while the fingers and thumb of the right hand are gently helping the head forwards by pressure on each side of the anus.

cannot be done the cord is clamped with two pairs of artery forceps and divided between them.

The shoulders usually follow with the next contraction after birth of the head, the anterior shoulder being delivered before the posterior. Even if the head has been born without perineal laceration the shoulders can cause damage unless they are carefully delivered.

If the shoulders do not descend after the birth of the head the mother should be exhorted to bear down. If the shoulders still do not move and the baby's head is becoming cyanosed birth must be assisted. If the shoulders have not rotated into the antero-posterior diameter of the pelvis they must be rotated by digital pressure. If there is then still delay attempts must be made to bring the anterior shoulder under the subpubic arch by bending the neck laterally (towards the anus). Once the anterior shoulder has passed the symphysis pubis the posterior shoulder can usually be delivered after pulling the head forwards. As little force as possible should be used, for fear of injury to the brachial plexus. An assistant can help by pressing on the fundus of the uterus at the same time.

After delivery of the shoulders the rest of the body quickly follows. As soon as the child is delivered it is held with its head downwards so that any liquor or mucus in the mouth can run out. The mouth and pharynx are sucked clear with a mucus extractor. A healthy baby breathes and cries very soon after it is born; if it fails to do so it is treated as described on p. 463. As soon as possible, and even before dividing the cord, the baby is placed on the mother's abdomen, or very close to her on the bed.

The cord should not be clamped in a normal case until the child has cried vigorously and pulsation in the cord has ceased. If it is clamped immediately the baby is deprived of about 50 ml of blood which would be drawn out of the placenta by the expansion of the lungs. It is best to keep the baby at about the same level as the placenta. It is best to avoid excessive placental transfusion by holding the baby too low or 'milking' the cord, which could overload the circulation. It is equally important to avoid the opposite effect of allowing blood to drain back into the placenta by holding the baby too high (particularly at Caesarean section), thus causing the risk of anaemia and hypovolaemia.

If resuscitation is necessary there should be no delay in clamping the cord and the baby is taken at once to the resuscitation table. At first the cord is divided between two artery forceps placed at 15 and 16 cm from the umbilicus, and as it is cut it is examined to see whether both umbilical arteries are present (see p. 500). Later, a plastic Hollister crushing clamp is placed on the cord 1 to 2 cm from the umbilicus and the cord is cut again 1 cm beyond it. The clamp gives continuous pressure, so that if the cord shrinks the clamp does not become loose. A sterile rubber band twisted tightly round the cord is otherwise a preferable alternative to the traditional pack thread ligature.

Management of the third stage

In a normal delivery, if oxytocic drugs are not injected, the uterus will generally remain quiescent for a few minutes after the delivery of the baby. Regular contractions then begin again and separate the placenta from the uterine wall and push it down into the vagina. The mother will become aware of its presence on the pelvic floor, and by straining expel it through the vagina.

The following signs indicate that the placenta has separated and been expelled from the upper uterine segment:
1. The cord moves down. It may be difficult to be sure of this, and in case of doubt the fundus of the uterus may be gently pressed upward by

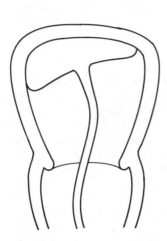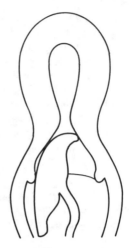

Fig. 12.6   Diagram to show signs of separation of the placenta. After separation the contracted upper segment is at a higher level and feels more rounded.

suprapubic pressure. If the placenta is still in the upper segment the cord will be drawn up with the uterus.

2. The uterus rises up because it is now perched on the lower segment which contains the placenta, and when it contracts the empty upper segment feels hard, round and movable from side to side.

3. There is often a small gush of blood when the placenta leaves the uterus.

The third stage of labour is a natural process which can be managed by simple observation and without interference unless bleeding or delay occurs, but even with such conservative management postpartum haemorrhage sometimes occurs if the uterus relaxes, and for that reason an intramuscular injection of ergometrine 0.5 mg is usually given after the placenta has been delivered. However, nearly all obstetricians now advocate an alternative and more active method of management of the third stage because this has been found to be safer.

Active management of the third stage. After 1935, when ergometrine became available as an effective and non-toxic oxytocic agent it was at first used for the treatment of postpartum haemorrhage after the uterus had been emptied, but it was soon found that by giving it at the time of the birth of the baby or immediately afterwards the number of cases of excessive bleeding (defined as a loss of more than 500 ml) was reduced. The ergometrine is injected intravenously as soon as the anterior shoulder of the fetus has passed under the subpubic arch and easy completion of the delivery is to be expected. The ergometrine causes a strong uterine contraction and almost immediate separation of the placenta. As soon as the delivery of the child is completed the obstetrician delivers the placenta by the Brandt-Andrews method, as described below. Ergometrine causes a prolonged contraction of the uterus without periods of relaxation, and while the uterus is contracting there is not likely to be any bleeding. However, there is a small risk that the placenta after separation may be grasped in the uterus or cervix, and with the active method there may be a slight increase in the number of cases in which manual removal of the placenta becomes necessary. This disadvantage is slight compared with the advantage of reduction in incidence of serious postpartum haemorrhage.

For this procedure ergometrine 0.5 mg may be injected intravenously but an alternative and generally accepted method is to use the preparation Syntometrine which contains 0.5 mg of ergometrine and 5 units of Syntocinon for intramuscular injection. The Syntocinon acts fairly quickly (although not so fast as intravenous ergometrine) and maintains its action for about 20 minutes. The ergometrine is effective after about 7 minutes (by which time the placenta will have been delivered) and it then maintains uterine contraction for about an hour.

The *Brandt-Andrews' method of delivering the placenta* is performed as follows. With the patient lying on her back the obstetrician places his left hand over the anterior surface of the uterus just above the symphysis pubis, at the presumed level of the junction of the upper and lower

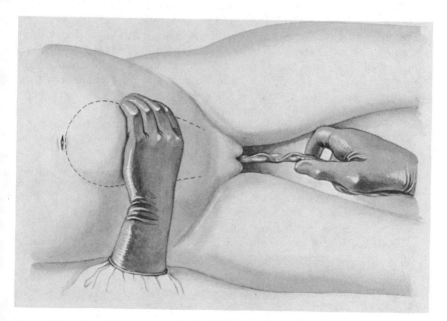

Fig. 12.7 Brandt-Andrews method of delivery of the placenta.

segments. An artery forceps is placed on the umbilical cord, which is held just taut but without strong traction with the right hand. The uterus is gently pushed upward with the left hand and if this can be done satisfactorily it means that the placenta is below the level of the lifting hand and is in the lower segment or vagina. Lifting is now discontinued and pressure made with the same (left) hand in a downward direction while the cord is still held taut until the placenta is seen at the introitus. After the placenta has been expelled the uterus is lifted out of the pelvis, as this is thought to diminish the tendency to haemorrhage. It will be noted that the principle of the method is not mainly of cord traction but rather of elevation of the uterus, which goes far to prevent acute inversion of the uterus (see p. 326) as a complication.

The membranes generally slip out after the placenta. If, however, they do not come away with gentle traction on the placenta they should be held with artery forceps and gently pulled, when they will usually be extracted.

Examination of the placenta, membranes and cord.   These must always be examined carefully as soon as possible. If the membranes have been inverted during delivery, as commonly happens, the placenta must be pushed through the hole in the bag of membranes so that its maternal surface will be seen to be divided into cotyledons, but these should all fit together when the maternal surface is made concave. If any part is missing a gap will be seen.

The membranes should form a complete bag except for the hole through which the fetus passed. The amnion and chorion can be separately examined after peeling the amnion off the chorion. An important but rare abnormality is that in which blood vessels run off the edge of the placenta to a small detached island of placental tissue called a *succenturiate lobe*. If this has come away with the main placenta and membranes it will be plainly seen, but if it is retained there will be a hole in the chorion corresponding to it, to which the vessels pass.

The cut end of the cord should be examined. A rare abnormality is absence of one umbilical artery, but this is important as it may be associated with other congenital abnormalities. POTTERS SYNDROME

If a piece of placenta is retained it is almost certain to cause postpartum haemorrhage, therefore it should be removed as soon as the diagnosis is made. If, however, a piece of membrane is retained within the uterus, be it large or small, it will not cause any complications and will come away in 2 or 3 days; uterine exploration is not necessary.

Examination of the perineum.   After the placenta is delivered the vulval outlet must be examined carefully for lacerations after separating the labia, with the patient on her back. Any tear other than a minute one must be sutured immediately.

13

The puerperium

The puerperium is the time following labour during which the pelvic organs return to their pre-pregnant condition. By convention the puerperium is said to last for 6 weeks, although it may take much longer for some of the organs to return completely to normal.

The management of the early puerperium consists in keeping careful watch upon the physiological processes during this time, and in being prepared to intervene if they should show signs of becoming pathological. Attention is given to the general mental and physical welfare of the mother and baby. Some special points of management are set out in the following sections.

Prevention of infection. Every precaution should be taken to prevent the implantation of exogenous pathogenic organisms into the birth canal during labour and the puerperium. The vulva and perineum should be kept clean and as dry as possible. Provided that there is no rise in temperature or pulse rate the patient may leave her bed to visit the lavatory and may have a shower or sitting bath. There is no need to swab the vulva or to pour antiseptic solution over it during delivery or in the puerperium. The vulva is simply kept covered with a dry sterile pad, which is changed by the nurse with clean hands whenever it is soaked or soiled.

Relatives, nurses, students or doctors who have septic foci due to streptococcal or staphylococcal lesions, or who may carry infection from recent contact with septic conditions or attendance at postmortem examinations, must be excluded from labour and lying-in wards. Patients who develop signs indicative of sepsis must at once be isolated from the normal cases until it can be established that any infecting organism is not pathogenic to others.

In order to reduce the risk of infection spreading, modern maternity units are designed with small wards of 4 to 6 beds. Ventilation should be by a system which introduces pure fresh air rather than one which draws in air from other parts of the hospital. Many organisms, in particular *Staphylococcus aureus* and the haemolytic streptococcus, are found in dust and blankets in hospitals. Only wet-dusting should be permitted in a maternity ward. Single rooms should be provided for suspect cases. The wide range of antibiotics now available should not justify lower standards in the prevention of infection.

Time of getting up.   After the physical and mental strain of pregnancy and labour a patient needs a period of rest from hard work and mental worry of at least 14 days. Not more than 5 to 7 days need be spent in hospital, however, and providing that steps are taken for adequate supervision by a midwife and doctor there is much to be said in favour of allowing the patient to return home 24 or 48 hours after delivery.

If the labour has been normal, and there has been no gross injury to the pelvic floor or other complications, the patient is allowed out of bed for short periods from the day after delivery, but she should limit her activities until the 10th day. This early ambulation must not be made an excuse for shortening the total time of convalescence. This period of rest will allow time for breast feeding to be comfortably established. Moderate exercise encourages recovery in the tone of the pelvic floor, the circulation is improved in the legs and the incidence of venous thrombosis is reduced. In abnormal cases it may be necessary to keep the patient in bed longer.

Temperature and pulse.   The temperature may rise to 37.8°C (100°F) briefly in the first 24 hours, but afterwards it should fall to normal and remain so. Provided that the patient feels and looks well the temperature need only be taken morning and evening.

The conventional definition of puerperal pyrexia is any febrile condition in which a temperature of 38°C (100.4°F) occurs within 14 days of childbirth or miscarriage. In the rules of the Central Midwives Board the midwife is bound to call in a qualified practitioner not only when there is puerperal pyrexia but also if the temperature reaches above 37.4°C (99.4°F) on 3 successive days.

It is strongly emphasized that when the temperature remains raised for more than a few hours, especially if there is a corresponding rise in the pulse rate, this should be regarded as due to infection arising in the genital tract until the contrary is proved. All cases of fever during the puerperium should be carefully investigated, as described on p. 417.

For the first few hours after a normal delivery the pulse rate is likely to be raised, but it should return to normal by the 2nd day. The pulse rate should be recorded at the same time as the temperature is taken. A rise in the pulse rate must be regarded as seriously as a rise in the temperature. It may indicate severe anaemia, venous thrombosis, infection of the birth canal, urinary tract or breast.

Onset of lactation.   During pregnancy there is considerable hypertrophy of the glandular tissue of the breasts, but secretion of milk does not start until after the birth of the child. With the stimulation of suckling and the release of prolactin the breasts become more active, and there is increased vascularity and engorgement. Up to the 3rd day only a little colostrum is secreted. By the 3rd or 4th day the breasts become tense, uncomfortable and tender, and there may be slight rise of pulse rate and temperature. After this engorgement the flow of milk begins and the discomfort is relieved by the child's suckling. Excessive engorgement of the breasts is discussed on p. 422.

Involution of the uterus. Immediately after delivery the fundus of the uterus lies about 4 cm below the umbilicus. The height of the fundus diminishes daily and it cannot normally be felt above the pubis after the 10th day. Any estimate of the height of the fundus should always be made when the bladder is empty. The uterus rapidly diminishes in size for the first week, then more slowly, being completely involuted in about eight weeks. At the end of labour the uterus weighs 1 kg, by the end of the first week about 0.5 kg, and by the end of the puerperium about 70 g. Involution is accomplished by autolysis of the muscle fibres, their protoplasm being broken down by enzymes, liquefied and removed in the blood stream. The end products are excreted in the urine. Delay in involution occurs in the presence of uterine infection, retention of placental products, or fibromyomata in the uterine wall, but in the absence of other signs of abnormality delay in shrinkage of the uterus is of no significance.

Retention of urine. A few patients have difficulty in passing urine for the first day or two after delivery. Retention is liable to occur after a difficult labour which causes bruising or lacerations in the vulva, after epidural anaesthesia, or when perineal stitches have been inserted. It is less likely with ambulant patients.

If the bladder is atonic residual urine accumulates and may become infected. Retention with overflow may occur with dribbling of urine. If retention occurs or residual urine in some quantity is suspected a catheter must be passed with careful aseptic precautions. Catheterization may have to be continued at regular intervals for a day or two, or a self-retaining catheter inserted.

Incontinence of urine. False incontinence, or retention with overflow, has just been mentioned.

True incontinence, now a rare event in Britain, results from a vesico-vaginal fistula, due either to a tear involving the bladder from instrumental delivery, or to pressure on the soft tissues from long labour and the formation of a slough involving the bladder. In the latter case incontinence does not appear until the slough breaks down some days after delivery.

Stress incontinence, or inability to hold water on coughing, laughing or sneezing, is not uncommon in late pregnancy and may worsen after delivery. It is caused by stretching and dislocation of the vesico-urethral junction from its attachments. If it occurs soon after labour it may be only temporary, but if it persists surgical treatment is required (See *Gynaecology by Ten Teachers*). The operation is not advised until several months have elapsed because in many cases improvement occurs with the help of active pelvic floor exercises and return of tone in the pelvic floor musculature.

Cystitis and pyelonephritis. Urinary tract infection with high fever may arise in the first week of the puerperium. Symptoms such as frequency and discomfort on micturition are often absent in puerperal infections, but tenderness over the kidneys may be found in the renal angles, more commonly on the right than the left. The infection is usually caused by coliform organisms, and may be an exacerbation of a preceding chronic infection of the urinary tract, or it may follow catheterization. It is difficult to obtain a satisfactory midstream specimen for bacteriological examination at this time, but one may be obtained by catheter or suprapubic aspiration. Treatment is by encouraging the patient to drink adequate quantities of fluid and by giving chemotherapy (e.g. sulphadimidine) or antibiotics (e.g. ampicillin).

Constipation.   This is common in the puerperium and is due to a combination of factors. The patient's food intake is interrupted, there may be dehydration during labour, the abdominal muscles are lax and perineal lacerations make defaecation painful. Constipation may need to be overcome by laxatives, suppositories or even an enema. Laxatives in vogue are Dorbanex, senna in tablets or granules, or a mixture of liquid paraffin and milk of magnesia. They are all transmitted in some degree to the child in the milk.

The lochia.   The lochial discharge comes from the large wound left in the uterus after separation of the placenta. For the first 3 or 4 days the lochia are red in colour. As the wound begins to heal the discharge decreases in amount and its colour changes to pink, finally becoming only serous. Although it has often been stated that the lochia disappear by the 10th day the average time before they become colourless is in fact usually 3 weeks. Lochia which remain red and excessive in amount indicate delayed involution, which may be associated with retention of a piece of placental tissue within the uterus. If placental tissue is retained the uterus may be enlarged and the internal os of the cervix remains open. The retained products can be 'seen' on ultrasonic examination. Curettage is not immediately required unless there is an increase in red loss or the passage of clots.

Offensive lochia may indicate infection of the uterus, although the organisms may only be saprophytes. Virulent infection with haemolytic streptococci is not accompanied by an offensive smell.

Sleep and avoidance of anxiety.   It is important to see that the patient not only gets a good night's rest, as free as possible from disturbance by the baby, but also that she has a rest in the afternoon. Pain from perineal stitches or engorged breasts are common causes of sleeplessness. If she is excitable and sleeping badly hypnotics such as nitrazepam (Mogadon) 5 mg should be given for the first few nights. After that sleeplessness, unless it is habitual, should arouse anxiety as it may be the first sign of the onset of mental disturbance.

Diet.   The day after a normal delivery the patient should be given a normal diet. During lactation she will need a considerable increase in her intake of protein and fat to compensate for that secreted in the milk. Once the flow of milk is established the fluid intake should be increased. At least a pint of milk a day should be taken. Animal fats, fruit and vegetables will supply necessary vitamins, and protein in the diet should be increased.

Perineal stitches.   Each day the perineum should be washed with soap and water and dried. A dry sterile vulval pad is then applied and changed frequently. Unabsorbed stitches are removed on the fifth day.

Care of the breasts. For antenatal care see p. 59.

To prepare for lactation and ensure an easy flow of milk along the ducts of the breast and nipple expression of colostrum from the breasts may be practised for 10 minutes daily in the last two months of pregnancy. It is held that patients who learn to express the breasts before delivery are better able to prevent milk engorgement by manual expression in the puerperium if this becomes necessary.

The nipple should stand out well when grasped between the finger and thumb, so that when the baby sucks he can get the whole nipple into his mouth with his jaws around the areola. If the nipple is flat or retracted the baby will be unable to do this and may bite on it, causing painful abrasions. A retracted nippled may sometimes be brought out if suitable nipple shells are worn under a well-fitting brassiere during the last three months of pregnancy.

During the first two or three days after delivery the breasts secrete colostrum only, but it is important that the baby is put to the breast in order to promote 'bonding' between the mother and baby, to stimulate the secretion of milk, and to teach the baby to suck. At first the baby should only be put to the breast every 6 hours and not allowed to remain there for more than 5 minutes. For further discussion of the details of breast feeding see p. 471.

If the mother cannot or does not wish to breast feed lactation is suppressed and she is helped to establish bottle feeding. Although oestrogens are effective in suppressing lactation their use has been given up because of the increased risk of thrombosis and embolism. By inhibiting the secretion of prolactin, bromocriptine in doses of 2.5 mg twice daily for 14 days is effective in suppressing lactation. It has the disadvantage of being expensive. Adequate support for the breasts and the administration of analgesics for the discomfort of engorgement is often all that is required.

Postnatal exercise. In many hospitals, patients who are confined to bed are given breathing exercises, exercises for the abdominal and pelvic muscles, and exercises to the legs to reduce the risk of thrombosis, but for most patients early ambulation has reduced the need for this. It is probably better to concentrate physiotherapy on the patients who have some special need for it.

Postnatal examination. This should be carried out at the end of the sixth week. Apart from discussing any problems or anxieties which the patient may present, and following up any complication of pregnancy or labour, the doctor enquires about her general health, whether the lochia have ceased, about bladder function, especially to exclude stress incontinence, and about any feeding problems.

The abdomen is examined and the state of the musculature noted. Pelvic examination is performed to check that any lacerations have healed normally, that there is no prolapse of the vaginal walls, and that the uterus has involuted normally. The uterus is not infrequently found to be retroverted. In most cases there are no symptoms from this, or the uterus is known to have been in this position before pregnancy, and no treatment is required.

A speculum is passed, and if a cervical smear was not taken in the antenatal period this is done. A cervical erosion is a common finding. Many of these heal spontaneously before the 12th week, and the patient should be seen again then. Only if the erosion persists and causes discharge which is sufficient to trouble the patient should it be treated (See *Gynaecology by Ten Teachers*).

Women not infrequently complain of backache at a postnatal visit. Most cases of lumbar backache are due to poor posture (persistence of the lordosis of pregnancy) or fatigue, and spontaneous recovery often occurs. Retroversion or other pelvic lesions will not cause backache at this level. Persistent backache, or of course any other disability discovered at the postnatal examination, may call for further investigation or treatment. Sometimes conditions such as hypertension or urinary tract infection call for prolonged follow-up.

Family planning advice.   Most women are anxious to space their pregnancies if not to limit them. Practical contraceptive advice should be made easily available at the time of the postnatal visit. The choice of method lies with the patient but it is necessary to discuss with her the pros and cons of the various methods. The patient may be prepared for family planning by discussion of the methods available while she is in the lying-in ward. If it is impossible for her to attend for advice in the postnatal period an intrauterine device may sometimes be inserted in the puerperium, or a prescription and instructions given for the use of the contraceptive pill. For a patient who has completed her family, and if she and her husband are certain that they will not change their minds later, sterilization may be performed in the early puerperium, but it is often better performed a few weeks later when the patient has had time to reflect whether or not she really wants it done.

Contraceptive pills containing oestrogen should not be given to women who are breast feeding because they may inhibit lactation. Progestogen-only pills do not inhibit lactation.

Details of contraceptive methods are given in *Gynaecology by Ten Teachers*.

14

Haemorrhage and pain in early pregnancy

Vaginal bleeding in early pregnancy is always a cause for concern. It may occur in cases of abortion or ectopic pregnancy, or with cervical lesions such as polypi or, rarely, carcinoma. In theory there may occasionally be slight bleeding from the uterine cavity before the decidua vera and decidua capsularis become fused together.

Abortion

The terms abortion and miscarriage are synonymous and denote the expulsion of the conceptus before the 28th week of pregnancy. After that date the fetus is considered viable and its expulsion is called premature labour. In the United Kingdom the delivery of the fetus before the 28th week is only notifiable if the fetus is born alive, whereas all deliveries after that date must be notified. There is no sharp demarcation in pathology between late abortion and early premature labour, and any discussion about late abortion passes on into that of antepartum haemorrhage.

The law relating to abortion and the indications for the therapeutic termination of pregnancy are not discussed in this chapter; for these topics see *Gynaecology by Ten Teachers*, p. 300.

The incidence of spontaneous abortion, leaving aside cases of legal or criminally induced abortion, is impossible to determine accurately; it is said to occur in between 10 and 15 per cent of pregnancies.

Causes of abortion

Despite a long list of aetiological factors, the cause cannot be determined in at least half the cases, and there is often more than one contributory factor. The causes include:

1. **Malformation of the zygote.** Many spontaneous early abortions are caused by defective development of the fertilized ovum. A large number of these are due to chromosomal abnormalities, for which either parent may be responsible, although they mostly arise from spontaneous mutation in the zygote itself. Most abortions of this type are not recurrent,

133

so that the prognosis in later pregnancies is good unless several abortions of identical pattern have already occurred.

Vesicular mole is a pathological condition of the chorionic tissues (see p. 146).

2. **General disease of the mother.**   Any acute illness with high fever may cause abortion. Maternal infection may involve the fetus, particularly in *rubella* and *syphilis*, but rarely in other diseases such as malaria and toxoplasmosis.

In a few cases of rubella abortion occurs, but more often the infected fetus is born alive. Syphilis does not cause early abortion, and it is an uncommon cause of late abortion; it is more likely to cause intrauterine death after the 28th week.

Diabetes is associated with a high incidence of malformation of the zygote, and abortion may occur if the disease is not adequately controlled.

Hypertension and renal disease. In these conditions intrauterine fetal death may occur, sometimes before the 28th week.

Acute emotional disturbances such as fright or bereavement may be followed immediately by abortion, presumably because strong uterine contraction occurs.

3. **Uterine abnormalities.**   Congenital abnormalities such as a *septate or double uterus* may predispose to abortion. Uterine *retroversion* is not a cause unless incarceration (p. 240) occurs and is left untreated. A submucous *fibromyoma* may cause abortion, but not tumours in other situations. *Incompetence of the internal os of the cervix* is usually the result of previous obstetric laceration or excessive surgical dilatation. It results in mid-trimester abortion if the membranes bulge through the cervix and rupture (see p. 140).

4. **Hormone imbalance.**   It has been claimed that inadequate production of progesterone by the corpus luteum before the placenta is fully formed will lead to inadequate development of the decidua and abortion (see p. 140).

Both thyroid deficiency and hyperthyroidism may be contributory causes.

5. **Irradiation** of the uterus during early pregnancy is a rare cause of abortion.

6. **Drugs.**   Cytotoxic drugs or poisoning with lead will cause fetal death and abortion. Oxytocic drugs have been used to procure abortion; quinine, derivatives of ergot and prostaglandins are sometimes successful in toxic doses.

7. **Trauma.**   Severe trauma to the uterus may cause partial detachment of the embryo, and this may also be caused by the insertion of instruments or foreign bodies through the cervix. Abortion may follow surgical operations, for example myomectomy. In normal pregnancy coitus has no ill effect, but it is unwise if there is a history of abortion in a previous pregnancy.

Pathological anatomy

In the first trimester of pregnancy the attachment of the chorion to the decidua is so delicate that separation may follow strong uterine contractions produced by any cause. The resulting haemorrhage into the choriodecidual space leads to further separation. In other cases fetal death precedes uterine contractions, which may occur some days later.

The decidua basalis remains in the uterus, and in the majority of cases the embryo with its membranes and most of the decidua capsularis is expelled. Sometimes the decidua capsularis is torn through, and only the embryo, surrounded by chorionic villi is passed.

By the 12th week the placenta is a definite structure and after that time the process of abortion is similar to that of labour. Bleeding and painful contractions are followed by dilatation of the cervix, rupture of the membranes and expulsion of the fetus and placenta. If all the conceptus is expelled (complete abortion) normal uterine involution follows, but frequently part of the placenta is retained with some blood clot (incomplete abortion). Rarely the uterine contractions mould the retained contents into a polypoid mass, described as a *placental or fibrinous polyp*.

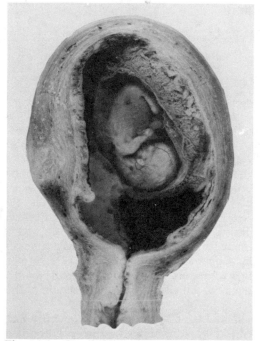

Fig. 14.1 Chorio-decidual haemorrhage.

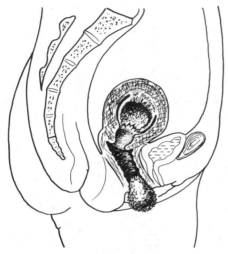

Fig. 14.2   Rupture of the decidua capsularis with escape of the embryo covered with chorionic villi through the rent.

Clinical varieties of abortion

The following terms are used to describe varieties of abortion:

1. Threatened
2. Inevitable
3. Complete
4. Incomplete
5. Septic
6. Missed (carneous mole)
7. Habitual

1. **Threatened abortion.**   In these cases haemorrhage occurs without dilatation of the cervix and with very little or no pain. The clinical distinction from inevitable abortion is based on the relatively slight degree of bleeding and the absence of cervical dilatation. If the bleeding is heavy or increases in amount the prognosis is bad, but the abortion should not be regarded as inevitable until the cervix begins to dilate. There may be repeated short episodes of bleeding without the abortion becoming inevitable, and if a slight red loss is followed for some days by old brown altered blood this may have little significance.

The patient is put to bed immediately, and rested until 5 days after all red loss has ceased. A gentle vaginal examination and the passage of a speculum will exclude any other unsuspected cause for the bleeding, such as a cervical polyp for example, and will also reveal any dilatation of the cervix.

There is no specific treatment and the essential task is to establish that the abortion is only threatened and is not becoming inevitable. Ultrasonic examination is most useful to determine the size of the fetus and to show that the fetal heart is beating. In normal pregnancy a gestation sac of about 1.2 mm diameter can be identified by the 6th week, and by the 8th week a crown-rump length of 20 mm can be measured. Repeated scanning is without risk to the fetus and can establish that growth is continuing. By the 14th week the crown-rump length averages 90 mm; thereafter growth can be monitored by measuring the biparietal diameter of the fetal head. Ultrasound will also help in the differential diagnosis; if the abortion becomes inevitable descent of the gestation sac into the cervical canal may be seen.

Serum progesterone levels can be measured, and decreasing levels may indicate that the attachment or the survival of the embryo is precarious, but administration of progesterone is of doubtful value (see p. 140).

If the pregnancy continues the mother may be anxious about the possibility that the fetus is abnormal; she can truthfully be told that this is very unlikely, especially if the ultrasonic scan is normal.

2. **Inevitable abortion.** The process is now irreversible. There is more bleeding and rhythmical and painful uterine contractions cause cervical dilatation.

In differential diagnosis other conditions need to be excluded. Inevitable abortion, ectopic pregnancy and vesicular mole all present with amenorrhoea, pain and bleeding. In abortion, haemorrhage is the dominant symptom; it often precedes the pain, and is profuse and bright red, with clots. In ectopic pregnancy severe abdominal pain usually precedes vaginal bleeding which is less severe, but rapid deterioration in the patient's general condition occurs if there is intraperitoneal bleeding. Examination under anaesthesia or laparoscopy may sometimes be required to exclude ectopic pregnancy. Ultrasound may also be helpful. In ectopic pregnancy a normal intra-uterine fetal echo will not be found and the cavity of the uterus will appear empty, but there will be an echo from an extra-uterine swelling. Vesicular mole gives a characteristic ultrasonic 'snow-storm' appearance.

In cases of inevitable abortion the uterus usually expels its contents unaided. All examinations are carried out with careful aseptic technique. Analgesics such as pethidine may be required. If haemorrhage becomes severe or the abortion is not quickly completed the uterus should be evacuated under anaesthesia with a suction curette.

3. **Complete abortion.** When all the uterine contents have been expelled spontaneously there is cessation of pain, scanty blood loss, and a firmly contracted uterus. If careful inspection of the products of conception confirms complete expulsion no further treatment is required.

4. **Incomplete abortion.** This term means that part of the products of conception, usually chorionic or placental tissue, is retained. Bleeding continues and may be severe. There is a danger of shock and of sepsis. If blood loss continues for more than a few days after an abortion it must be assumed that there are retained products, particularly if the uterus is still

found to be enlarged and the cervix is open. The products can be seen on ultrasonic scanning. The chief dangers are haemorrhage and sepsis, so that the placental débris must not be left in the uterus for any length of time.

Severe bleeding associated with shock may necessitate blood transfusion by a mobile emergency unit before the patient is moved from home to hospital. Intramuscular ergometrine 0.5 mg is given immediately, and any placental débris in the cervical canal is removed under direct vision, using a speculum and ring forceps. The foot of the bed is raised, and transfusion is continued until the blood pressure reaches a level safe enough for transfer of the patient to hospital. There the uterus is evacuated under anaesthesia with the suction curette or ring forceps. Postoperatively a prophylactic antibiotic such as ampicillin is given.

In some cases of incomplete abortion the bleeding is not severe but it continues intermittently for several weeks and the uterus remains enlarged. Surgical evacuation of the uterus is then essential, with histological examination of the products. Some of these cases are due to a placental polyp (p. 135).

5. **Septic abortion.**   Infection may occur during spontaneous abortion but it more often occurs after illegal induced abortion. Blood clot and necrotic débris in the uterus form an excellent culture medium, and if placental tissue blocks the cervical canal pus and blood collect above it. Infection may spread rapidly to surrounding structures, causing pelvic peritonitis, pelvic cellulitis and salpingitis, sometimes with septicaemia. There is fever and a raised pulse rate, and there may be lower abdominal pain. Permanent blockage of the Fallopian tubes may occur from salpingitis.

The commonest infecting organisms in cases of septic abortion in Britain now are *Staphylococcus aureus*, coliform bacteria, bacteroides organisms and *Clostridium welchi*, and of these the most dangerous are the Gram-negative and anaerobic organisms which produce endotoxic shock.

The patient must be admitted to hospital and isolated from other obstetric and surgical patients. High vaginal swabs and blood specimens are sent for bacteriological culture, while treatment is started with wide spectrum antibiotics. There is much debate about the best choice; one that has been recommended is penicillin 1200 mg 6-hourly intravenously, with gentamycin 160 mg followed by 120 mg 6-hourly intravenously, together with metronidazole 500 mg 8-hourly intravenously. When the bacteriological report is received the antibiotic treatment is modified according to the sensitivities of the organisms discovered.

Anaemia may occur from haemolysis as well as from haemorrhage, and the haemoglobin level must be determined. Blood transfusion may be necessary.

The uterus must be emptied, but if the bleeding is not of serious degree evacuation is best postponed until 24 hours after the start of antibiotic treatment. In cases with serious bleeding it cannot be deferred. In most cases evacuation is performed under anaesthesia with a suction curette or ring forceps. In cases of more than 14 weeks gestation in which a dead fetus is retained its expulsion may be achieved by administration of an oxytocic infusion and vaginal insertion of prostaglandins.

Some patients are gravely ill, especially if anaerobic infection has occurred, with high swinging fever, anaemia and sometimes haemolytic jaundice. Endotoxic shock may be superimposed on hypovolaemic shock, with circulatory failure due to peripheral vasodilatation caused by endotoxins released from coliform organisms which have invaded the blood stream. Before surgical intervention massive doses of intravenous penicillin and metronidazole are given, sometimes with isoprenaline infusion to maintain the central venous pressure. Oxygen is often necessary. The urinary output must be carefully watched, since oliguria may indicate renal cortical or tubular necrosis (see p. 164).

6. **Missed abortion.** This occurs when the embryo dies but is retained in the uterus for weeks or months. Haemorrhage occurs into the choriodecidual space and extends around the gestation sac. The amnion

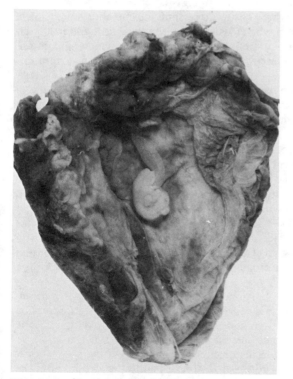

Fig. 14.3 Carneous mole surrounding early embryo.

remains intact and becomes surrounded by hillocks of blood clot with a fleshy appearance, hence the term *carneous mole*. Mild symptoms like those of threatened abortion are followed by absence of the usual signs of progress of the pregnancy. The uterine size remains stationary, and the cervix is often tightly closed. Urinary gonadotrophin pregnancy tests remain equivocal for weeks, but repeated ultrasonic scans will show no growth of the fetal crown-rump measurement and absence of fetal heart movements.

All carneous moles would eventually be expelled spontaneously, but there may be a delay of weeks or months and many patients become distressed once the diagnosis is made, so that active treatment is often chosen. In a few late cases there is a risk of hypofibrinogenaemia after retention of a dead fetus for some weeks, probably caused by thromboplastins from the chorionic tissue entering the maternal circulation.

Successful evacuation of the uterus is usually achieved in late cases with a combination of intravaginal prostaglandins and an intravenous Syntocinon infusion. In early cases the uterus may be emptied surgically with ring forceps or a suction curette after dilating the cervix.

7. **Habitual abortion.**   By convention this term refers to any case in which there have been three consecutive spontaneous abortions. Unless each successive abortion has occurred at about the same time and in similar fashion it should not be assumed that there is an underlying and continuing cause. Repeated miscarriages can occur by unlucky chance from different causes.

Early habitual abortion has been attributed to progesterone deficiency. It has been claimed that examination of vaginal smears shows this. In a smear from a normal pregnant woman the vaginal squamous cells have their edges rolled over (navicular form) and are clumped together; these changes are said to be less evident if there is progesterone deficiency. Another test is to examine the cervical mucus by allowing it to dry on a microscope slide; it shows a fern-like pattern of salt crystals if there is progesterone lack. However, neither estimations of serum progesterone nor controlled clinical studies have shown any significant improvement from treatment with progestogens in these cases. Advocates of this treatment give twice weekly intramuscular injections of 17α hydroxyprogesterone caproate (Primolut-Depot) 250 mg. Other progestogens are contra-indicated because they are partly androgenic and may have a virilizing effect on a female fetus.

Repeated mid-trimester abortions may result from *incompetence of the internal os of the cervix*, which is usually caused by previous obstetric trauma, injudicious surgical dilatation, cone biopsy or cervical amputation. In the non-pregnant state this condition may be diagnosed by a hysterogram or finding that a dilator 1 cm in diameter can be passed. During pregnancy it is suspected from a history of repeated, almost painless, abortions after the 16th week, or sometimes by observing the membranes bulging through the partly dilated cervix.

It is treated by insertion of a purse-string suture of non-absorbable material in the thickness of the wall of the cervix before the 14th week (Shirodkhar operation). This is removed shortly before term.

When a definite cause for habitual abortion cannot be established simple general advice is given. Any defect of general health is rectified if possible. Coitus is forbidden during pregnancy, and the patient may be rested in bed, especially at the time at which previous abortions occurred. In all cases the patient will need constant encouragement and support.

Ectopic pregnancy

An ectopic or extrauterine pregnancy occurs when the fertilized ovum embeds in some site other than the uterine decidua. Nearly all ectopic implantations are in the Fallopian tube, but very rarely the ovary or the peritoneal cavity is the site of origin of an abdominal pregnancy. In Britain the incidence of ectopic pregnancy is about 1 case to 300 mature intrauterine pregnancies, but much higher incidences are found in countries where pelvic infection is common, e.g. 1 in 28 in the West Indies.

Aetiology

Fertilization of the ovum normally occurs in the ampulla of the Fallopian tube, and the ovum takes about 5 days to reach the uterine cavity where it implants at the blastocyst stage in the prepared endometrium.

Delay or arrest in transit along the tube may be caused by a number of factors. Previous salpingitis may have destroyed part of the ciliated epithelium, or formed pockets of epithelial folds within the lumen; peritoneal adhesions may kink or compress the outside of the tube. Rarely a congenital diverticulum or abnormal length of the tube may be causative factors. There is a higher incidence of ectopic pregnancy in women using an intrauterine contraceptive device, possibly due to interference with normal tubal peristalsis or to ascending infection.

Pathological anatomy

The ampulla is the commonest site of implantation of the fertilized ovum. In less than a quarter of the cases the embryo is lodged in the isthmus; the other sites are very rare. The process of embedding is similar to that in an intrauterine pregnancy but, because the tube has no decidua, after the endothelium is penetrated by the trophoblast the embryo burrows directly into the thin muscular wall, where it grows and distends the tube. Tubal blood vessels are eroded with resulting haemorrhage around the embryo which then bursts either into the lumen of the tube (*intratubal rupture*) or through the wall (*extratubal rupture*) into the peritoneal cavity or occasionally between the layers of the broad ligament.

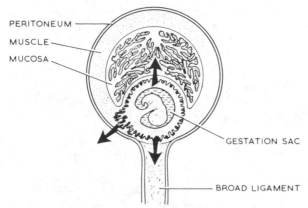

PERITONEUM

MUSCLE

MUCOSA

GESTATION SAC

BROAD LIGAMENT

Fig. 14.4 Tubal pregnancy. Diagram to show that the embryo becomes embedded in the muscular wall of the tube. The gestation sac may then rupture into the lumen of the tube, through the wall of the tube into the peritoneal cavity, or between the layers of the broad ligament.

The uterus also hypertrophies and the endometrium undergoes normal decidual changes. After death of the embryo the decidua is shed either in fragments or as a decidual cast, with some external bleeding.

Clinical course and management

Symptoms most commonly arise after one menstrual period is missed, but they may occasionally begin before this. On the other hand it is rare for ectopic pregnancy to advance beyond 8 weeks without the occurrence of pain or bleeding, a point which is sometimes helpful in differentiating between a uterine abortion and an ectopic pregnancy.

The dominant feature is low abdominal pain, often acute and severe, and this is followed by slight irregular bleeding from the uterus. Profuse intraperitoneal haemorrhage and severe pain may result in sudden shock and collapse of the patient, which may be fatal unless immediate transfusion and laparotomy are undertaken.

A tubal pregnancy may terminate in the following ways:

1. **Tubal mole.** Bleeding around the embryo kills it, and it is retained in the tube surrounded by clot. The patient complains of pelvic pain, sometimes unilateral, and slight dark vaginal blood loss. On bimanual examination a very tender swelling is palpable beside a bulky uterus. Lateral displacement of the cervix causes pain. The diagnosis from salpingitis or torsion of a small ovarian cyst may be difficult. An immunological test for pregnancy is often positive for a time. Ultrasonic scan and laparoscopy may be helpful, but if there is a pelvic mass

PERITUBAL HAEMATOCELE

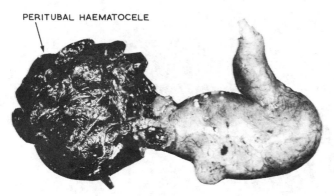

Fig. 14.5 Tubal mole, with bleeding through the ostium of the tube.

exploratory laparotomy is usually performed, and the damaged tube is removed.

2. **Tubal abortion.** As the name implies, this occurs when separation of an ampullary ectopic gestation is followed by its expulsion through the ostium of the tube into the peritoneal cavity. Blood escapes from the tube to collect in the recto-vaginal pouch as a *pelvic haematocele*. This blood becomes walled off by adhesions, producing a tender cystic swelling behind the uterus. With a large haematocele the cervix is pushed forwards and upwards, and occasionally retention of urine may occur. Later on, when absorption of the blood has begun, an untreated haematocele may have a lumpy and uneven consistence. There is often slight fever. Rectal pain and tenesmus may occur.

Surgical removal of the damaged tube and the haematocele is required.

3. **Tubal rupture.** This usually follows implantation in the isthmus of the tube. In this narrow part of the tube early rupture occurs into the peritoneal cavity, sometimes provoked by pelvic examination.

The patient rapidly develops signs of severe intraperitoneal bleeding, with pain, fainting or collapse, pallor, rapid pulse and low blood pressure, and signs of an 'acute abdomen'. The whole lower abdomen is extremely tender, and there may be some distension. Shifting dullness can sometimes be demonstrated. When the patient lies down the blood tracks up the paracolic gutters to reach the diaphragm and causes referred shoulder-tip pain. On pelvic examination there is exquisite tenderness, but no mass will be felt as the ruptured tube is now empty.

Immediate blood transfusion is required, followed without delay by laparotomy to clamp the bleeding points and remove the damaged tube and the blood clot.

In rare instances the rupture occurs downwards between the layers of the broad ligament to form an *intraligamentous haematoma*. The management

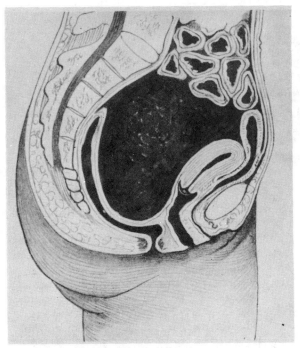

Fig. 14.6 Drawing to show a large pelvic haematocele pushing the intestines upwards and displacing the uterus forwards.

is similar to that of a tubal mole, since the differential diagnosis may be impossible before laparotomy.

4. **Tubal erosion and secondary abdominal pregnancy.** Intraperitoneal rupture, as described above, is occasionally accompanied by relatively little bleeding. The embryo is then partially extruded into the peritoneal cavity and may continue to grow, developing partial placental attachment to surrounding structures. If the amnion remains intact the pregnancy may progress to term, the patient then experiences a mock labour which is followed by death of the fetus and thrombosis of vessels going to the placental site. This very rare condition is known as *secondary abdominal pregnancy*. Ultimately mummification of the fetus occurs with subsequent calcification, forming a *lithopaedion*. If infection does not occur this may be retained for many years in the abdominal cavity, only to be discovered if the patient presents with intestinal obstruction or an abdominal mass.

In advanced abdominal pregnancy removal of a live fetus is seldom technically difficult at laparotomy, but there is a risk of severe haemorrhage when the placenta is separated from its attachment to other structures. It may sometimes be best to leave the placenta in situ and to close the abdomen, allowing spontaneous absorption to occur.

5. **Interstitial (cornual) pregnancy.** The site of implantation is in the part of the tube which lies in the uterine wall. The pregnancy may continue until about the 12th week, but sooner or later there is extensive rupture of the uterine cornu with very free bleeding from the vascular myometrium. This will necessitate enucleation of the gestation sac and wedge resection of the cornu, or even hysterectomy if there is uncontrollable bleeding.

Occasionally rupture of the sac into the uterine cavity is followed by abortion.

Ovarian pregnancy is exceedingly rare and clinically indistinguishable from a ruptured tubal pregnancy. The diagnosis can only be proven by careful histological examination of the gestation sac and ovary after removal.

Rupture of a pregnant rudimentary horn of a bicornuate uterus is not strictly an extrauterine pregnancy, but it is a serious accident with intraperitoneal bleeding. This occurs later than rupture of a tubal pregnancy, often at about the 14th week. The diagnosis is usually made at laparotomy, when the horn is removed.

Other causes of haemorrhage during early pregnancy

Bleeding may come from lesions of the cervix:

1. **Cervical erosion** is very common during pregnancy, when the high level of oestrogens causes proliferation of the columnar epithelium of the cervical canal, so that this extends outwards on the vaginal aspect of the cervix, forming a velvety red area around the external os, with well-defined edges. Such erosions occasionally cause a slight blood-stained discharge, but with any bleeding the possibility of malignancy must be considered. So long as a cervical smear is examined and found to be normal no treatment is required during pregnancy, and most erosions resolve after delivery.

2. **Cervical adenomatous polypi** may be found during pregnancy as small soft red tumours, attached by a stalk to the cervix near the external os. If they are not causing more than a slight blood-stained discharge, and a smear arouses no suspicion of malignant disease, they may be left alone during pregnancy; otherwise they are easily removed for biopsy.

3. **Carcinoma of the cervix.** See p. 248.

15

Vesicular mole and other abnormalities of the placenta and cord

Vesicular mole

A vesicular or hydatidiform mole consists of a large number of vesicles of varying size resulting from abnormal development of the chorionic villi. The vesicles are arranged on stalks which arise from the chorion, and each stalk represents an original villus. These villi branch, and the branches show the same vesicular formation, so that they come to resemble strings of beads. Usually all the villi are involved, but in rare instances vesicular change has occurred in only part of the placenta of a healthy fetus. It has been seen with extrauterine pregnancy, and accompanying a normal twin.

In Europe vesicular mole occurs about once in 2500 pregnancies, but it is much more common in China, the Philippines, Singapore and parts of West Africa and South America. The reason for this geographical distribution is not known.

Pathology

Vesicular mole has to be regarded as a potential chorionic neoplasm. The change in the villi begins in early pregnancy when the whole chorion bears villi. The amniotic sac is usually indistinguishable and an embryo cannot be found.

Owing to enlargement of the villi, the chorion takes up as much room as the whole of a normal gestation. In many cases the size of the uterus is greater than that of a normal pregnancy of the same duration. This increase in size is because of the large mass of vesicles present. Bleeding may occur around the vesicles and cause further distension of the uterus with pain. In a few cases the uterus is normal or smaller in size than would be expected.

Vesicles vary in size from microscopic to about 3 cm in diameter. Histologically they have the usual structure of a chorionic villus, but show excessive proliferation of both layers of the trophoblast, with hydropic degeneration of the central connective tissue. Simultaneous proliferation and degeneration is therefore taking place. In the smaller vesicles the connective tissues of the villus can still be recognized, but in the larger vesicles nothing remains but the cyst wall composed of chorionic epithelium surrounding clear fluid.

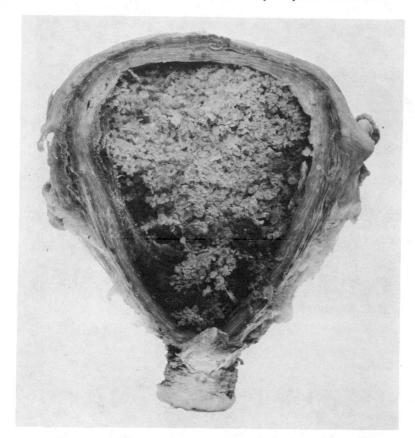

Fig. 15.1 Uterus containing a vesicular mole.

Both the syncytiotrophoblast and the cytotrophoblast proliferate, form-ing massive buds. Such masses of chorionic epithelium attached to some of the vesicles are almost indistinguishable from the cell masses which characterize the malignant growth known as *choriocarcinoma*, which may sometimes follow abortion of a vesicular mole. This active proliferation of the chorionic epithelium is the essential feature of the condition, and it gives the mole a much increased power of eroding the uterine wall and signifies its potential malignancy. In some cases the villi penetrate com-pletely through the decidua and perforate the uterine muscle. Even the peritoneum may be broken through, so that haemorrhage occurs into the peritoneal cavity. This power of deep penetration is the distinguishing feature of the so-called invasive or penetrating mole (*Chorio-adenoma destruens*). Every gradation from a simple vesicular degeneration for the

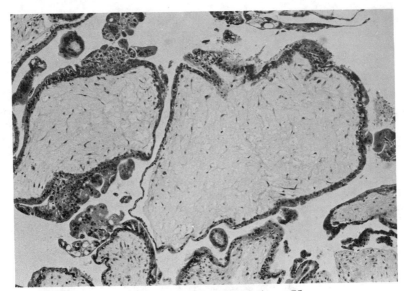

Fig. 15.2   Microscopical section of vesicular mole. × 75.

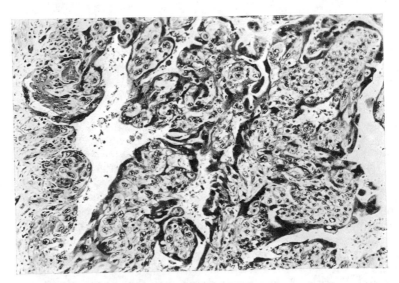

Fig. 15.3   Microscopical section of choriocarcinoma.

chorion up to the penetrating mole can be found. Histologically it is difficult to distinguish the simple from the penetrating mole.

As a result of stimulation by the chorionic gonadotrophin which is secreted in large amounts by the chorionic epithelium, bilateral thecalutein cysts are often present in the ovaries, and may be quite large. They disappear after the mole is removed.

Symptoms and signs

The chief symptom is bleeding. This usually begins between the 12th and 16th week, but may start sooner. The abnormally large size of the uterus may be noticed, and after the 20th week the absence of fetal movements. The uterus is generally larger than in a normal pregnancy of the same duration, but not invariably so; sometimes it is smaller. It may be tense or of normal consistency. There may be abdominal pain, especially if the mole is complicated by concealed haemorrhage. Fetal parts cannot be felt, nor can fetal heart movements be detected with ultrasound.

Vomiting may be persistent or excessive, and often the patient does not look or feel well. There may be slight pyrexia. Signs of pre-eclampsia such as hypertension or proteinuria are often present with large moles, and even eclampsia may occur.

On vaginal examination watery brown discharge ('prune juice') may be discovered. If abortion of the mole is in progress the cervix may be dilated and there will be free bleeding. Sometimes vesicles are seen. Bilateral ovarian tumours may be palpable.

Diagnosis

A vesicular mole has to be differentiated from threatened miscarriage of a normal or twin pregnancy. The main points are the size of the uterus, the absence of any signs of the presence of a fetus, and the discovery of bilateral ovarian tumours. A rise of blood pressure or proteinuria first appearing in mid-pregnancy might suggest the diagnosis.

An ultrasonic scan will immediately provide the correct diagnosis. A fetus is not seen and there is a characteristic 'snow-storm' appearance on the screen.

Quantitative assay of urinary gonadotrophin excretion may be diagnostic, because the levels are abnormally high in cases of vesicular mole, usually higher even than in twin pregnancy. (The ultrasonic scan would also exclude twins). If the usual immunological test for pregnancy is performed it will be found positive even if the urine is in a dilution of 1:100 or 1:200. Blood levels can also be estimated by radioimmunoassay, when high concentrations will be found.

Prognosis

Danger to life may arise from haemorrhage during expulsion of a mole and still more during surgical evacuation. The uterus may not retract well, and vaginal evacuation when the uterus is not contracting is a dangerous procedure. Sepsis may also occur because the mole may be incompletely evacuated.

When the villi penetrate deeply haemorrhage may occur into the peritoneal cavity, or the uterus may rupture. There is a risk of perforating the uterine wall during evacuation of a mole.

Choriocarcinoma. This rare malignant growth occurs more often after vesicular mole than after any other type of pregnancy. In the West it follows about 10 per cent of molar pregnancies, but the incidence seems to be higher in Asiatic countries. It used to be inevitably fatal, but now if it is recognized early it can be successfully treated with methotrexate combined with other cytotoxic drugs.

Treatment

The treatment of vesicular mole is to empty the uterus and to promote its contraction and retraction. If the cervix is already dilated spontaneous expulsion of the whole or greater part of the mole may be achieved. The uterus should be encouraged to expel the mole itself, provided that haemorrhage does not become excessive. An intravenous infusion of Syntocinon is given and, provided that the dose is increased gradually while the uterine response is observed, much larger doses can be given than would be used during induction of labour with a living fetus. Prostaglandins can also be used.

If it is found necessary to extract the mole an intravenous infusion of Syntocinon or ergometrine is started before the operation. This will greatly reduce the bleeding. A suction curette is used, but with great care as the uterus is easily perforated when the villi have penetrated deeply. Abdominal hysterotomy is now seldom necessary; with the suction curette and an oxytocic infusion even large moles can be safely removed. Many obstetricians advise that the uterus should be curetted 5 days after evacuation of a mole.

If the patient is nearing the menopause or already has the family she wants, hysterectomy with the mole *in situ* should be performed, particularly as the incidence of choriocarcinoma may be higher in women over 40.

If red loss continues for more than 3 weeks after surgical or spontaneous evacuation of a mole the uterus should be curetted and any material found should be examined histologically for choriocarcinoma. In every case regular estimation of blood levels of chorionic gonadotrophins must be made by radioimmunoassay afterwards, first at 6 weeks and then two-monthly for three years. Only when this test has been persistently negative for that time, further pregnancy having been avoided, should the patient be regarded as cured.

For the diagnosis and treatment of choriocarcinoma the reader is referred to *Gynaecology by Ten Teachers* p. 202.

Other abnormalities of development of the placenta

Anomalies in weight

The average weight of the placenta at term is 500 g. The weight varies according to whether the umbilical cord has been clamped early or late, thus imprisoning less or more of the fetal blood. In cases of diabetes and erythroblastosis fetalis the placental weight may increase up to half the weight of the fetus.

Site of implantation of the placenta

The placenta is usually attached to the uterine wall near the fundus, and either on the anterior or posterior surface. Anterior implantation may play a part in causing an occipito-posterior position of the fetus, as the fetal back cannot then be easily accommodated in the anterior position.

In about 1 in 250 pregnancies the placenta is implanted wholly or partially on the lower segment of the uterus (*placenta praevia*). This is a serious abnormality as it may cause severe haemorrhage in pregnancy or labour (see p. 166).

Abnormalities in the shape of the placenta

The chorionic villi at first cover the whole surface of the chorion, and a discrete placenta is only formed after the 12th week of pregnancy, by which time villi related to the decidua capsularis which have a relatively poor blood supply have atrophied, whereas those related to the decidua basalis continue to proliferate. Various placental anomalies occur, which are thought to be due to some abnormality of vascularization at an early stage.

Bipartite and tripartite placenta

Instead of a single disc the placenta may consist of two or three lobes, usually partly fused, but sometimes completely separate except for their vascular attachments. Such abnormalities are of no significance.

Placenta succenturiata

This anomaly is not uncommon. One or more accessory lobes of placental substance are found on the chorion at a distance from the edge of the main placenta. They are united to the placenta by arteries and veins. Placenta succenturiata is of clinical importance because it is liable to be retained in the uterus after the placenta proper has been expelled, causing postpartum haemorrhage. The abnormality should be discovered when the membranes and placenta are inspected after delivery, when a round defect will be seen in the membranes, with a leash of vessels running from the edge of the placenta to end abruptly where they have been torn across at the edge of the defect. In such a case the uterine cavity should be explored immediately, and the succenturiate lobe removed.

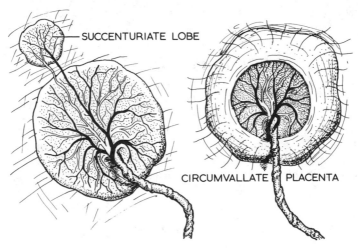

Fig. 15.4   Placenta succenturiata and circumvallata.

Placenta circumvallata

This is due to a late outward proliferation of chorionic villi because the original area of the chorionic plate was unduly small. As a result the chorionic villi proliferate outwards into the decidua, beneath the ring of attachment of amnion and chorion. A white ring is seen on the fetal aspect of the placenta, and this bounds a central depression, from which the fetal vessels radiate and disappear under the white ring. This abnormality does not usually interfere with placental function, but it may be associated with antepartum or intrapartum haemorrhage.

Placenta accreta or increta

In the third stage of labour the placenta normally separates through a plane which runs through the thickness of the maternal decidua. The superficial part of the decidua comes away with the placenta, and the deeper part remains on the uterine wall. The layer of separation is in the stratum spongiosum of the decidua. Normally the chorionic villi only penetrate as far as this.

If the chorionic villi penetrate more deeply the placenta is abnormally adherent and the condition is called placenta accreta or increta. In the former condition there is a solid fusion between the placenta and the decidual tissues, the spongy layer is absent and there is no plane of cleavage. In the latter the chorionic villi penetrate the uterine muscle, so that the placenta and the uterine wall become continuous. Sometimes the area of adhesion is limited to part of the placental site, but in rare cases the entire placenta is firmly attached. Morbid adhesion of the whole placenta occurs about once in 20 000 deliveries.

There is delay in the third stage of labour, and the abnormality is only discovered when an attempt to remove the placenta manually is made, and no plane of cleavage is found. If the whole placenta is adherent there can be no bleeding, but with partial adherence or after attempts at removal severe bleeding may occur. If adherence is only partial it is usually possible to remove the placenta, but there is risk of leaving part of it behind.

In cases of complete placenta accreta it may be possible to remove the placenta piecemeal, but this is a dangerous procedure. Unless haemorrhage has been caused by attempts to remove the placenta or the uterus has been torn, when hysterectomy is inevitable, it is justifiable to leave the placenta *in situ* and await its separation by necrosis. Antibiotics should be given during this time.

Diseases of the placenta

Infection of the placenta

The placenta may be invaded by bacteria during prolonged labour, or after fetal death if the membranes are ruptured.

Tuberculosis of the placenta. Tuberculosis in the fetal portion of the placenta is very rare. Local lesions may be found in the decidua and chorion when the mother has miliary tuberculosis.

Syphilis of the placenta. The syphilitic placenta is sometimes heavier than normal. Histological examination of the placenta is of no value in excluding or confirming syphilis of the newborn. The presence of *Treponema pallida* may be demonstrated, but not easily.

Placenta in erythroblastosis fetalis (haemolytic disease)

In mild degrees of this condition no abnormality may be evident, although the placenta may be stained yellow with bile pigment. In cases of hydrops fetalis the placenta is oedematous, large, pale and friable, and often as heavy as the fetus itself. There is abnormal persistence of the cytotrophoblast (Langhans' cells) of the chorionic villi; the reason for this is not known.

Degenerative changes in the placenta

The placenta has a limited life span; it grows actively for about 30 weeks, and after that time degenerative changes are commonly found in it. In the past any degenerative change in the placenta was called a placental 'infarct', but this term should be given up, as the abnormalities included under it bear no resemblance to the ordinary infarct of general pathology, which is due to occlusion of the artery supplying part of an organ. The chorionic villus is nourished by maternal blood flowing in the intervillous space, which bathes its entire surface, and obstruction of the central fetal arteriole will not cause its death.

Fibrinoid degeneration.   In nearly every mature placenta white fibrinoid areas may be found near the periphery, under the chorionic plate, or in the septa between cotyledons ('white infarcts'). Such areas are due to fibrinoid degeneration of trophoblast. Not all the trophoblast becomes effectively vascularized and these 'infarcts' are merely areas in which surplus trophoblast, which has never been effectively organized into villi, has degenerated. Such lesions do not interfere with fetal nutrition.

Intervillous thrombosis.   Another more important type of lesion is due to coagulation of maternal blood in the intervillous space. A 'red infarct' is formed, consisting of coagulum enclosing villi whose blood supply has been cut off. In time such a lesion becomes organized, and forms a 'white infarct' consisting of a mass of fibrin surrounding the degenerating villi. The cause of intervillous thrombosis is not always evident, but it may be due to occlusion by internal thickening and thrombosis of the arteriole which supplies a lobule of the placenta. The maternal blood supply to the lobule is impaired and necrosis of the trophoblast covering the involved villi occurs. The maternal blood in contact with the damaged trophoblast then clots. The blood flow in the intervillous space is not enough to remove small clots, so that the thrombosis may extend. Small lesions are unimportant, and can probably be found in any placenta, but if large areas of the placenta are involved the fetal oxygenation and nutrition are disturbed.

Calcification of the placenta.   Calcification is often to be seen on the maternal surface of the mature placenta in the form of numerous scattered gritty areas. Other small deposits may occur in areas of degeneration in the substance of the placenta. The common deposits on the maternal surface

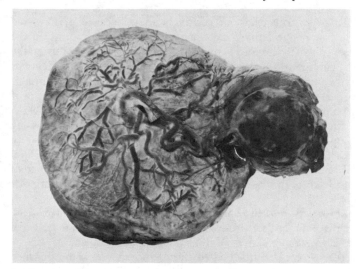

Fig. 15.5   Placenta showing chorio-angioma.

are in the decidua, and they do not interfere with the blood flow in the intervillous space. Such lesions are of no importance, but sometimes show the position of the placenta in a radiograph.

Cysts of the placenta.   Small cysts may occur in the chorionic plate of the placenta or in other sites, due to liquefaction of an area of fibrinoid degeneration. They are of no importance.

Tumours of the placenta

Apart from choriocarcinoma tumours of the placenta are rare, and consist of masses of chorionic villi with hypertrophied blood vessels. Such vascular tumours are termed *chorio-angiomata*. The tumour is usually single and the rest of the placenta is normal. Such a tumour is a rare cause of hydramnios, due to exudation of fluid from the surface of the tumour.

Very rarely metastases from a maternal carcinoma or melanoma may occur in the placenta.

Anomalies of the umbilical cord

Abnormal length.   The usual length of the cord is about the same as that of the fetus, 50 cm at term, but considerable variations occur. Excessive length predisposes to descent of the cord below the presenting part and prolapse (see p. 348), and to the formation of loops round some part of the fetus and knots.

The cord may be truly short or relatively short because it is twisted around some part of the fetus. This may cause intrauterine death in the very rare cases in which the cord is pulled tight. In labour delay during the second stage, rupture of the cord, premature separation of the placenta or inversion of the uterus have rarely occurred. During delivery the treatment for a loop round the neck is to slip it over the head after that is born, or if this cannot be done to divide the cord between clamps.

Knots in the cord may be formed by fetal movements, the fetus passing through a loop which later forms a knot. Knots are rarely tight enough to obstruct the circulation, but they do occasionally cause intrauterine fetal death. Local protuberances of Wharton's jelly may give an appearance of knotting, and have been described as false knots; they are of no importance.

Abnormal insertion of the cord.   The cord is usually attached to the centre of the placenta, but sometimes it is eccentric or attached to the edge of the placenta (*battledore placenta*). This is of no importance.

In rare cases the cord is attached to the membranes at some distance from the edge of the placenta, and at this point the vessels may divide into branches which run on the membranes for some distance before reaching the edge of the placenta (*velamentous insertion of the cord*). This can be dangerous to the fetus if the vessels happen to pass across part of the chorion that lies below the presenting part (*vasa praevia*), as a branch may be torn when the membranes rupture.

Single umbilical artery.   This is an uncommon finding but it may be associated with other abnormalities of the fetus. The cut end of the cord should always be inspected after delivery, and if only one artery is seen the child should be carefully examined for any other defect.

16

Antepartum haemorrhage

The term antepartum haemorrhage is applied to bleeding from the vagina occurring at any time after the 28th week of pregnancy and before the birth of the child.

As defined above, antepartum haemorrhage may be divided into three classes:

1. Haemorrhage due to the partial separation of a placenta normally situated on the upper segment of the uterus. This is called *accidental haemorrhage*, or *abruptio placentae*. In these cases labour may progress without further bleeding.
2. Haemorrhage due to the partial separation of a placenta abnormally situated on the lower uterine segment. This is termed *placenta praevia*. In this class of case haemorrhage is inevitable when the lower segment becomes dilated in labour. The haemorrhage here is the reverse of accidental, it is unavoidable. The term 'accidental' does not refer to trauma, although trauma may be one cause of haemorrhage.
3. Haemorrhage due to a lesion of the cervix or vagina such as an erosion, a polyp or a carcinoma. This may be called *incidental haemorrhage*.

Accidental haemorrhage

Varieties

Owing to the separation of a portion of the placenta from its uterine attachment, part of the wall of the intervillous space is removed and maternal blood escapes from the opened sinuses. This blood may track down between the membranes and the wall of the uterus and so escape at the cervix (*revealed accidental haemorrhage*), or may remain inside the uterine cavity (*concealed accidental haemorrhage*). In fact the distinction is more clinical than anatomical; in nearly all cases there is some external bleeding, but in concealed cases the shock is out of proportion to the external loss.

Cause and pathology

In many cases no cause can be discovered. About 25 per cent of the cases are associated with pre-eclampsia, essential hypertension or (rarely)

157

chronic nephritis. It is not certain that the hypertension or proteinuria is the cause of the haemorrhage; in a few cases proteinuria follows and does not precede the haemorrhage.

It has been claimed that accidental antepartum haemorrhage is caused by folic acid deficiency. The disease is more common with advanced parity and in lower income groups. There is also said to be an association with cases of megaloblastic anaemia, which is due to folic acid deficiency. Studies of folate levels and of the bone marrow have given some support to the theory. However, accidental haemorrhage is not especially common in Nigeria, where megaloblastic anaemia is common; and there has been little evidence that folic acid supplements during pregnancy reduce the incidence in this country.

A few cases of placental separation are due to trauma during external version.

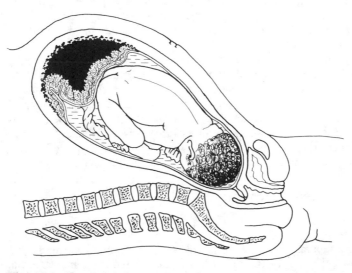

Fig. 16.1   Concealed accidental haemorrhage.

The bleeding in cases of accidental haemorrhage may be of any degree from a small retroplacental haematoma, which may not affect the fetus and which may only be discovered after the placenta is delivered, to a large collection of blood which distends the uterus and kills the fetus by separating the placenta.

In severe cases blood is extravasated into the substance of the uterine wall and may be seen under the peritoneal surface (Couvelaire uterus).

It is usually stated that such haemorrhage interferes with uterine contraction, and that it explains the continuing haemorrhage which occurs in some of these cases, even after delivery of the fetus and placenta. In fact this is improbable as the uterus is tense from spasm, rather than relaxed, before delivery. In concealed cases the whole uterus may be tense and tender, but in revealed or less severe cases there is more localized tenderness over the site of haemorrhage. If a postpartum haemorrhage occurs it may be due to hypofibrinogenaemia and failure of blood clotting rather than to atony of the uterus.

Hypofibrinogenaemia may occur because thromboplastins are forced into the maternal circulation, defibrinating the blood. Severe antepartum or postpartum blood loss may then occur because the blood does not coagulate. (See p. 430.)

There is some evidence to show that there is a uterorenal reflex, and that severe accidental haemorrhage of the concealed type causes spasm of the renal arterioles. This may be sufficiently widespread and prolonged to cause bilateral renal cortical necrosis, which results in anuria.

Symptoms and signs

Revealed accidental haemorrhage. With or without any obvious exciting cause the patient notices blood coming from the vagina. There may be slight abdominal discomfort and tenderness over the placental site.

The initial diagnosis is between accidental haemorrhage and placenta praevia. Tenderness over the placental site, engagement of the fetal head (in late pregnancy), and fetal death or fetal distress suggest that the symptoms are due to accidental haemorrhage. However, in many slight cases the fetus is not adversely affected, and in multiparae the fetal head may not engage until the onset of labour, even in normal cases. If the head is not engaged the placenta may be localized by ultrasonic scan (see p. 169).

It is dangerous to attempt to exclude the presence of a placenta praevia by vaginal examination and the passage of a finger through the cervix. If the placenta should prove to be low-lying such an examination may cause very severe bleeding, and even if the placenta is not within reach there is the risk of starting labour. In exceptional cases in which the diagnosis is in real doubt and the degree of bleeding is such that investigation cannot be delayed, vaginal examination must be made in the operating theatre, with the patient anaesthetized and all preparations made for Caesarean section, which could then be performed immediately if a placenta praevia was found.

On vaginal examination, friable smooth blood clot may fill the vagina and cervix, but the placenta cannot be felt. The amount of blood lost varies from a slight show to a violent flooding.

Concealed accidental haemorrhage. The symptoms and signs naturally vary with the severity of the case. In the extreme cases, the gravity of the patient's condition may be out of all proportion to the amount of blood effused into the uterus. Shock is due not only to the

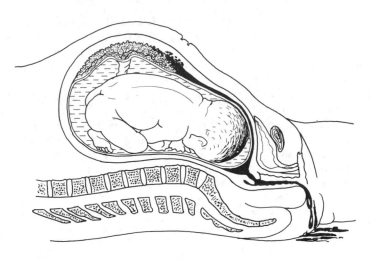

Fig. 16.2   Revealed accidental heamorrhage.

haemorrhage but also to the painful uterine distension. In spite of severe shock with a low blood pressure the pulse rate may not be raised, at least for a time, and this may be misleading.

The overdistension of the uterus gives rise to severe and constant abdominal pain. The uterus may be larger than would be expected for the period of gestation reached and more globular in outline. It has a hard wooden consistence and is extremely tender. Contraction or relaxation cannot be detected, the fetal outlines cannot be made out, and the fetal heart cannot be heard. Vaginal examination is not usually indicated, but revealed haemorrhage and dilatation of the cervix will occur with the onset of labour.

Should the loss of blood be smaller, the symptoms are correspondingly less severe. The patient complains of a sudden attack of abdominal pain and at the same time feels faint and suffers from nausea. She looks ill, her mucous membranes are pale, and the pulse-rate is raised. No abnormality may be discovered on abdominal examination, except that palpation of the uterus elicits tenderness, usually localized to the placental site, and if a sufficient area of placenta has been detached, the fetal heart is often inaudible. A correct diagnosis is important as such a patient is likely to have a recurrent and more serious haemorrhage. Protein may be present in the urine.

Mixed concealed and revealed accidental haemorrhage.   The symptoms and signs may be those of concealed haemorrhage with some external loss, and generally some dilatation of the cervix; or there may be external haemorrhage with little or no evidence of distension of the uterus by retained blood, although after delivery a quantity of dark blood found behind the placenta and membranes will show that concealed bleeding has occurred.

The severity of a case with external haemorrhage must never be judged solely by the amount of blood lost *per vaginam* but by the general condition of the patient. A trifling external loss may be accompanied by serious internal haemorrhage.

Diagnosis

Revealed accidental haemorrhage. Revealed accidental haemorrhage simulates placenta praevia, and in many cases an immediate distinction is not possible. Placenta praevia is suggested by a history of recurrent attacks of bleeding, by the absence of hypertension or proteinuria, by a malpresentation or an unduly high presenting part. If the fetal head becomes engaged or investigation by ultrasound shows that the placenta is certainly situated in the upper uterine segment a firm diagnosis of accidental haemorrhage can be made.

The danger of vaginal examination, except in the operating theatre with all preparations made for Caesarean section, has already been emphasized.

After delivery the diagnosis can be confirmed by examining the membranes, as the hole through which the child is delivered is within 5 cm of the placental edge if the case was one of placenta praevia.

Concealed accidental haemorrhage. The diagnosis must be made from cases of intraperitoneal haemorrhage, caused by advanced ectopic gestation, spontaneous rupture of the uterus, or acute hydramnios. These, although very rare complications of pregnancy, closely resemble accidental haemorrhage of the concealed variety. They must be diagnosed by the history and on the physical signs present in each case. Other conditions complicating pregnancy, such as torsion of the pedicle of an ovarian cyst, volvulus, intestinal obstruction, acute apendicitis or peritonitis from any other cause, may have to be considered during the early stages of a concealed accidental haemorrhage.

Prognosis

The most important factor in the prognosis is the degree of shock and its duration. The amount of blood lost will obviously be important. If the uterus starts to contract rhythmically, instead of remaining in spasm, the prognosis is improved, even if the external bleeding increases temporarily when the patient goes into labour. The sooner the uterus is emptied the sooner will bleeding be arrested, and the risks of hypofibrinogenaemia or renal cortical necrosis are reduced.

In cases of revealed haemorrhage the maternal risk is small, but in severe cases of concealed haemorrhage the mortality may exceed 10 per cent.

The prognosis for the child is bad. The mortality is over 50 per cent.

This is due to (*a*) asphyxia from placental separation; (*b*) pre-eclampsia; (*c*) prematurity.

Treatment

All cases of antepartum haemorrhage should be admitted to hospital. In severe cases this is essential, in less severe cases the diagnosis is often uncertain and placenta praevia cannot always be excluded. A vaginal examination should not be made before the transfer of the patient to hospital. In cases with severe shock a blood transfusion and an injection of morphia should be given before moving the patient.

Revealed accidental haemorrhage.   Since this term includes cases which vary in severity from a slight loss of blood to a profuse flooding no single method of treatment will be applicable to all cases.

Cases with slight bleeding.   If the amount of bleeding is only slight and the pregnancy is still some weeks short of term there is no need to do more than put the patient at rest. In many cases no further bleeding occurs and the pregnancy continues to term. The eventual appearance of the placenta will show that part of it has been detached, being brown, shrunken, and more solid than the rest, and having old blood clot adherent to it.

Cases with more severe bleeding.   This group includes cases in which the amount of bleeding is sufficient to be dangerous or there is any degree of shock. In most severe cases the fetus is already dead and need not be considered. The object of treatment is to get the uterus empty, contracted, and retracted with as little bleeding as possible and without added risk to the mother. This end can best be achieved by allowing the uterus to empty itself; Caesarean section is seldom indicated if the fetus is dead. A blood transfusion should be given if the loss is more than slight or there are any signs of shock. If the patient is not already in labour that should be induced by low rupture of the membranes under anaesthesia. This should be done without delay. If regular contraction do not follow an oxytocin drip may be given; only in a few exceptional cases in which profuse bleeding persists should the uterus be emptied by Caesarean section.

Many cases are already in labour, and labour usually follows induction in the other cases. The second stage of labour may be shortened with the aid of the forceps or the vacuum extractor. The third stage should be conducted with care, an intravenous injection of ergometrine (0.5 mg) being given immediately after the birth of the head.

Caesarean section is sometimes justified if the fetus is alive, but it should never be performed in the presence of severe maternal shock. It would be justifiable in a case with a viable fetus and fairly severe bleeding. Caesarean section is not required in cases with slight bleeding unless there is evidence of fetal distress. Fetal blood sampling may be useful in these cases to assess the degree of hypoxia; sometimes it will show that the fetus is so severely affected that section is not justifiable.

Concealed accidental haemorrhage. Most cases of concealed accidental haemorrhage are very serious, because the patient is collapsed as a result of the loss of blood and the painful distension of the uterus. The first essential is to treat the shock and not to attempt to deliver the child before this has been done. An emergency obstetric unit should be called.

The patient must be given an immediate injection of morphia, 15 mg. She should not be moved until severe shock has been treated by blood transfusion and the injection of morphia, but transfer to hospital will be required, and should not be long delayed. If the patient's condition is poor and facilities for blood transfusion are not available, dextran or other plasma substitute may be used, or failing that, intravenous saline, but dextran should not be used until blood has been taken for grouping. A note is made of the girth of the abdomen and the height of the fundus is likewise marked upon the skin. Following these steps the condition of the patient is observed, hour by hour, and she must not be left. A further injection of morphia 10 mg is given if the pain is not relieved.

In a severe case several litres of blood will be needed. The pulse and blood pressure are not always reliable indices of need; the speed of transfusion is best judged by monitoring the central venous pressure with a catheter inserted through the external jugular vein.

As the state of shock passes off improvement usually occurs. Treatment will be influenced by the parity of the patient and by the duration of the pregnancy. The majority of these patients are multiparous women, and as the fetus is small and premature, an easy quick delivery is to be expected if labour is established. After the initial treatment for shock the membranes should be ruptured. It was formerly taught that the membranes should not be ruptured until the uterus had lost its wooden hardness, as it was feared that further loss of blood would occur from an atonic uterus. There is little ground for this fear, and continued bleeding is more often due to hypofibrinogenaemia, and the danger of this or of renal necrosis is reduced by early rupture of the membranes and consequent reduction of intrauterine tension.

Surgical treatment by Caesarean section is now being recommended in some of these cases. The results in the past were poor, because the operation was performed in desperate cases, some of which had received inadequate transfusion, and in some of which hypofibrinogenaemia was present so that bleeding could not be checked even by hysterectomy. If section has any place it must be performed .before irreversible shock is established. Most cases respond rapidly to artificial rupture of the membranes; and the operation should only be considered in those in which the patients' condition is deteriorating in the absence of uterine contractions, especially in the case of a primigravida with a tight cervix.

The possibility of *hypofibrinogenaemia* as a result of concealed accidental haemorrhage should be borne in mind. It should be suspected in any case of delayed or absent clotting. A fibrinogen estimation should be made and a critical level is considered to be 100 mg per 100 ml. It can be treated by giving 2 to 10 g of fibrinogen in solution. If fresh blood is available this will provide approximately 1 g in each 500 ml. However, the fibrinogen level is often less important than the circulatory condition. See p. 427 for further discussion.

Treatment after the labour is over.   The fact that the patient has been delivered after accidental haemorrhage and that there is no great amount of postpartum haemorrhage does not necessarily mean that she will do well. In the absence of efficient treatment some of these patients die a few hours after delivery from heart failure. The patients should not be left until recovery from shock is complete, as will be indicated by the general condition, the pulse rate and blood pressure. An amount of postpartum haemorrhage which would be trifling in the case of a robust woman may be of grave consequence in the case of a patient who has had severe antepartum haemorrhage, and it is always prudent to obtain a generous amount of cross-matched blood for these patients.

It is important to continue with blood transfusion until the patient's condition is restored to normal or until the total blood loss has been made good. Bleeding in the third stage must be controlled by ergometrine intravenously during delivery and intramuscularly afterwards.

Renal cortical necrosis and lower nephron nephrosis

A rare but serious complication of accidental haemorrhage, particularly of the concealed variety, is renal failure or extreme oliguria. (Anuria may also occur as a very rare complication of eclampsia, abortion, or traumatic delivery and postpartum haemorrhage.)

Pathology.   In fatal cases one of two pathological conditions is found, either renal cortical necrosis or lower nephron nephrosis. In *renal cortical necrosis* both kidneys show uniform symmetrical necrosis of almost the entire cortex; only a thin layer under the capsule survives. The zone of necrosis involves nearly all the glomeruli and a large part of the tubular structure. In *lower nephron nephrosis* the kidneys may appear normal to the naked eye, but microscopical examination reveals widespread necrosis and degeneration of the distal convoluted tubules and collecting tubules. The glomeruli are not involved.

The mode of production of these two pathological conditions has been much disputed, and it is still uncertain whether they are not different degrees of one pathological change. Renal cortical necrosis is due to ischaemia; the blood flow through the cortex ceases. Trueta has brought evidence to show that there is an arterial shunt in the kidney which regulates the blood flow through the cortex. When the shunt is closed the blood flows through the intralobular vessels to supply all the cortex (except a thin lamina which gains its blood supply from the capsule). When the shunt is open the blood returns to the veins by an alternative pathway which diverts it from the cortex. It is suggested that this shunt is brought into operation in cases of concealed accidental haemorrhage by toxic substances which pass into the bloodstream, and perhaps also by nervous stimuli from the uterus along sympathetic pathways. Although the details of this theory are not universally accepted, it is at least certain that cortical necrosis is due to ischaemia. The changes are irreversible and lead to permanent renal failure which has to be treated by dialysis or renal transplant.

The cause of the changes of lower nephron nephrosis is less certain. The changes have been attributed to the direct action of a toxin, or alternatively to ischaemia. It is difficult to explain the escape of the glomeruli and the selective effect on the distal convoluted tubules on either hypothesis. It is believed that regeneration of the damaged tubules can occur, and that the cases of obstetric anuria which recover are of this nature.

Clinical features The initial clinical features of anuria due to cortical necrosis and lower nephron nephrosis are identical. After recovery from shock, or after delivery, the first danger sign is the passage of a few millilitres of bloodstained urine. Complete, or nearly complete, anuria follows and only a small quantity of very dilute urine is passed. The patient remains well for several days, during which time the blood urea rises progressively. In fatal cases, after about ten days, drowsiness and twitching movements appear, and death quickly follows the appearance of these signs. In other cases, spontaneous diuresis occurs after about a week, and rapid and apparently complete recovery occurs. It is believed that the cases in which the kidneys recover are those due to lower nephron nephrosis.

Treatment. In the early stages of anuria the osmotic diuretic mannitol, 100 ml of a 25 per cent solution, given intravenously over 10 minutes, may prevent renal failure. If there is evidence of disseminated intravascular coagulation (see p. 430), with failure of the shed blood to clot and a lowered plasma fibrogen level, heparin given intravenously may prevent deposition of fibrin in the glomeruli, which is one of the suggested causes for renal failure in these cases.

In established renal failure there is no means of distinguishing the lethal cases of cortical necrosis from the cases of lower nephron nephrosis in which recovery may occur, the only possible course is to treat all cases alike, and hope that spontaneous diuresis will occur. Many patients have been lost by injudicious treatment, particularly by giving large volumes of fluid intravenously. Diuretics are useless and harmful, and such surgical procedures as decapsulation of the kidneys or splanchnic block only add further pain and disturbance to the patient's illness. Although some cases treated surgically have recovered, they might well have done so in any event, and equally frequent and dramatic recoveries follow the simple treatment now to be described.

In anuric patients the only loss of water which is taking place is in the breath, sweat and faeces, and this is less than 1 litre per diem. Unless there is additional loss by vomiting the total fluid intake should never exceed this. Since the metabolism of fat in the body provides as much as 400 ml of water a day the intake should be restricted to about 500 ml. Disturbance of electrolyte balance also occurs, but in the absence of normal renal function it is highly dangerous to give electrolytes which can so easily be given to excess. The temporary disturbance of balance will neither interfere with spontaneous diuresis, nor will it be of a degree to endanger the patient before spontaneous diuresis occurs.

If the patient is able to take food by mouth she is given enough carbohydrate and fat to provide 1500 calories per day and 75 g of protein to prevent wasting.

If food cannot be taken by mouth intravenous infusion of glucose should be given into a large vein to avoid the common difficulty of thrombosis of small veins with glucose infusion. A catheter inserted into an arm vein may be advanced so that the tip lies in the superior vena cava. Amino acids and fat may also be given in this way.

Anuric patients are best treated in special centres where dialysis may be undertaken if necessary. Dialysis is indicated if:
1. There is overhydration as shown by pulmonary oedema.
2. There are convulsions or coma.
3. The blood urea level persists at 200 mg per 100 ml.
4. The blood potassium concentration exceeds 7 mmol/litre.
5. The serum bicarbonate concentration is less than 12 mmol/litre.
Peritoneal dialysis is usually successful and allows some freedom in the diet. In some centres haemodialysis is preferred.

If diuresis occurs renal recovery is often surprisingly complete; otherwise the patient has to remain under the care of a renal unit for dialysis or renal transplantation.

Placenta praevia (unavoidable haemorrhage)

A placenta is described as praevia when it is wholly or partly attached to the lower uterine segment.

Degrees of placenta praevia

The degree of encroachment onto the lower uterine segment is important because both treatment and prognosis are determined by it. Figure 16.3 illustrates the classification which is now often used.

Type I. The placenta is only partly attached to the lower segment. Its lower margin dips into the lower segment but is at a little distance from the internal cervical os. This is sometimes called a lateral placenta praevia.

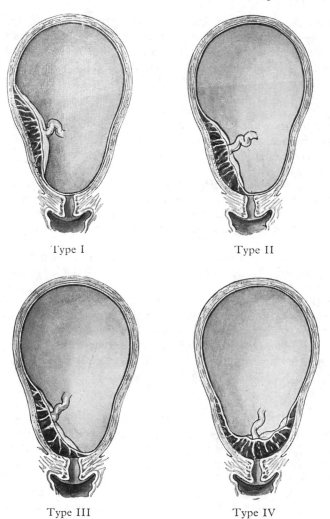

Type I   Type II

Type III   Type IV

Fig. 16.3 Classification of degrees of placenta praevia.

Type II. A greater part of the placenta is attached to the lower segment so that its lower margin reaches down to the internal os.

Type III. The placenta overlies the undilated internal os, but if a finger was passed through the cervix it would be able to reach the margin of the placenta.

Type IV. The placenta overlies the undilated internal os, but if a finger was passed through the cervix it could not reach the margin of the placenta.

This classification may be useful for descriptive purposes, but most unfortunately it gives the impression that the diagnosis of placenta praevia and its degree is made by passing a finger through the cervix. *This method of diagnosis can be disastrous and is to be avoided* (see also p. 171).

Pathology

Placenta praevia occurs about once in 250 pregnancies, and is slightly more common in women who have had a number of children.

A placenta praevia is often irregular in shape and variable in thickness. It may cover a larger area than normal, and is often pathologically adherent in part. These changes are explained by the comparatively poor blood supply which the placenta obtains from the non-vascular lower segment. The cord frequently has a low marginal insertion. The lower segment of the uterus and the cervix are more vascular and softer than usual; in consequence they will tear readily.

The haemorrhage comes from maternal vessels which are opened up by separation of the placenta as the uterine contractions dilate the lower segment. The separation during pregnancy may be slight, but it is inevitably greater during labour, when severe bleeding occurs. Except in cases in which the placenta is torn there is little loss of fetal blood, but in severe cases fetal oxygenation will be impaired because of placental separation or compression during labour, or because maternal haemorrhage causes anaemia and hypotension with reduced blood flow on the maternal side of the placenta.

Symptoms and course of labour

During the last 12 weeks of pregnancy (and occasionally earlier) the patient notices slight haemorrhages from the vagina. These occur without evident cause, perhaps during sleep, but they may also follow hard exercise or any local disturbance such as coitus. There are usually repeated slight 'warning' haemorrhages, but occasionally the first bleed may be a severe one, and in a few cases there is no bleeding until labour starts. There is no pain and the fetal heart sounds are usually normal.

During labour severe haemorrhage is inevitable as the cervix dilates.

In the third stage of labour there may be postpartum haemorrhage because the placental site is larger than normal and lies on the lower segment which may not retract efficiently. Any cervical tear will bleed freely because of the increased vascularity.

Diagnosis

A history of repeated losses of blood in late pregnancy, small in amount at first but usually increasing, is strongly suggestive of placenta praevia.

On abdominal examination the fetal head may be high and freely mobile, or the breech may be presenting or the lie oblique, because the placenta occupies the lower segment and prevents the head entering the pelvis. There is no tenderness and the fetal heart sounds are present.

On vaginal examination the presenting part may be obscured, or felt plainly through one fornix and indistinctly through the other, but a certain clinical diagnosis can only be made by feeling the placenta with a finger passed through the internal os. *This may be followed by furious bleeding*, and today such dangerous digital examination can nearly always be avoided because the placental position can be determined by ultrasound.

In cases with slight bleeding it is safe to inspect the cervix by gentle passage of a speculum to exclude any incidental cause of bleeding. However, if a cervical erosion is found this does not exclude placenta praevia, and only if any cervical lesion is actually bleeding should it be accepted as a possible cause of antepartum haemorrhage.

Hypertension or proteinuria are not found unless there is some other cause for them.

Placental localization

Unless the patient is bleeding so profusely that immediate treatment is essential an attempt should be made to determine the position of the placenta. Several techniques have been tried in recent years but only two are now in common use, the ultrasound scan and (less often) soft-tissue x-ray placentography.

Other methods have disadvantages. Pelvic arteriography gives the best outline of the placenta but has potentially dangerous complications and is painful. Scanning with a counter after intravenous injection of a radio-isotope such as technetium to find the vascular placenta does not delineate the lower edge of the placenta well, and requires access to a radio-isotope laboratory.

Ultrasound scan is now available in many maternity units in Britain. It is without risk to the patient or fetus and is the method of choice. If a scan is performed at any stage of pregnancy for other reasons placental localization should always be undertaken at the same time. Performed in this way, in a recent series 28 out of 42 cases of placenta praevia were diagnosed before any antepartum haemorrhage had occurred.

The characteristic mottled shadow on the screen may not outline the lower edge of the placenta accurately, but repeated scans can safely be performed if necessary. The placenta sometimes appears to be low-lying before the 32nd week, but re-examination later in pregnancy after the lower segment has formed may not confirm this.

A fundal placenta is easy to outline, and this immediately excludes placenta praevia.

Soft-tissue placentography. If the ultrasound examination is inconclusive a single standing lateral radiograph of the pelvic soft tissues may be helpful. The principle of the method is to look for any significant displacement of the fetal head away from the symphysis pubis or the sacral promontory. Displacement of the head indicates that placental tissue is interposed between it and the bony pelvic inlet.

Prognosis

Maternal. The chief causes of death in cases of placenta praevia are haemorrhage and shock, and without efficient and modern treatment the danger is great. The amount of bleeding will be least with a Type I (lateral) placenta praevia, but progressively greater with the more central types. Both antepartum and postpartum haemorrhage may occur. Some hazards arise from Caesarean section, which is the necessary treatment. Sepsis is now rare; it used to be common when vaginal manipulations were carried out near the low-lying placental site.

The essential measure to reduce the risk of placenta praevia is to transfer any patient with slight antepartum haemorrhage to hospital at once, so that accurate diagnosis and preparation for treatment can be made before severe haemorrhage occurs. The maternal mortality in cases managed in this way is less than 1 per cent.

Fetal. Unless Caesarean section is performed or unless the placenta praevia is of minor degree the outlook for the child is bad. Fetal death may occur from hypoxia caused by separation or pressure on the placenta, or by maternal hypotension and anaemia. Prematurity used to be a common cause of neonatal death, but with modern management it is less frequent.

Treatment

If there is any possibility of placenta praevia the patient must be admitted to hospital as soon as possible. In what is now an exceptional case, if the patient is first seen when bleeding severely in her own home she should be given morphine 15 mg intramuscularly and the doctor should send for the obstetric emergency team, the members of which will be able to give a blood transfusion. *It is most important that no vaginal examination is made before transfer to hospital,* as such an examination may cause further serious haemorrhage. The patient's condition may allow her to be moved by ambulance immediately or only after blood transfusion.

In all cases with severe bleeding immediate active treatment is required and delay is perilous, but in the most common type of case seen today the patient is admitted when the bleeding has only been slight, there is time for investigation, and it is usually possible to make a diagnosis by clinical and ultrasound examination. The chief cause of fetal mortality used to be prematurity, but it was found that if the bleeding was only slight and the fetus was some weeks premature, then the risk of keeping the patient in bed while the fetus grew was justifiable, provided that she was in a hospital where treatment by blood transfusion and operation was immediately available should severe bleeding occur. This expectant attitude greatly reduced the fetal mortality without increasing the maternity mortality. If severe bleeding starts while the patient is in hospital Caesarean section is immediately performed. The exact position of the placenta is of no importance and digital examination is dangerous and unnecessary.

In a few cases the diagnosis is still uncertain after ultrasonic and radiological examination, and in these *few exceptional cases* when the pregnancy is near term it may be justifiable to make a pelvic examination, provided that it is done in the operating theatre with the patient anaesthetized and the instruments sterilized and ready for Caesarean section. A finger is passed very gently through the cervix. If a placenta of Type II, III or IV is encountered Caesarean section is performed, but if the placenta is of Type I low rupture of the membranes is done, which allows the presenting part to descend and compress the lower margin of the placenta and so to control the bleeding. If no placenta praevia is felt it is still wise to rupture the membranes, as the finger has now been inserted into the cavity of the uterus.

If the patient is shocked Caesarean section should not be performed until this has been corrected by transfusion. Section should still be performed if there is severe bleeding and the fetus is premature or dead; the primary purpose of the operation is to control the bleeding by emptying the uterus and allowing it to retract.

If the placenta lies anteriorly a few obstetricians recommend upper segment Caesarean section as there may be severe bleeding from large vessels in the lower segment and from the placenta during a lower segment operation, but it is found in practice that the lower segment operation can be safely performed, with the advantage of a much safer uterine scar.

In all cases blood transfusion should be freely employed, for although the patient may recover from the initial haemorrhage the possibility of further bleeding in the third stage must be anticipated.

Other methods of treatment.　In the United Kingdom other forms of treatment are now hardly ever employed because these older methods are less effective than Caesarean section in controlling the bleeding, are more often followed by infection, and give worse fetal results. The principle of controlling the bleeding in these methods is to compress the placental site by the presenting part. The simplest method is low rupture of the membranes, which has a place in the treatment of a Type I placenta praevia, particularly in a multipara.

Willett's toothed scalp forceps may be used to grasp a fold of fetal scalp, and then traction of about 0.5 kg may be applied to the handles of the forceps. This is simple, but seldom used now.

If the patient is in labour with the cervix half dilated and the breech presenting it is possible to pull down a leg to plug the lower segment while the uterus contracts to complete dilatation of the cervix. This carries a very high fetal mortality.

Plugging the vagina with gauze is useless. It often fails to control the bleeding and merely hides the blood loss. The plug causes pain and increases the risk of sepsis.

17

Polyhydramnios and oligohydramnios

Polyhydramnios

In this condition (which is usually simply termed hydramnios) there is an excess of liquor amnii. It is difficult to define exactly how much is excessive; the average volume of liquor at term is 800 ml, but a range of 400 to 1500 ml is accepted as normal. Probably only volumes in excess of 2000 ml would be noticed as abnormal on clinical examination. For theories about the mode of formation of amniotic fluid see p. 24.

In most of the cases the excess fluid accumulates gradually (*chronic hydramnios*) and is only noticed after the 30th week. In a few exceptional cases hydramnios occurs earlier and more quickly (*acute hydramnios*), and many of these cases are associated with uniovular twins. The composition of the fluid in cases of hydramnios does not usually differ from normal.

Aetiological factors

Hydramnios occurs more often in multiparae than in primigravidae. It may have fetal or maternal causes.

Fetal causes. (1) Hydramnios may occur with *twin pregnancy* of either type. Usually only one sac is distended. The association of acute hydramnios with uniovular twins has been mentioned.

(2) *Fetal abnormalities.* With anencephaly hydramnios often occurs. There may be some exudation from the exposed brain, but a more likely explanation is that the fetus does not swallow normally.

Hydramnios occurs with oesophageal atresia, when inability to swallow is certainly the explanation. In all cases in which there has been an excess of liquor the newborn infant must be examined to exclude oesophageal atresia (p. 490).

Hydramnios may also occur with other fetal abnormalities, including spina bifida.

(3) A rare cause is *chorio-angioma of the placenta* (p. 155).

(4) There may be excess of fluid in cases of *hydrops fetalis*.

Maternal causes. Hydramnios may occur with maternal diabetes. Not only is there an excess of amniotic fluid, but the placenta and fetus are large. There may be an excess of glucose in the liquor, but this is only

173

found in a proportion of the cases and does not explain the hydramnios.

There is a clinical association of hydramnios and maternal hypertension, but the hypertension is probably the result and not the cause of the hydramnios.

Clinical features

The patient may notice that her abdomen is unduly enlarged and that the fetus is unusually mobile. If the uterus is very much enlarged she may have dyspnoea and flatulent dyspepsia. However, it is extraordinary how tolerant the abdomen may be of even an enormous accumulation of fluid, provided that it has formed slowly. In the rare cases of acute hydramnios there is abdominal pain and vomiting.

The physical signs depend on the amount of liquor. The abdomen is larger than expected for the duration of pregnancy, and the abdominal muscles may be stretched and the recti divaricated. It may be difficult to feel the fetus, and the fetal heart sounds may be muffled or inaudible. A fluid thrill can be elicited. The fetus is unduly mobile and malpresentations may occur. Oedema of the abdominal wall and vulva is sometimes seen. The tightness of the uterus varies, but in cases of acute hydramnios the uterus is very tense.

Diagnosis

Chronic hydramnios has to be distinguished from multiple pregnancy. This may be difficult, especially as hydramnios may complicate multiple pregnancy; in such a case the diagnosis of twins is easily missed. If the twin pregnancy is not complicated by hydramnios the essential clinical observations are the discovery of more than one head, or more than two fetal poles and an unusual number of small parts. The fetal heart sounds may be heard, or heart movements recognized with ultrasound, in more than one place, beating at different rates. Ultrasonic scan or radiological examination must be a routine in all cases of hydramnios to exclude multiple pregnancy or fetal abnormalities such as anencephaly.

If pregnancy coexists with a large ovarian cyst the diagnosis from hydramnios can be difficult. Ultrasonic scan will show two sacs, only one of which contains a fetus.

Acute hydramnios may simulate concealed accidental haemorrhage, but in most cases of accidental haemorrhage there is at least a little external bleeding. If fetal heart movements can be detected a severe concealed haemorrhage is very improbable.

Vesicular mole may also cause a tense enlargement of the uterus with tenderness. Ultrasound will show the absence of a fetus and the presence of vesicles.

If there is much vomiting, intestinal obstruction must be considered, but with this the uterus itself is not distended.

Effects on pregnancy and labour

Spontaneous premature labour may occur. The membranes may rupture suddenly and there is a risk of prolapse of the umbilical cord. Because the fetus is unduly mobile malpresentations may occur. If a large quantity of liquor escapes suddenly the placental site may diminish in area, and this may lead to separation and antepartum haemorrhage. After delivery there is a risk of postpartum haemorrhage.

The perinatal mortality is greatly increased with hydramnios because there may be a fetal abnormality, and because of the possibility of premature labour, cord prolapse and malpresentation.

Treatment

There is no known method of controlling the production or absorption of amniotic fluid. Hydramnios without symptoms and without any evidence of fetal abnormality requires no treatment.

If ultrasonic or radiological examination shows a gross fetal abnormality labour should be induced by rupturing the membranes and setting up a Syntocinon infusion.

In cases near term in which the patient is in serious discomfort labour should be induced. When there is a great deal of liquor under tension there is some risk of placental separation after rupturing the membranes, and some obstetricians would draw off part of the liquor by abdominal amniocentesis before the induction.

Abdominal amniocentesis is particularly suitable in cases in which the pregnancy is not sufficiently advanced for safe induction but the patient is in discomfort, and there is no evidence of fetal abnormality. After the patient has emptied her bladder the abdomen is palpated to find a point away from the fetus, and ultrasonic examination may also be used for this. After injection of a local anaesthetic a 16 gauge Tuohy needle, with some rubber tubing and a clip attached to it, is inserted into the amniotic cavity. Up to 2 litres of fluid may be removed provided that it is only allowed to escape slowly. Although there is some risk of labour starting after this operation, a few patients will continue in comfort to term. Unfortunately in most cases the fluid quickly returns, but amniocentesis may be repeated. There is always a slight risk of perforating a fetal vessel and causing bleeding into the amniotic sac.

Oligohydramnios

This means deficiency of amniotic fluid. It is a rare abnormality. In most of the cases there is some abnormality of the fetal urinary tract, of which *renal agenesis* is the most common. In this condition the fetus has a typical facies called Potter's syndrome. The nose is hooked the lower jaw is underdeveloped and the ears are set low. The amnion is studded with tiny white nodules. Microscopical examination shows these to be islands of degenerate squamous epithelium resting on a bed of flattened amniotic cells. It is thought that the squamous cells have been rubbed off the dry skin of the fetus. The fetus invariably dies within about 48 hours after birth.

In a few cases of oligohydramnios there is no renal or any other demonstrable abnormality. The fetus has little room to move and if it presents by the breech in early pregnancy it will be unable to alter its position and version is impossible. Deformities of the limbs such as talipes, and ankylosis of joints, may be caused by pressure, and amniotic adhesions may form bands which can constrict a limb.

There is a fall in the volume of liquor, which is not in itself of serious significance, if pregnancy continues beyond term.

18

Multiple pregnancy

In Caucasian women twin conceptions occur spontaneously about once in 90 pregnancies, triplets about once in 8000, and quadruplets about once in 500 000. (Helin stated that these incidences were in the ratios 89, 89^2 and 89^3, but there is no biological basis for this rule, which is far from accurate.) The spontaneous occurrence of the higher multiples up to septuplets has been reliably recorded.

The spontaneous incidence of twins is greater in the negro race (1:70) and lower in the mongol race (1:150). A tendency to multiple pregnancy is inherited, and it occurs more frequently in certain families. A woman who has given birth to twins is said to be 10 times more likely to have a multiple conception in a subsequent pregnancy than a woman who has not previously had twins.

The incidence of twin pregnancy rises slightly with increasing maternal age up to 40, and (independently) with increasing parity. All these factors of race, family tendency, parity and age affect binovular rather than uniovular twins.

Pregnancies following artificial induction of ovulation with clomiphene or gonadotrophins are not infrequently multiple unless the dosage is carefully controlled by hormone assays. From this cause there have been several quintuplet and sextuplet pregnancies, and recently a woman in Naples gave birth to octuplets, only 3 years after she had a sextuplet pregnancy.

In multiple pregnancies the normal sex ratio at birth, with a slight preponderance of males, is altered to a female preponderance.

Varieties of twins

Twins may be binovular or uniovular.

Binovular twins are developed from two ova arising in a single Graafian follicle, or from two follicles which may or may not be in the same ovary. This variety of twins is three times more common than the uniovular variety. The children may be of the same or of different sex, and are not more alike than is usual with members of the same family. As they are developed from separate ova and separate spermatozoa their genetic material will differ. They have separate and distinct placentae. Sometimes

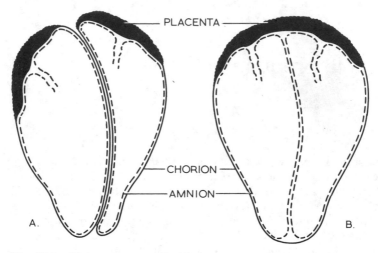

Fig. 18.1   Twin pregnancy.   **A.** Binovular twins. The placentae are separate and each fetus has its own amnion and chorion. Even if the placentae are more closely related there is no anastomosis between the fetal circulations.   **B.** Uniovular twins. Each fetus usually has its own amnion, but the chorions are fused and the placentae are anastomosed.

these are loosely joined at their margins but there is never any anastomosis between their blood vessels. Each fetus has its own amnion and chorion.

Uniovular twins are developed from a single ovum, which after fertilization has undergone division to form two embryos. Division may occur in the early stage of segmentation, or later when two germinal areas are formed in one blastodermic vesicle. Uniovular twins are always of the same sex and are often remarkably alike in their physical and mental characters. The arrangement of genes in the chromosomes is identical, and inherited characteristics such as blood groups are necessarily the same. Uniovular twins which arise from very early division each have a complete set of membranes (chorion and amnion); those which arise by later division have only one chorion but usually have separate amniotic sacs. Mono-amniotic twins are rare; this type is associated with a higher fetal loss from cord entanglement. The umbilical cords are usually separate, but the fetal circulations always communicate by anastomoses in the placenta. This communication may cause unequal development of the fetuses, and occasionally death of one fetus. If one fetus perishes early in pregnancy it is retained until term, when the small fetus is discovered compressed flat on the membrane (*fetus papyraceous*).

When the process of division of a single germinal area is incomplete some form of *conjoined twins* may occur. Many varieties have been described; they may be joined by the sternum, the pelvis or the head, and the degree of union varies from fusion of skin and soft tissues to formation of a double monster in which head, trunk, viscera or limbs may be shared or duplicated.

Diagnosis of twins

With twins all the early symptoms of pregnancy such as morning sickness may be more pronounced, and in late pregnancy pre-eclampsia is common. If the patient has already borne children she may notice an unusual rate of abdominal enlargement, and excessive fetal movements. In late pregnancy she may have discomfort and shortness of breath because of the large size of the uterus. The patient is more likely to become anaemic. Apart from the fact that there is a greater increase in plasma volume than in a single pregnancy, there is a double fetal demand for iron. As well as iron deficiency anaemia megaloblastic anaemia is more common with twins. It is

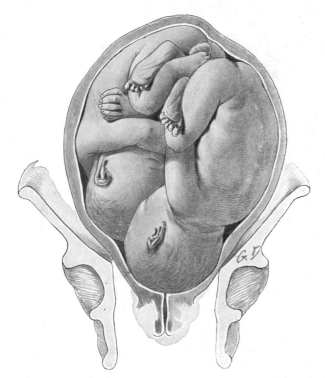

Fig. 18.2 Twin pregnancy. Both presenting by the vertex. Fetuses lying alongside one another. Both heads could probably be felt, one at the brim and the other above it in the iliac fossa. One back and an unusual number of small fetal parts would be recognised and possibly two breeches in the fundus.

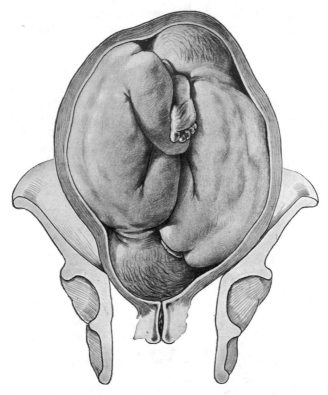

Fig. 18.3 Twin pregnancy. First presenting by the vertex, second by the breech: fetuses lying alongside one another. This offers the easiest diagnosis. One head would be felt at the brim and one at the fundus; two backs with the small parts in the groove between would be palpable and two points of maximal intensity of the fetal heart-sounds could be made out, one on the right and below the umbilicus and the other on the left and above.

important to ensure that the patient has an adequate diet and supplements of iron and folic acid. Oedema of the legs is common, and any tendency to varicose veins of the legs or haemorrhoids is accentuated.

On examination the uterus is found to be larger than expected from the duration of gestation. Hydramnios may occur with twins, adding to the size and confusing the diagnosis. The diagnosis is simple if two fetal heads can be felt. Both backs and both breeches may be identified, and an unusual number of small parts. The diagnosis is more certain if fetal heart sounds are heard in two separate areas, and sometimes the rates will differ. If heart movements are detected with the ultrasound apparatus in two separate areas or directions the diagnosis of twins is almost certain.

Multiple pregnancy can be diagnosed from about 12 weeks by ultrasonic scan, when two separate sacs and two heads may be seen. It is wise to add radiological examination after the 32nd week to exclude any fetal abnormality or conjunction of the twins.

If antenatal supervision is poor the diagnosis of twins is sometimes missed until after the birth of the first twin. The high position of the fundus, abdominal palpation of the second fetus, and discovery of a second bag of membranes and fetal parts on vaginal examination will make the diagnosis clear.

Complications and prognosis

The risk to the mother is increased for the following reasons:

1. *Pre-eclampsia and eclampsia* occur at least three times more often than in single pregnancies, although pre-eclampsia often seems to run a mild course.

2. *Malpresentations* are common with twins. In about 45 per cent of cases both twins present by the head; in about 35 per cent one fetus presents by the head and the other by the breech; in about 10 per cent both present by the breech; and in about 10 per cent of cases a transverse lie is associated with a vertex presentation, a breech or a second transverse lie. It is very rare for both fetuses to lie transversely.

3. *Hydramnios* may occur, and hypertension may be associated with it.

4. *Uterine action in labour* may be inefficient because of the overdistension of the uterus. This is seldom of importance in the first stage, but assistance is often required in the second stage, especially for the second twin, and there may be poor retraction in the third stage.

5. *Postpartum haemorrhage* may occur, both because the uterus does not contract well and because the placental site is large. The incidence of *placenta praevia* is increased because the large placental site may encroach on the lower segment. Because of the risk of haemorrhage the treatment of *anaemia* during pregnancy is very important.

The fetal risk is much higher than in single pregnancies, and the perinatal mortality may exceed 15 per cent for the following reasons:

1. Twins are often of *low birth weight*, and this is the most important factor in causing the increased perinatal mortality. Not only may labour begin before term, but the rate of growth of a twin after the 28th week is slower than that of a singleton fetus; the reduced rate of growth begins when the total weight of the twins is in the region of 3500 g. The cause for this is not related to the size of the placenta; for at any given placental weight a single fetus will be larger than a twin. The duration of twin pregnancy is variable, but about 20 per cent only reach the 36th week and 9 per cent only the 34th week.

2. *Complications of labour* including malpresentations, prolapse of the cord and placenta praevia may occur, and one twin may interfere with the

descent of the other. The second twin may be endangered by retraction of the uterus after the birth of the first twin, and premature separation of the placenta. As a reflection of these complications of labour it is found that among patients with cerebral palsy there are between 4 and 10 per cent more twins than in the general population.

3. Intrauterine death of one or both twins may be caused by *pre-eclampsia* or *cord accidents*.

4. *Congenital malformations* occur twice as often among twins as among singleton pregnancies.

Management of twin pregnancy

The antenatal care of a patient with a twin pregnancy should be intensified so that pre-eclampsia, anaemia, hydramnios, antepartum haemorrhage, malpresentations and premature labour can either be avoided or discovered and treated. The patient is seen more often than usual from mid-pregnancy onwards. It is important that she should have adequate rest. The practice of admitting patients with twins to hospital from the 30th to the 35th week is now less common, but it may be advisable if the home conditions are poor. It is by no means certain that rest will prevent premature labour, but it may increase the placental blood flow and so improve fetal growth. In addition many patients are uncomfortable when carrying twins and need more rest on that account.

Some obstetricians recommend that labour should be induced at the 38th week to avoid the theoretical risk of placental insufficiency, but there is little to prove the advantage of this. However, it is reasonable to suggest that no twin pregnancy should be allowed to go beyond term.

Management of twin labour

All preparations should have been made for the resuscitation and special care of babies of low birth weight. Because this can only be effectively done in hospital, and because other complications of labour may occur, all cases of twin labour should be in hospital units.

The first stage of labour is managed in the ordinary way. Sometimes painful contractions occur before labour is truly established, but once labour has begun it is not often prolonged. Epidural analgesia is very suitable for these cases, and an intravenous glucose drip should also be set up. The former will allow any necessary operative intervention without delay, and the latter will permit an oxytocic infusion to be started at any time. Because of the changing relationships of the fetuses it may be difficult to hear both fetal hearts, but an effort must be made to locate them. Provided that one can be heard at a normal rate no interference should be contemplated for fetal distress, but Caesarean section might be performed for prolonged delay in the first stage which did not respond to a careful trial of oxytocin, and rarely in cases in which both twins were lying transversely or the twins were conjoined.

The second stage is also managed in the usual way unless some complication arises. As in other cases the indications for delivery with the forceps or vacuum extractor, or for breech extraction, are undue delay, fetal distress or maternal distress. Unless the perineum is very lax an episiotomy should be performed routinely for the protection of a small baby's head, under local anaesthesia if an epidural injection has not been given. After the first twin is delivered the maternal end of its cord must be clamped or tied, because if the twins are uniovular bleeding from the cord might exsanguinate the second twin through the anastomosis in the placenta.

It is after the birth of the first twin that any problems usually arise, and it is the second twin which is mainly at risk. It may have to be delivered without delay and therefore an anacsthetist must be ready in the labour ward during all twin dcliveries. The advantages of epidural analgesia have already been pointed out. A doctor skilled in fetal resuscitation should be available in addition to the obstetrician conducting the delivery.

Usually both twins are delivered before the placentae, but rarely with binovular twins the placenta of the first twin will come away before delivery of the second fetus.

Soon after the delivery of the first twin the abdomen is palpated to determine the lie of the second fetus. If it is oblique or transverse external version is immediately performed to bring one pole of the fetus over the cervix. It is preferable to make the breech present because if extraction of the second twin should become necessary this is often easier by bringing down the legs of a breech than by application of forceps or the vacuum extraction to a very high head.

The fetal heart rate is counted every few minutes, for if the fetus is distressed immediate delivery is required. Distress may occur because the volume of the uterine cavity is reduced after delivery of the first twin, and there may be separation of the placenta on which the second twin depends. It may also be caused by prolapse of the cord, and a vaginal examination to exclude this should always be performed when the second sac of membranes ruptures.

Uterine contractions are often in abeyance for a few minutes after delivery of the first twin. When they start again delivery of the second twin is usually rapid as the birth canal has already been fully dilated. Delivery is conducted in the ordinary way, whether the head or the breech comes first.

If the uterine contractions do not return in about 5 minutes after the delivery of the first twin the second sac of membranes is ruptured with Kocher's forceps. In the past it was customary to wait some time before rupturing the second sac, unless fetal distress occurred. During this interval the cervix sometimes partly closed down, and experience has proved that fewer babies are lost after early rupture of the membranes, which is usually followed by rapid delivery of the second twin.

If the second twin shows signs of distress or its cord prolapses it must be delivered with reasonable expedition. The head may be found presenting but lying high above the pelvic brim, and application of forceps at that level can be very difficult. If forceps delivery is attempted the head should be pressed down as far as possible by abdominal pressure from an assistant, but in many cases vacuum extraction would be safer. Alternatively it is possible to pass a hand into the uterus to find the feet and to perform internal version and breech extraction. If the breech already presents it is comparatively easy to bring down a leg (or both legs) and extract the baby.

Locked twins.   This is a very rare complication of twin delivery. If there is unexplained delay in the second stage or difficulty in extracting a first breech it should be considered, and the possibility of conjoined twins should not be forgotten. The diagnosis is made by examination under anaesthesia.

Locking may occur when the first twin presents as a breech and the second as a vertex. The aftercoming head of the first twin is caught above

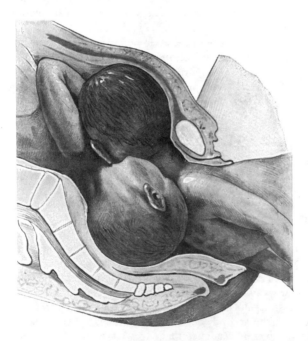

Fig. 18.4   Aftercoming head of the first twin locked with the forecoming head of the second.

the chin of the second twin, and if disengagement is not quickly achieved the first twin dies. Any attempt at disengagement requires deep anaesthesia, perhaps with fluothane. If it fails the neck of the dead fetus is divided and its head pushed up into the uterus to free the head of the second twin. The decapitated head is delivered later with forceps.

Delay can also occur if both heads are in collision at the brim, with the head of the second twin pressed against the neck of the second. Disengagement may be possible, but otherwise Caesarean section is performed.

Third stage of labour. There is an increased risk of postpartum hacmorrhage because of the large size of the placental site, which may encroach on the lower segment where the contraction of the muscle is relatively ineffective in closing blood sinuses. A prophylactic injection of ergometrine, preferably 0.5 mg intravenously, should be given with the birth of the second twin and the placenta delivered in the usual way. If haemorrhage occurs it is treated as described on p. 336.

Triplets and higher multiple births

The exact diagnosis is only likely to be made by ultrasonic or radiological examination. All the fetal hazards already described are accentuated, and some of the babies are likely to be very small. The perinatal mortality is high. Delivery of triplets is usually managed in the same way as twins, by vaginal delivery unless some complication necessitates Caesarean section. Delivery of higher multiples is generally best managed by Caesarean section. Obviously special arrangements for the provision of adequate expert paediatric help must be made.

19

Pre-eclampsia and eclampsia

The fact that some pregnant women had epileptiform fits was known to Hippocrates, who wrote in about 500 B.C. The word eclampsia does not refer to fits, for the original Greek word meant 'flash out', in the sense of a sudden event. Little more was known about eclampsia until in 1843 Lever of Guy's Hospital found that many of the women who had fits also had albumin in their urine. It was not until early in this century when the sphygomanometer was introduced that it came to be recognized that eclampsia was associated with hypertension. The fact that albuminuria and hypertension could precede the onset of fits gave rise to the concept of pre-eclampsia.

For many years it was postulated that a toxin was liberated from the pregnant uterus and the disorder became known as toxaemia of pregnancy. All efforts have so far failed to demonstrate any such toxin, and it is therefore inaccurate to employ the term toxaemia in this condition. It will be easier to discuss the numerous theories of the aetiology of eclampsia and pre-eclampsia after describing the clinical and pathological features of these conditions (p. 196).

Pre-eclampsia is a disease of signs, not symptoms. This is important because it means that early diagnosis is only possible if the pregnant woman is examined regularly. Early recognition and treatment of pre-eclampsia can almost always prevent eclampsia, which is a serious danger to the life of both mother and fetus. The signs that a pregnant woman has pre-eclampsia are excessive weight gain, oedema, hypertension and pro-teinuria. They usually appear in that order over a period of several days, but they can appear in any order or all together in less than 24 hours. It has been customary to say that at least two of the signs must be present before a diagnosis of pre-eclampsia can be made, but from the point of view of prac-tical management, if hypertension alone occurs the condition should be regarded as pre-eclampsia until the contrary is proved. Some discussion of each of the signs is required.

Weight gain. During normal pregnancy the average weight gain is about 12 kg. Sometimes there is a loss of weight during the first trimester if nausea and vomiting are prominent. After the 12th week there is an average weight gain of about 0.5 kg per week until term, when the weight

186

gain becomes less; indeed there may be a loss of about 0.5 kg in the week before delivery. There are great individual variations and the pattern may be distorted by dieting, overeating and vomiting. The weight gain is made up of the weight of the fetus, placenta and liquor, the increase in size of the uterus and breasts, the increased blood volume and some expansion of the extracellular fluid, and a fat store (see p. 40).

In pre-eclampsia there is often, although not always, a large increase in salt and water retention in the extracellular space. This causes a sudden above-average weight gain. An increase of weight of 1 kg or more in a week should arouse the suspicion that pre-eclampsia may be developing. As all the components of pregnancy weight gain depend upon the efficient functioning of the placenta, and as there is frequently a degree of placental insufficiency associated with pre-eclampsia, the total picture of weight fluctuations during pregnancy may be difficult to interpret. There is no evidence that women who are overweight before pregnancy or have an above-average weight gain throughout pregnancy are more likely to develop pre-eclampsia than their slimmer sisters (although a fat arm may lead to an incorrect diagnosis of hypertension when the pressure is measured with a standard sphygomanometer).

Oedema during pregnancy. A woman of average weight (55 – 60 kg) normally increases her extracellular fluid by about 6 litres during the course of pregnancy. Osmotic equilibrium is maintained by the retention of about 850 mmol of sodium. This degree of fluid retention may cause slight thickening of the skin, rings on the fingers will be tighter and, if the carpal tunnel is restrictive, oedema of the sheath of the median nerve may cause paraesthesia of the fingers.

Excessive fluid retention eventually gives rise to oedema. This can usually first be detected over the lower subcutaneous surface of the tibia by gentle sustained pressure, but ultimately the feet and ankles are obviously swollen. Oedema of the feet and ankles may also be caused by pressure of the uterus on the pelvic veins, or associated varicose veins. This non-significant dependent oedema is particularly common at the end of the day, especially when the woman has to spend much time standing or sitting, and during warm weather. Dependent oedema of moderate degree is so common that it is usually disregarded as a sign of pre-eclampsia unless it is accompanied by one of the other signs. Oedema of the fingers or face is more significant because gravity has little effect upon the accumulation of fluid in these places, but even here it does not establish a diagnosis of pre-eclampsia.

Blood pressure during pregnancy. Most younger women have a resting blood pressure of 110 – 120 mm Hg systolic, and 60 – 70 mm Hg diastolic. There is wide variation in healthy women, and the response to stress adds to the differences found at the first visit to a clinic or to the doctor. Ideally, to assess the changes observed during pregnancy the pressure before pregnancy should be known, but as this is rarely the case it is necessary to take the readings made during the first trimester as the indicator of the normal state.

The control of blood pressure is affected by normal pregnancy. Pooling of blood in the legs and splanchnic area may result in transient cerebral ischaemia when the pregnant woman stands up suddenly or stands still for a time. The faintness that results is often regarded by lay folk as an indication of pregnancy. The pulse pressure is slightly higher during pregnancy than in the non-pregnant state because the diastolic pressure is lower. In the mid-trimester some patients have a slight fall in both systolic and diastolic pressure, a change that reverts before term. In late pregnancy another factor causes variability; the pressure of the uterus on the large pelvic veins and the inferior vena cava brings about a diminished return of blood to the right side of the heart and induces a low-output hypotension. This most commonly occurs when the patient is lying on her back, especially if she is under an anaesthetic, and is termed the *supine hypotensive syndrome*.

There is some disagreement as to what may be regarded as a normal blood pressure during pregnancy. In most clinics 140/90 mm is taken to be the dividing point between physiology and pathology. Some will diagnose hypertension in pregnancy at any level above 130/80 mm, but the majority think that this is overcautious and leads to the inclusion of too many patients in the category of pre-eclampsia and hypertension, especially when it is realized how relatively inaccurate the clinical measurement of blood pressure is.

The standards of hypertension used in general medicine are not appropriate in obstetrics. A pregnant woman with a blood pressure of 140/90 mm may be running into danger; and at 160/110 she might develop eclampsia. Pregnant women are in a young age group; during pregnancy the blood pressure may sometimes rise very quickly, the fetus may be at risk with relatively slight hypertension, and the physiopathology of eclampsia differs from that of essential hypertension, whether benign or malignant.

If the blood pressure rises acutely, with the diastolic reading above 100 mm, the patient may complain of a severe and persistent frontal headache, and may vomit. These are warning signals of the possibility of eclampsia. But of course many pregnant women develop headache for other reasons such as migraine, and in the absence of hypertension a headache during pregnancy is not to be attributed to pre-eclampsia.

The patient who has an abnormally high blood pressure before pregnancy requires special consideration. In her case a rise in the diastolic pressure of 20 mm Hg is usually required before a diagnosis of superimposed pre-eclampsia can be made.

Proteinuria during pregnancy.   The term proteinuria is more accurate than albuminuria. Although at first the protein is largely albumin, the molecules of which are among the smallest of the plasma proteins, as pre-eclampsia worsens larger molecules, including globulins, appear in increasing proportions. Proteinuria is most easily detected with test paper strips although older methods, including boiling the urine, remain satisfactory. The test paper strips are very sensitive and indicate a degree of proteinuria which would not be detected by older methods. Nevertheless proteinuria during pregnancy is always potentially serious and demands investigation. Besides pre-eclampsia, the main causes are contamination from vaginal discharge, urinary tract infection and chronic renal disease.

Most patients produce a urine specimen when they attend the antenatal clinic or doctor's surgery without particular care, and often bring it in any jar that is at hand. Before accepting that proteinuria is present contamination must be excluded by obtaining a 'clean catch' midstream specimen, after cleansing the vulva with sterile water or saline.

Urinary infection can be excluded by examining the urine microscopically. When infection is present pus cells and bacteria can be seen. Bacteriological examination must also be used to confirm the diagnosis and to indicate the most appropriate treatment.

Proteinuria associated with chronic renal disease rarely presents a diagnostic problem because there is usually a history of the disease predating the pregnancy. Even if there is no such history it is likely that the proteinuria will be present throughout pregnancy, while pre-eclampsia is very uncommon before the third trimester.

After excluding these other causes of proteinuria it is reasonable to attribute it to pre-eclampsia. It is then always a sign of serious significance. The risk of intrauterine death of the fetus and of eclampsia is increased many times over when proteinuria occurs, even when there is only a slight increase in blood pressure.

There are other causes of proteinuria besides those just mentioned, but they are much rarer. One of the more interesting is *orthostatic proteinuria*. Orthostatic means 'standing straight', and the proteinuria only occurs after the patient has been on her feet for some time. At night in the recumbent position the proteinuria disappears. It is not peculiar to pregnancy, and is not uncommon in adolescents. It can be provoked in a number of pregnant women by having them stand in extreme lordosis for some time. It is thought that in this posture the left renal vein is compressed where it crosses the vertebral column in front of the aorta and beneath the superior mesenteric artery. This presumably raises the venous pressure in the left kidney, and it has been shown that in this condition most of the protein in the urine comes from the left kidney. The diagnosis is most improbable in a fully ambulant pregnant woman. Unexplained proteinuria necessitates admission to hospital, but in some women the proteinuria promptly disappears; then the diagnosis of orthostatic proteinuria can be made by testing the urine before and after activity.

Sometimes other uncommon causes of proteinuria during pregnancy such as acute nephritis or disseminated lupus erythematosus, may need consideration.

Clinical features of pre-eclampsia

Pre-eclampsia occurs in between 3 and 10 per cent of all pregnancies, depending on the population from which the statistics are drawn and the strictness of the criteria for diagnosis. As has been seen, each of the signs requires careful evaluation in individual patients.

Primigravidae develop pre-eclampsia more than twice as frequently as multiparae. Those multiparae who develop the condition almost always have a history of a similar event in the preceding pregnancy or pregnancies. Unless there is some underlying vascular disease pre-eclampsia usually becomes less severe from one pregnancy to the next.

Pre-eclampsia is more common in women over 35, especially in relatively infertile primigravidae. Those who have essential hypertension are more likely to develop superadded pre-eclampsia than normotensive women, but they do not invariably do so. However, in patients with hypertensive renal disease pre-eclampsia almost always occurs. It is more common in patients with diabetes mellitus, and almost invariably occurs when there is diabetic vascular disease.

There is an increased incidence of pre-eclampsia in association with multiple pregnancy, with polyhydramnios, with severe rhesus incompatibility and in cases of vesicular mole (p. 149). The last association is of interest because the pre-eclampsia is frequently severe, occurs early in pregnancy (usually 16 – 20 weeks), and in the absence of a fetus. One other condition deserves mention, although it is extremely rare. This is abdominal pregnancy, where the placenta has become attached to structures outside the uterus, but has succeeded in maintaining the fetus into the third trimester. In these cases pre-eclampsia almost invariably occurs.

Management of pre-eclampsia

Although the aetiology of pre-eclampsia is still obscure, empirical management has achieved considerable improvement in the prognosis for both mother and baby. It is possible that the severity of the disease has also declined in recent years. As a result the incidence of eclampsia in countries where there is comprehensive antenatal care has fallen from 1 to 1000 to 1 in 5000 births.

The most important factor in management is early diagnosis. Because pre-eclampsia becomes more likely as pregnancy nears term, antenatal attendances should be more frequent at this time. In the first 28 weeks of pregnancy visits are usually made monthly, from 28 to 36 weeks fortnightly, and after that weekly. At each visit the patient is weighed, oedema is sought at the ankles and in the fingers, the resting blood pressure is recorded and the urine tested for protein. Excessive weight gain, moderate oedema, and a rise of blood pressure not exceeding 130/80 mm Hg may be dealt with by advising rest at home. A check on the effectiveness of this advice must be made within a week.

A rise of blood pressure to 140/90 mm, or a rise of 20 mm in the diastolic pressure above the booking pressure, is an indication for admission to hospital, and if there is protein in a clean specimen of urine the need for admission is urgent.

The aim of treatment is to obtain a live baby, as mature as possible, while preventing injury to the mother. It is desirable to maintain the pregnancy until the 37th week, always providing that the placental function remains adequate and the mother's blood pressure is under sufficient control to minimize the risk of eclampsia, cerebral haemorrhage and accidental antepartum haemorrhage. Pre-eclampsia will not be cured until the fetus is delivered, and however well controlled it may appear to be, it is usually necessary to keep the patient in hospital until this time.

The most important component of treatment is rest in bed. This will usually result in stabilization of the blood pressure and, because uterine blood flow is relatively greater when the patient is at rest, better fetal growth. Sedatives are sometimes employed, and have a marginal effect upon the blood pressure. Diazepam (Valium) should not be used for mild cases as it can have a depressant effect on the baby if it is born prematurely. Hypotensive agents and diuretics should only be used in special circumstances. Reduction of the blood pressure to normal values can often be attained by the use of potent hypotensive agents, but this is often at the expense of placental function, which in many cases seems to depend on the raised blood pressure, in the same way as a damaged kidney may depend upon an increased blood pressure to maintain a tolerable function.

Routine observations in hospital will include blood pressure recording at least twice daily, and more frequently if the condition is worsening. Oedema may be sought in the sacral region, but it is difficult to detect there, and checking daily on the tightness of rings on the fingers is more profitable. A record should be kept of fluid intake and urinary output in all but the slightest cases, for reduction in urinary output almost always precedes eclampsia. Each urinary specimen should be tested for protein.

Regular palpation of the uterus to detect growth failure or diminishing liquor volume is helpful in judging placental function. These observations should be supplemented by ultrasonic measurements of the biparietal diameter of the fetal head, and some centres also measure the abdominal circumference of the fetus.

Urinary oestriol assays and other biochemical tests for placental function (see p. 57) are useful in cases of pre-eclampsia in which fetal growth is suspected of being impaired, especially cases in which the duration of gestation is too short to permit the easy solution of induction of labour without anxiety.

Another indication of fetal well-being is its activity. This can be assessed by the mother counting the number of fetal movements over a given time (a 'kick count'), by recording fetal breathing movements with ultrasound, or by observing the variation in fetal heart rate that accompanies fetal activity or occurs in response to uterine contractions.

A time may come in any pregnancy complicated by pre-eclampsia when the fetus is safer delivered and in a cot, even in the premature nursery, rather than in the unhealthy environment of the uterus. The purpose of all these investigations is to decide when this moment has arrived. In some cases labour starts prematurely, and in most cases there is a ready response to induction. In any event the patient should not be allowed to pass her expected date of delivery.

The worsening situation—imminent eclampsia.   If the diastolic blood pressure remains above 100 mm Hg in spite of rest in bed, or if proteinuria persists, and the duration of gestation is more than 36 weeks labour should be induced without hesitation. During labour the fetal heart rate should be continuously monitored (p. 352). Units without equipment for monitoring should not be conducting such labours.

If the fetus is very immature, between 28 and 33 weeks, hypotensive agents may be used to prevent further elevation of the blood pressure. However, the diastolic pressure should not be reduced to less than 90 mm, as this can reduce placental perfusion and lead to fetal death. No one agent seems to be better than another among the many powerful drugs on the market today. It is sensible to become familiar with one agent, and methyldopa is often chosen, used perhaps in conjunction with a diuretic. If control of the blood pressure cannot be achieved, or the amount of protein in the urine is increasing or heavy, or if there is evidence of placental failure then early delivery is advisable, often by Caesarean section, in spite of the risks of prematurity.

In cases between 33 and 36 weeks judgment is exercised. In all cases of doubt about the decision to induce labour or perform Caesarean section a test for the maturity of the fetal lung may be useful. Liquor amnii is obtained by amniocentesis for measurement of the lecithin-sphingomyelin ratio (p. 369).

Signs that an eclamptic fit is imminent include a continually rising blood pressure, increasing oedema of the face and hands, heavy proteinuria, oliguria, headache and disturbances of vision. Vomiting and epigastric pain, with tenderness over the liver, indicate hepatic haemorrhages or necrosis. Urgent action is required to prevent fits, to reduce the blood pressure, to promote diuresis and to deliver the fetus.

An intravenous injection of diazepam (Valium) 10 mg is given at once, followed by a slow infusion containing 40 mg in a litre of 5 per cent dextrose solution. This acts as a sedative and raises the threshold at which fits occur. The blood pressure can be most promptly reduced by intravenous administration of hydrallazine (Apresoline). While monitoring the blood pressure closely, hydrallazine 10 mg is injected intravenously over a period of 15 minutes. The initial dose is usually followed by a continuous slow infusion of 50 mg of hydrallazine in a litre of 5 per cent dextrose solution. The rate of infusion is adjusted to keep the blood pressure just above 140/90 mm; if the pressure falls below this the infusion is stopped.

Frusemide (Lasix) 40 mg intravenously will produce a diuresis within minutes which helps to reduce the blood pressure and appears to protect the kidney from possible damage caused by a vascular shutdown. An indwelling catheter will avoid the discomfort of a full bladder or the disturbance of frequent micturition.

External stimuli are liable to trigger off a fit, therefore undue noise, bright lights and painful procedures should be avoided.

The method of delivery will depend upon the parity of the patient, the stage of pregnancy and the state of the cervix. In all but the most severe cases, and cases in which placental function is notably poor, vaginal delivery should be the aim. If delivery has to be effected before the 34th week, when induction is less certain, Caesarean section may be considered, and it would be advised if there was not an immediate response to induction, or if labour was not progressing quickly.

During labour the maternal blood pressure must be recorded frequently. Painful uterine contractions may raise the blood pressure and trigger off a fit. Good control of pain is therefore essential, and this can be best achieved with an epidural anaesthetic. The progress of the first stage of labour should be checked by vaginal examination at 2 – 3-hourly intervals, and the condition of the fetus monitored by continuous fetal heart rate recording.

The second stage should be short because of the risk of raising the maternal blood pressure. With an epidural anaesthetic a low forceps delivery or vacuum extraction is easy, and ensures the minimal risk.

The third stage of labour is potentially dangerous in the pre-eclamptic patient because there is usually a transient rise in blood pressure when the uterus contracts down and the vascular space is reduced. This rise in pressure is greater if an oxytocic drug is used, especially with ergometrine which causes peripheral vasoconstriction. These patients seem to be particularly prone to this vasoconstrictor effect and it is therefore sensible to avoid the routine use of ergometrine in the third stage of labour. If anything is needed to treat postpartum haemorrhage Syntocinon 5 units intravenously is usually effective, and its hypertensive effect is minimal and brief.

Because of the possibility of postpartum eclampsia, the blood pressure is carefully watched after delivery, and the urinary output recorded. Drugs should be withdrawn gradually over the course of 3 or 4 days, depending on the progress of the patient.

Eclampsia

Eclampsia remains one of the most serious complications of pregnancy. It may occur before, during or shortly after delivery. Postpartum eclampsia is usually less severe than ante- or intrapartum eclampsia. The mortality varies with the number of fits and the quality of treatment and the speed with which it is made available. A maternal mortality of 2 to 3 per cent and a perinatal mortality of 30 per cent still occur, even in countries with modern obstetric services.

Eclampsia is characterized by the occurrence of major epileptiform convulsions in patients with signs and symptoms described above under 'imminent eclampsia'. Four stages in the fits are described; the aura, the cry, the tonic phase and the clonic phase. In eclampsia if there is an aura it is visual—flashes of light and spots before the eyes. Spasm of the respiratory muscles and larynx causes the cry, which is not usually noticeable. The tonic and clonic phases are similar to those which occur in epilepsy. During the tonic phase the patient loses consciousness, has generalized muscular spasm and becomes cyanosed. The fetus may show signs of hypoxia. During the clonic phase of violent movements the tongue may be bitten, vomiting and inhalation of vomit may occur. In severe cases recurrent fits occur, and the patient remains deeply unconscious between them. The risks of hypoxia, of inhalation of vomit, and of cerebral haemorrhage caused by elevation of the blood pressure during the fits are considerable. Accidental separation of the placenta, disseminated intravascular coagulation and renal necrosis are other serious dangers.

Treatment.   The whole emphasis of this chapter has been on prevention of eclampsia by vigilance during pregnancy, during labour and soon after labour. It is especially important to recognize cases of worsening and fulminating pre-eclampsia, so that they can be prevented from further development by delivery followed by full sedation for at least 48 hours.

If eclampsia does occur the aim is to prevent further fits. The greater the number of fits the worse is the prognosis for the mother and baby. Any stimulus may precipitate another fit, so the excitability of the central nervous system must be reduced by sedatives or anaesthesia, and everything done to cut down external stimuli such as noise, bright light and discomfort, arising especially from a full bladder or a strained position in bed.

Immediate heavy sedation with diazepam (Valium) is given. Because the patient is comatose or else heavily sedated there is a risk of both asphyxia and hypostatic pneumonia. A clear airway must be maintained and oxygen may be required. Provision must be made for aspiration of any vomit. False teeth must be removed, and a gag may be placed between the jaws. The patient may need restraint to prevent her injuring herself during the fits. An indwelling catheter will both prevent the stimulus of an overfull bladder and allow accurate observation of the urinary output.

Hypotensive agents, as already described on p. 192 may reduce the risk of cerebral haemorrhage or of accidental antepartum haemorrhage.

The patient will not be safe from the possibility of further fits until she is delivered, and the risk of hypostatic pneumonia is another reason to urge early delivery. The mode of delivery will depend to some extent on the prognosis for the fetus. If it is dead or very small Caesarean section may not be justified, but with a fetus of reasonable size the risk of labour with a poorly functioning placenta may not be acceptable. If Caesarean section is not chosen labour must be rapid and easy. Forceps or the vacuum extractor are often used for delivery, and with any additional obstetric problem section is advised.

Remote prognosis of pre-eclampsia and eclampsia

After pre-eclampsia or eclampsia approximately one-third of women will be found to have 'residual hypertension'. The question is whether these conditions caused this hypertension. At present it is held that these women would eventually have developed hypertension even if they never had a pregnancy. The evidence that supports this view is that the incidence of deaths from cardiovascular disease are the same at all comparable ages in nulliparous women and in women who have borne children.

Some women have hypertension in every successive pregnancy and most of these will later be found to have essential hypertension.

Pathology of pre-eclampsia and eclampsia

It is fortunately uncommon nowadays to have an opportunity to study the postmortem features of pre-eclampsia or eclampsia. The available evidence throws scant light upon the aetiology of the disease or of the mechanism by which the hypertension, oedema and proteinuria are produced. Most of the lesions observed result from the hypertension rather than provide an explanation for it.

Cerebral lesions. Because of the raised intracranial pressure the brain is oedematous and the convolutions are flattened. There are small haemorrhages scattered throughout its substance which may become confluent. Massive haemorrhage in the brain may be a cause of death. Haemorrhage and oedema may also occur in the retina.

Hepatic lesions. The lesions found in the liver in eclampsia are diagnostic of the disease. There is no other disorder which produces similar changes. Macroscopically the liver is enlarged and there are patchy focal red and yellow areas, of which the red are caused by haemorrhage and the yellow by necrosis of the liver cells. The red and yellow patches are visible under the capsule and throughout the cut surfaces. On microscopical section the haemorrhages are mainly grouped around the portal canals, but they may be so extensive that they completely disrupt the liver architecture. By interrupting the blood supply they cause necrosis in the periphery of the lobules with fatty change, which is responsible for the yellow colour. The extravasated blood shows many fibrinous thrombi.

The epigastric pain and liver tenderness which may occur in eclampsia probably arise from distension of the capsule. The interference with liver function is caused by destruction and damage to liver cells, and if this is severe it will result in jaundice. This is therefore a very serious sign. The damage to the liver may be so great that death occurs from hepatic failure.

Renal lesions.   The primary renal lesion is in the glomeruli which show swelling of their cells and of the underlying basement membrane. The whole glomerulus appears to be so stuffed with its own swollen cells that it looks as if there is no room for blood to flow through the capillaries, although in fact a greatly diminished flow continues. It is generally held that the reduced renal blood flow is caused by vascular spasm, although the cause of the spasm is uncertain. Beyond the glomerulus the rest of the nephron which is supplied by the afferent arteriole is starved of oxygen. The result is necrosis of the proximal and distal convoluted tubules. This may be of any degree of severity from simple cloudy swelling up to death.

Depending on circumstances, large or small areas of the kidney may be involved. In extreme cases the cortex of the kidney may be destroyed almost entirely, the condition of bilateral cortical necrosis (p. 164). This is less common in eclampsia than in cases of concealed accidental antepartum haemorrhage, when the degree of renal ischaemia may be extreme. In eclampsia the ischaemia is usually less severe and causes areas of patchy necrosis which affect the tubules rather than the glomeruli. Such lower nephron necrosis may be reversible, so that spontaneous recovery occurs. Whether the glomeruli or the tubules are chiefly affected, there is always some degree of renal failure, which in severe cases may progress to anuria.

These pathological changes explain the proteinuria by damage to the glomerular cells, and the oliguria by reduction of glomerular filtration. Sometimes the amount of glomerular filtrate may be very little diminished but the tubules are incapable of concentrating the fluid which reaches them.

Pathology of oedema.   Oedema is due to an increase in fluid in the extracellular extravascular compartment of the body. Normally fluid flows out of the capillaries into the tissue space because of the hydrostatic pressure at the arterial end. Fluid flows back at the venous end of the capillary because of the high osmotic pressure brought about within the capillary by the outflow of fluid and the retention of protein molecules within it. One likely mechanism of production of oedema in pre-eclampsia is the forcing out of fluid by increased blood pressure. Loss of protein in the urine might accentuate this effect.

Aetiology of pre-eclampsia and eclampsia

There are many theories of the cause of pre-eclampsia and eclampsia but none is entirely satisfactory. This is probably because there are a number of different ways in which the mechanism that produces the various signs of pre-eclampsia can be activated. The mechanism itself is also unexplained.

Certain clinical observations must be fitted into any theory, however complex:

1. Pre-eclampsia is a disease of pregnancy. There is no instance of it occurring outside pregnancy, although a number of other diseases have some similarities to it. It resolves completely when the pregnancy is over unless some structural damage has been caused by the hypertension.

2. Pre-eclampsia occurs more commonly in first than in subsequent pregnancies.

3. The incidence is high when there is pre-existing vascular disease or long-standing hypertension.

4. Pre-eclampsia tends to be less severe in successive pregnancies unless there is pre-existing vascular disease.

5. It occurs more frequently as pregnancy advances but its progress can often be slowed or even arrested. However, the only cure of the disease is the ending of the pregnancy.

6. Intrauterine death of the fetus is often associated with considerable improvement in the signs of the disease.

7. It is not necessary for a fetus to be present. With a vesicular mole severe pre-eclampsia may occur early in pregnancy.

8. Pre-eclampsia is commoner in multiple than in singleton pregnancy.

9. It is commoner in women who have diabetes mellitus, especially if there is diabetic arterial disease, nephropathy or retinopathy.

10. It may occur in haemolytic disease with a hydropic placenta and fetus.

11. The fetus is frequently light in weight for its period of gestation and shows signs of intrauterine malnutrition which has often preceded the development of the signs of pre-eclampsia.

12. Hypertension sometimes appears or becomes worse after delivery, even to the stage of eclampsia. This has not occurred so often since the risk of the pressor effect of ergometrine in pre-eclamptic patients has been recognized.

The most satisfactory way of considering the aetiology of pre-eclampsia at present is to think of the placenta as being at the centre of the problem. If the placenta is unable to carry out its essential function of supporting the fetus adequately, either because the maternal perfusion of the placenta is insufficient, because there are excessive demands upon the placenta, or because the placenta is itself abnormal, then a mechanism is activated to attempt to alter this placental inadequacy. The maternal blood pressure is raised to increase the placental perfusion. Many of the other signs of pre-eclampsia result from this acute rise in blood pressure, and eclampsia itself is due to intracranial hypertension and oedema.

Observations which suggest that the inadequate placenta is of fundamental importance are that poor intrauterine growth often precedes the development of hypertension, and that in some cases placental function tests indicate a failing placenta before signs of pre-eclampsia develop. The high risk of intrauterine death, the tendency to premature labour and the ready response to induction of labour all support the view that the placenta is inadequate, but without pointing to it as the basic cause of the syndrome.

Why should the placenta be inadequate? What indeed is meant by placental inadequacy? The placenta must be deemed inadequate when it cannot sustain the fetus or fetuses *in utero* long enough for them to reach a degree of maturity which will enable them to survive after birth. There is circumstantial evidence that all placentae become inadequate eventually, and that this somehow triggers labour. The intrauterine growth of the fetus declines shortly before term in normal pregnancy, and most placental function tests show a levelling off of placental efficiency.

Clearly the greater the demands upon the placenta the more likely is failure to occur. Thus in multiple pregnancy there is a higher incidence of pre-eclampsia than in singleton pregnancies.

Alternatively placental function may be inadequate because the maternal blood supply to the placental site is inadequate. This could explain the high incidence of pre-eclampsia in primigravidae, while the relatively improved uterine blood flow in subsequent pregnancies would explain its comparative infrequency in them, and also the fact that in general babies get heavier in pregnancies after the first. The concept of a uterine blood flow incapable of matching the demands of pregnancy would explain the high incidence of pre-eclampsia in patients with vascular disease. In diabetic patients there is frequently early vascular degeneration, and to this may be added the excessive demands of a large fetus in poorly controlled diabetic pregnancy.

The placenta may also be inadequate because part of it has been lost during threatened abortion or accidental antepartum haemorrhage, or there may be a fibrinoid barrier to the transfer of essential substances from mother to fetus (see intervillous thrombosis, p. 154). The cause of this laying down of fibrinoid material over the chorionic villi is unknown, but theoretically it could be a partial breakdown of the immunological suppression which enables the feto-placental unit (which is genetically half incompatible with the mother) to maintain its situation in the uterus as a 'transplant'.

If it is granted that the inadequate placenta is the basic cause of the pre-eclamptic syndrome, it remains to explain the mechanism by which the various features of it are produced. Most of them can be attributed to acute hypertension, and it is necessary to look first at ways in which the rise in blood pressure may be brought about.

One of the earliest theories of the aetiology of pre-eclampsia was that 'placental infarcts' (a term of very loose meaning, see p. 154) produced degradation products which acted as toxins and caused widespread vascular spasm. No direct evidence for this has been found, although the normal placental cells contain many substances which, if generally released, could have widespread pressor effects.

More recently it has been suggested that the ischaemic uterus and placenta produce substances which increase general vascular tone, and thus increase placental perfusion. There are suggestions that the renin-angiotensin system, which operates in the case of the damaged kidney, may operate in a similar way in pre-eclampsia. As yet this remains unproven.

It has recently been shown that in some cases of severe pre-eclampsia there is a depression of plasma fibrinolytic activity, an increased level of fibrin degradation products, and a reduced platelet count. The increase in fibrin degradation products is even greater after eclamptic fits. These observations suggest that intravascular coagulation is taking place. If the disturbed balance between coagulation and lysis of clot was localized to certain organs, for example the placenta, kidneys and liver, some of the manifestations of pre-eclampsia and eclampsia could be explained. Fibrin deposition in vessels supplying the placenta would cause placental insufficiency; fibrin in the renal vessels would cause glomerular damage and proteinuria, and renal ischaemia might be related to hypertension.

Surveys of diets have purported to implicate various deficiencies and excesses in the genesis of eclampsia, but none have yet been of help in understanding aetiology. There is no evidence that restricting protein intake will reduce the incidence of the disease. It is difficult to accept a dietary cause for eclampsia in view of the fact that it is more common in first than in subsequent pregnancies, and that the incidence is not increased in women suffering from calorie deprivation, although it is more common in some deprived areas of the world.

Clearly much remains to be determined about pre-eclampsia and eclampsia. The theories we have about its aetiology are inadequate but empirical management gives increasingly satisfactory results. Careful consideration of the treatment advocated and the propositions made about the aetiology of the disease will show that these are compatible.

20

Essential hypertension and renal diseases in pregnancy

Essential hypertension in pregnancy

The definition of essential hypertension is a matter of controversy and its significance is even more hotly disputed. In the early stages of the disease the blood pressure is raised above the average normal pressure but there are no gross pathological changes in the arteries supplying the kidneys, heart or brain. It may be that those people who have such a raised blood pressure are representatives of the higher end of a normal distribution of blood pressure levels in the population but, whether or not this is so, it does seem that in time the higher blood pressure causes arterial disease. For the obstetrician the importance of essential hypertension is that women starting pregnancy with a raised blood pressure are more likely to develop pre-eclampsia than those who are normotensive. However this only occurs in a proportion of the cases, and two out of three women who have a mild or moderate degree of hypertension at the start of pregnancy do not develop the disease and have babies of normal birth weight.

If a pregnant woman is not seen until after the 12th week of pregnancy an accurate base-line pressure reading may not be obtained because of the tendency of the pressure to fall slightly in the middle trimester. This tendency is most marked in those who have mild hypertension of recent origin, and it is of good prognostic significance because the incidence of superadded pre-eclampsia is lower in this group of patients than in those hypertensive patients who do not show such a fall.

Management

A resting blood pressure of 140/90 mm Hg or more during the first 24 weeks of pregnancy is usually deemed to be significantly raised, and at that time in pregnancy is unlikely to be due to pre-eclampsia.

If hypertension is found an effort must be made to discover any underlying cause for it such as chronic pyelonephritis, chronic nephritis, polycystic disease of the kidneys, coarctation of the aorta or phaechromocytoma. The femoral pulses must be palpated; absence of pulsation would suggest the possibility of aortic coarctation. The urine is examined for protein and casts, and bacteriologically examined if any pus cells are found. The blood urea may be estimated and other renal function tests may be required.

Proteinuria is of serious prognostic significance when found with hypertension, for it implies that there is both renal and cardiovascular disease. Which of these is primary is not of immediate importance in obstetric practice, and fortunately most cases of essential hypertension have not progressed far enough to cause renal damage during the childbearing years. However, proteinuria may be due to chronic pyelonephritis, chronic nephritis or to relatively rare diseases such as systemic lupus erythematosus involving the kidney. This may be diagnosed by the discovery of LE cells in the blood.

The retina should be examined in all patients with hypertension, abnormal signs being nipping of the veins where they are crossed by the arteries, narrowing of the arteries, and occasionally haemorrhages or exudate. Such findings may show that the hypertensive disease is of long standing and preceded the pregnancy.

In all cases of mild essential hypertension (less than 150/100 mm) the patients must be seen more frequently than usual because of the risk of pre-eclampsia being added. A rise in diastolic pressure of 20 mm, or the appearance of proteinuria, is an indication for admission to hospital. Careful watch must be kept on the growth of the fetus both by clinical observation and with the help of ultrasound.

With moderate or severe hypertension (above 150/100 mm) the patient should be admitted to hospital for rest. She may also be given a mild sedative such as phenobarbitone 30 – 60 mg twice daily. The effect of rest gives a valuable indication of the prognosis, for if the blood pressure is thereby reduced a favourable outcome can be expected. Such a patient may be sent home, but weekly checks of blood pressure and fetal growth must continue.

If the blood pressure does not fall with rest in bed and sedation, thought should be given to the use of hypotensive drugs. In using such drugs the prime consideration is the protection of the mother from the dangers of high blood pressure such as cerebral haemorrhage and left heart failure. Artificial lowering of the blood pressure will not improve the chance of survival of the fetus; indeed it may diminish the blood flow to the placenta and affect the fetus adversely.

Our preference among the many hypotensive drugs is at present for methyldopa. It is started at a dosage of 250 mg twice daily and then slowly worked up towards a maximum dose of about 4 g daily, depending on the response of the blood pressure. It has the special advantage that its effects are not dependent upon the patient standing up; with some other drugs a hypotensive effect is only seen when the patient is on her feet and then the pressure may fall so precipitously that she feels faint. A thiazide diuretic may also be given, together with a potassium supplement to guard against depletion when this element is lost with sodium in the urine.

Some patients are already taking hypotensive drugs before they become pregnant; these drugs should be continued, adjusting the dose if necessary.

Obstetric treatment in essential hypertension is exactly the same as for pre-eclampsia. It is essentially that of securing delivery at the best time to avoid serious maternal complications and to prevent fetal death in utero. When the diastolic pressure is 90 mm or more the perinatal loss will be about 7 per cent (as compared with a loss in normotensive pregnancy of about 1.5 per cent), and if the systolic pressure is above 160 mm the loss is about 13 per cent. When the blood pressure is regularly 170/100 mm or more the fetal loss is about 30 per cent. Much of this fetal loss occurs in the last few weeks of pregnancy, so that it is often best to secure delivery before term. The best time for this will depend on the particular case, but in general the higher the pressure the earlier the delivery should be. Placental function tests, ultrasonic measurement of fetal growth and fetal heart monitoring may all play a part in determining the optimum time for delivery. Assessment of the maturity of the fetal lung by measurement of the lecithin-sphingomyelin ratio in the liquor amnii may be helpful in deciding whether to induce labour.

The method of induction or delivery depends on the particular case. In the milder case amniotomy may be aided by the use of an intravenous oxytocin drip. There would be some hesitation in using such a drip for more severe cases, in which Caesarean sections might be performed if there was not a quick response to amniotomy. Elderly primigravidae, and patients with evidence of placental insufficiency, may be treated by Caesarean sections without any attempt at induction.

Accidental antepartum haemorrhage and hypertension during pregnancy. In about 25 per cent of cases of accidental antepartum haemorrhage moderate hypertension or proteinuria (or both) are discovered. It was at one time believed that pre-eclampsia or essential hypertension were common causes of accidental haemorrhage. However, in 90 per cent of cases of accidental haemorrhage there is no record of any *preceding* hypertension. It is certain that in some cases the hypertension and proteinuria *follow* the bleeding, perhaps as a result of a utero-renal reflex.

It seems likely that both events may occur, i.e. that hypertension may occasionally lead to placental separation, and that placental damage may sometimes cause hypertension.

Pyelonephritis during pregnancy

In pyelonephritis there is inflammation of the renal pelvis and renal parenchyma.

Acute pyelonephritis has long been known as a common and apparently transient complication of pregnancy, but it is only relatively recently that it has been recognized that it is a potentially dangerous disease which, if it persists and becomes chronic, may progress to cause hypertension and ultimate renal failure. The obstetrician is in a particularly favourable position to prevent this, not only by effective treatment during pregnancy, but by securing for his patients proper subsequent investigation and care.

Aetiology

Bacteriuria. Acute pyelonephritis in pregnancy is sometimes just an episode in a long-standing disease process, which began in childhood or even during early infancy. Repeated attacks of urinary infection may occur throughout childhood, and often there is an exacerbation with the beginning of sexual activity and during pregnancy. Infection in childhood may produce renal scarring with irregular narrowing of the renal cortex. The infecting organisms, usually *Escherichia coli*, probably invade the bladder from the urethra and if the uretero-vesical sphincter is incompetent they may ascend and proliferate in the upper urinary tract.

If women are examined early in pregnancy about 6 per cent of them will be found to have significant bacteriuria in two or more separate fresh midstream specimens of urine. A 'significant' level is conventionally taken as more than 10^5 organisms per ml in a midstream specimen. This level was chosen empirically; it is believed that higher counts indicate that the bladder or higher urinary tract is colonized; lower counts may only indicate colonization of the urethra. (In a specimen obtained by suprapubic bladder aspiration any bacterial growth is regarded as significant.)

A few of the patients with bacteriuria have had evident infection in childhood, with recurrent clinical attacks, but in many the time of invasion of the upper urinary tract is unknown, and the bacteriuria is completely asymptomatic. However, if asymptomatic cases are investigated by intravenous pyelography, particularly those cases in which the bacteriuria is not quickly eradicated by sulphonamides or ampicillin, many of the patients are found to have renal abnormalities such as chronic pyelonephritis or congenital malformations.

Women who are found to have bacteriuria are far more likely than others to develop acute pyelonephritis during pregnancy. If the bacteriuria responds to treatment during pregnancy the risk of acute pyelonephritis is largely prevented, but if the patients are not treated or if there is no response to treatment the incidence of pyelonephritis during pregnancy is as high as 30 per cent.

These facts show that all antenatal patients should be˙screened for bacteriuria, and those who have bacteriuria should be treated in an attempt to eradicate it. However, this will not eliminate all acute urinary infections in pregnant women because some attacks occur in patients who have no preceding bacteriuria.

To screen a large number of antenatal patients makes a heavy demand on the time of nurses, in collecting the midstream specimens, and on laboratory facilities. One solution is to use 'dip-slides' which have a thin coating of culture medium. One of the slides is dipped into each specimen of urine and the batch of slides is easily incubated. Subcultures are made from any positive slides, and the fixed area of the medium on the slide allows a rough colony count.

About 75 per cent of cases of bacteriuria are cured by a single course of sulphadimidine (0.5 g 6-hourly for 8 days). A similar percentage of success is obtained with ampicillin (500 mg 8-hourly for 8 days), but the cases which respond are not the same in the two groups. Put in another way, most patients will be cured by one or the other of these two drugs, and only a few cases by neither of them. Some other antibiotic may then be tried; but in many of the cases in which the infection cannot be eradicated intravenous pyelography after delivery will show scarring due to chronic pyelonephritis, some congenital abnormality of the renal tract, or some other lesion such as a calculus.

Some have advised giving a long continuous course of treatment during pregnancy, but there is no evidence that this is better than a short course.

Changes in the renal pelvis and ureter in normal pregnancy. Intravenous pyelography, which was freely performed during pregnancy in the past before the possible fetal hazard was recognized, shows that dilatation of the ureters and renal pelves occurs during pregnancy, and in about 80 per cent of pregnant women there is marked stasis in the right ureter and to some extent in the left ureter also. The dilatation extends down as far as the brim of the bony pelvis; below that level the ureter often appears normal. The ureters often appear tortuous, and may be kinked. There is at present little evidence that ureteric reflux from the bladder occurs during pregnancy, but this is a possible explanation of ascending infection. The dilatation may be caused in part by pressure of the enlarged pregnant uterus on the ureter at the brim of the pelvis. The right ureter is more likely to be involved on account of the tendency of the uterus to incline towards the right side.

In addition to mechanical factors causing dilatation of the ureter, there may be reduced tone in the ureteric musculature during pregnancy. Although the ureter is dilated the intra-ureteric pressure is not increased. It has further been suggested that this atony is caused by the inhibitory effect of progesterone.

The infecting organism.   An organism of the *Escherichia coli* group is present in nearly 80 per cent of cases. The organism has been obtained not only from the bladder, but directly from the kidney by ureteric catheterization. Other organisms are occasionally found, such as the *Streptococcus faecalis*, *Bacillus proteus* or *Staphylococci*.

The path of infection.   Although it has been suggested that organisms may reach the kidney from the blood stream or by the periureteric lymphatics it is more likely that they do so by upward spread from the bladder by proliferation of organisms in the lumen of the ureter. Urine containing bacteria can enter the urethra if there is reflux at the uretero-vesical junction, and during pregnancy stasis of urinary flow makes upward spread more likely.

Morbid anatomy

In the rare cases in which death occurs the following changes are found:

The kidney is of a pale colour and softer than the normal. It is usually enlarged by the distension of the pelvis. The epithelium of the pelvis and ureter is injected, thickened, and roughened. Within the renal cortex small abscess cavities are frequently discovered and streaks of pus may be seen radiating outwards in the medulla from the renal pelvis. Histological section shows acute inflammatory reaction which extends to a greater or less degree into the renal parenchyma. It is the fibrosis which follows this infection of the parenchyma which may ultimately destroy the function of the involved areas.

Symptoms

(a) **Acute pyelonephritis.** The patient, usually at least 16 weeks pregnant, is suddenly seized with an acute attack of abdominal pain, which is felt in the lumbar or iliac region of one or both sides. In 50 per cent of cases the infection is confined to the right side and in 16 per cent to the left; in 34 per cent of cases both kidneys are involved. The temperature rises suddenly to levels such as 39.5°C (103°F), and may be accompanied by a rigor; the pulse rate is rapid and often remains at about 120 per minute for several days. The patient who is untreated, frequently appears profoundly ill, and complains of severe vomiting and sometimes of constipation. It is a characteristic of the disease, however, that the patient improves rapidly in appearance after the rigor is over. The abdomen may be distended and is tender, especially over the region of the affected kidney.

In severe cases at first the urine is diminished in amount and of high specific gravity. Later the amount is much increased, owing to the large amount of fluid given in the course of treatment. The urine in the earliest stages contains only bacilli but soon it becomes turbid and contains pus and flocculent débris; the reaction is almost invariably acid. It is seldom offensive. A pure culture of the coliform bacillus is usually obtained. The centrifuged deposit contains large quantities of these organisms, pus cells, epithelial cells, some red blood corpuscles, and albumin. Macroscopic haematuria is occasionally seen.

(b) **Subacute pyelonephritis.** In this form the symptoms are not so characteristic, and the mode of onset is variable. There may be a gradual onset with malaise and increasing lumbar pain, frequency, vomiting, or symptoms suggesting pleurisy and pneumonia. The temperature is slightly raised and irregular; on palpation the kidney may be tender and feel enlarged. The tenderness of the kidney often subsides after the free passage of pus in the urine, and there is a tendency for the pain to subside in one lumbar region and later to develop upon the opposite side. The attack in some cases is extremely mild; there may be pain but no other symptom, or the patient may have rigors without any apparent cause.

Diagnosis

The diagnosis is based upon the occurrence of a raised temperature, bacilluria, pyuria, and the presence of abdominal pain and tenderness in the situation of the kidney or down the line of the ureter. It should always be thought of when there is renal tenderness during pregnancy. Care must be taken, when examining the kidney, that the affected side is uppermost, the patient being on her side, so that the uterus does not obscure the palpation of the kidney. The diagnosis is confirmed by examination of a midstream specimen of urine. Part of the specimen is sent to the laboratory for bacteriological examination, including the testing of any organism found for sensitivity to the various antibiotics. The rest of the specimen may be examined immediately under the microscope for pus cells. The discovery of pus cells is sufficient for preliminary diagnosis and will permit treatment to be begun while the laboratory report is awaited.

The differential diagnosis may include:

(1) Other conditions causing acute abdominal pain during pregnancy, such as appendicitis, torsion of an ovarian cyst, red degeneration of a fibromyoma and concealed accidental antepartum haemorrhage. The onset of pyelonephritis may sometimes be very acute with vomiting, and there may be tenderness in the right iliac fossa or even rigidity, so that the clinical picture may closely simulate that of appendicitis. However, in acute pyelonephritis the temperature is often higher (39°C or more) than is seen in appendicitis, and rigors often occur which are rare in appendicitis. Fetor of the breath does not usually occur, and the tongue is cleaner than in appendicitis. If the urine is properly examined a mistake is unlikely.

In cases of torsion of an ovarian cyst or of red degeneration of a fibromyoma a tender swelling can usually be felt. In accidental haemorrhage it is the uterus which is tender, there is often at least a little vaginal bleeding and the fetal heart may not be heard.

Cases of pneumonia or pleurisy occasionally give rise to diagnostic difficulty, for in these conditions pain arising from the right lower lobe or related pleura can be confused with renal pain. In all cases the chest should be properly examined. Epidemic myalgia affecting the diaphragm (Bornholm disease) may also cause confusion, but in all these conditions the urine does not contain pus cells.

(2) Vomiting may be the predominating presenting symptom in cases of pyelonephritis, and dysuria may be absent. In any case of vomiting in pregnancy after the first trimester the urine should be examined for pus cells.

(3) The differential diagnosis of proteinuria is discussed on page 189. There is unlikely to be confusion in cases of acute pyelonephritis; it is more likely that chronic pyelonephritis will be mistaken for pre-eclampsia or nephritis.

(4) A few cases will present with pyrexia and little else, and the urine should be examined carefully in any case of undiagnosed febrile illness.

(5) In chronic pyelonephritis anaemia frequently occurs, and in cases of anaemia which do not respond to treatment this possibility should be remembered.

Treatment

The patient must be put to bed in order to obtain rest and for the relief of pain. If one kidney is chiefly affected, she will obtain more relief if she lies mainly upon the unaffected side, with the knees flexed to relax the abdominal muscles.

As soon as a specimen of urine has been obtained for bacteriological examination, including testing the sensitivities of any organisms to antibiotics, treatment is started with ampicillin, 500 mg 6-hourly. As soon as the bacteriological report is available it may justify continuation of treatment with ampicillin; otherwise some other appropriate drug is chosen. If the correct antibacterial drug is given in adequate doses a clinical response is to be expected within two or three days, but treatment must be continued for at least three days after the fever and symptoms have subsided, and checked by repeated urinary cultures.

A large fluid intake will increase urinary flow and therefore reduce the time during which organisms can proliferate in the urine, but at the same time it will dilute any antibiotic in the urine. On balance, the advantage of an adequate urinary flow has been shown to outweigh the disadvantage of diluting the antibiotic.

Prognosis

Maternal prognosis. In the majority of patients with suitable treatment an immediate improvement takes place, and within a few days the pain subsides, the temperature falls, and the urine contains less pus. In the past, before sulphonamides and antibiotics were available, there were occasional cases of pyonephrosis and of multiple small abscesses in the renal parenchyma. Although such events are now rare, we have come to realize that the acute infection is often followed by further attacks which may continue for many years, and that sometimes chronic pyelonephritis may be an insidious, progressive and persistent disease, leading to gradual destruction of the renal parenchyma. Interstitial fibrosis occurs, and the kidney shows irregular scarring and contraction. Histological examination shows patchy areas of fibrosis and of round cell infiltration in which both glomeruli and tubules may show ischaemic atrophy, and other nephrons are distended from obstruction. The important sequel is hypertension, when further arteriolar changes occur in the kidney, and eventually uraemia may occur.

Follow-up after delivery. It is important that recurrent or persistent pyelonephritis should be treated effectively. In any suspicious case, and indeed in any patient who has had pyelonephritis during pregnancy, the urine should be examined repeatedly for pus cells and organisms. If these are found an intravenous pyelogram should be carried out after the pregnancy, but in fact impairment of structure or function will seldom be found until the disease has continued for some years.

If excretion of pus cells or bacilli continues, even intermittently, every attempt must be made to give adequate treatment with antibiotics or long-acting sulphonamides. In rare instances of severe unilateral disease nephrectomy may eventually be necessary to prevent or treat hypertension.

Fetal prognosis. If severe pyelonephritis with high fever is untreated abortion or intrauterine fetal death may occur. With less severe infection, and even in cases of asymptomatic bacteriuria, there may be fetal growth retardation or premature onset of labour, so that the perinatal mortality is increased. It is claimed that effective treatment will prevent this.

Sulphonamides, if given for prolonged periods during pregnancy, may interfere with protein-binding of bilirubin, so that the risk of kernicterus (see p. 497) would be increased if premature delivery occurred.

Chronic renal disease during pregnancy

Pregnancy in association with chronic renal disease is often viewed with concern. The fetal outlook has been regarded as poor, and there has been anxiety in case pregnancy should cause serious deterioration in renal function, which may already be impaired.

When chronic renal disease is suspected, because of the past history or the discovery of hypertension and proteinuria in the first half of pregnancy, it is best to admit the patient to hospital for investigation. Observation will determine the effect on her hypertension of rest and sedation, and renal function can be investigated. A blood urea concentration of over 30 mg per 100 ml or a creatinine clearance of under 60 ml per minute are taken as evidence of impaired renal function, although these can only be regarded as crude tests.

It is always important to try to determine the nature of the renal disorder; chronic glomerulonephritis and chronic pyelonephritis are the most common lesions. In some cases there is a history of previous investigation and an accurate diagnosis. Rarely it is justifiable to carry out a single-film pyelogram or a renal biopsy during pregnancy, but usually these are part of the more extensive investigations to follow in the puerperium.

If renal function is impaired the perinatal mortality is increased, and intrauterine fetal death may occur without warning.

The same principles of management apply to all patients with chronic renal disease. First, there must be early assessment and investigation. Then frequent antenatal visits are essential, and these will have to be weekly during pregnancy. The patient should be readmitted to hospital at the least sign of deterioration. Rest in bed for a large part of each day may be necessary. A high protein diet to offset the loss of protein in the urine and a low salt diet are recommended. In most cases it is advisable to admit the patient to hospital from the 30th week, and from this time on daily observations are made, as in cases of pre-eclampsia. The advice of a nephrologist may be required about the use of hypotensive drugs and diuretics.

The growth of the fetus is carefully watched, and placental function tests performed. By such means the optimum time for delivery of the fetus can be chosen. It is unlikely to be later than 38 weeks and may have to be much earlier. The mode of delivery will depend on the circumstances of the case, and Caesarean section is to be considered if the pregnancy has not reached the 35th week.

There is seldom any medical reason for terminating a pregnancy for chronic renal disease. There is no evidence that pregnancy causes any permanent deterioration in the renal or cardiovascular condition of these patients—a few will do badly, but probably these would have done badly if they had not become pregnant.

Glomerulonephritis

Physicians seldom agree on the classification of cases of nephritis. Acute glomerulonephritis is a very rare coincidental illness during pregnancy, and is treated in the same way as if the patient was not pregnant. If corticosteroids are given it must be remembered that they suppress normal adrenal activity, and the patient may need supplementary doses of hydrocortisone during labour. They also cross the placenta and depress the fetal adrenals, and there is therefore a low output of oestriol. The output of oestriol in the mother's urine cannot be used as an index of placental function.

If a patient merely gives a history of a previous attack of acute nephritis and has no residual hypertension or proteinuria no problem is to be expected during pregnancy.

If, after nephritis, there is only a little proteinuria and slight hypertension which does not increase during pregnancy the prognosis is good for both mother and child. The urine may contain casts, but the precise diagnosis may only be made after pregnancy. However, in cases in which there is exacerbation of the hypertension the fetus is at considerable risk.

In a few cases, and sometimes without a history of acute nephritis at the onset of the illness, the patient will present with massive proteinuria, oedema and low plasma protein levels, but with relatively little hypertension. In these cases of nephrosis the prognosis is already serious, but if the blood pressure rises during pregnancy the fetal risk is much increased.

On the whole the later stages of chronic nephritis are seldom seen by the obstetrician because the patients are too ill to become pregnant.

Chronic pyelonephritis

This condition may be distinguished from the history (see p. 205 above) from urine cultures, and possibly by a pyelogram, a single film being taken. Renal biopsy later will confirm the diagnosis.

In these patients it is extremely important to maintain a constant watch for any exacerbation of urinary tract infection, which must be treated energetically and over a prolonged period. The outlook for the fetus is better than in cases of glomerulonephritis, but there is a still an increased perinatal mortality and a tendency for the fetus to be underweight.

Lupus erythematosus

Systemic lupus erythematosus affecting the kidney is dealt with on the same general lines as given for chronic nephritis. Its course during pregnancy is unpredictable. Hypertension may develop and there is always proteinuria. Treatment is with adrenal corticosteroids or their derivatives. Pregnancy is managed according to the course of the disease.

Various other renal lesions

Polycystic disease of the kidneys

A few patients with this congenital disease of the kidneys become pregnant. The problems are similar to those of chronic nephritis; the outcome depends on the degree of renal failure or of superadded hypertension.

Renal tuberculosis

This offers no special problems to the obstetrician except those of diagnosis. It is rarely severe enough in women who become pregnant to cause any serious impairment of renal function or hypertension. It is treated with anti-tuberculous drugs.

Renal artery stenosis

This is a rare cause of hypertension during pregnancy, and will only be diagnosed after delivery by intravenous pyelography and renal angiography. Such investigations should be considered for all patients with unexplained persisting hypertension after delivery.

Previous nephrectomy

If the remaining kidney is normal there need be no concern during pregnancy.

Pregnancy after renal transplantation

An increasing number of women who have had successful renal transplants are becoming pregnant. If the function of the transplanted kidney is good, as it will usually be if the patient has proved that her fertility is normal, there are no unusual problems.

21

Intercurrent diseases during pregnancy

Anaemia during pregnancy

Physiological changes in the blood during pregnancy

During pregnancy the blood volume is increased by about 30 per cent, but there is a relatively greater increase in the volume of the plasma than of the red cells. This leads to a fall in the red cell count and the haemoglobin concentration during pregnancy, although the total mass of haemoglobin in the body is increased by about 15 per cent. The increase in blood volume is maintained until shortly before term when there is a fall, but the original non-pregnant level is not reached until about 6 weeks after delivery. The degree of increase in the blood volume varies greatly; some patients show only a slight change whereas in others it may reach 50 per cent.

Although haemodilution occurs, in many cases a more important explanation for the fall in haemoglobin concentration is relative iron deficiency. A haemoglobin level of 11 g/100 ml is regarded as the lower limit of normal during pregnancy, but if the diet is adequate or if additional iron is given to pregnant women the haemoglobin concentration often does not fall below 12.5 g/100 ml.

The usual daily dietary intake of iron by a non-pregnant woman is about 12 mg, of which 10 per cent is absorbed. This balances the loss in the urine and faeces and from desquamation of the skin (amounting to about 0.5 mg daily) and the menstrual loss. Menstrual loss varies greatly, but averages 12 mg per month.

If a woman is to maintain her iron balance during pregnancy she needs to retain about 800 mg of iron to provide 350 mg for the fetus, 100 mg for the placenta, and 350 mg for her own increased haemoglobin mass. She will save about 100 mg of iron because menstruation ceases, so that the total absorption during pregnancy must *exceed* her normal uptake by about 700 mg. Since about 0.5 mg is still excreted daily, this works out to a daily requirement of about 3 mg. The increased requirement is not spread uniformly over the whole of pregnancy, but rises from zero at 20 weeks to 8 mg daily at term.

There will be a loss of iron from blood loss during delivery and in the lochia of say 150 mg, and a further deficit of about 150 mg during lacta-

212

tion, and these losses will use up the increased haemoglobin mass which has been built up during pregnancy.

A very good diet contains 15 mg of iron daily, of which about 1.5 mg is absorbed. During pregnancy the ability of the duodenum and jejunum to absorb iron and the iron-binding capacity of the serum are increased to meet the added need. If the diet is less well supplied with iron the intake may be inadequate. About 30 per cent of the body iron (1000 mg) is in the cells of the reticulo-endothelial system in the form of haemosiderin, and this forms a reserve. Only when the iron stores are depleted will the serum iron fall. Not only may there be a deficiency of iron in the diet during pregnancy but many women start pregnancy with poor iron reserves. Several pregnancies in rapid succession will accentuate any deficiency.

Women who are taking a well-balanced diet with a high iron content do not need supplemental iron during pregnancy. Women on less adequate diets need additional iron, which is often combined with a small dose of folic acid in a single tablet. Although simple ferrous sulphate 200 mg three times daily is the cheapest form of supplement it does tend to cause constipation. A slow-release preparation containg ferrous sulphate 150 mg with folic acid 0.5 mg is to be preferred, and this has the advantage that the woman is only required to take one tablet a day. If ferrous sulphate causes gastro-intestinal upset a good alternative is ferrous fumarate 300 mg daily. It is best to postpone prophylactic iron administration until any nausea or vomiting of early pregnancy has passed.

Blood tests for anaemia during pregnancy. All patients should have an estimation of haemoglobin level and simple examination of a blood film at the initial antenatal visit, and again at 30 and 36 weeks. More frequent examination will be required if anaemia is found.

Iron deficiency anaemia

In Britain by far the commonest type of anaemia during pregnancy is that due to iron deficiency as a result of a poor diet, or of the patient failing to take the tablets which are prescribed for her. In many of the slighter cases the patient makes no complaint and anaemia is only discovered after routine examination of the blood. In a severe case the patient may look pale (although this is a most unreliable sign), and she may have noticed tiredness, breathlessness, palpitation or fainting. Apart from the adverse effect on the health of the mother during pregnancy, anaemia greatly increases the risk should haemorrhage occur unexpectedly during pregnancy or labour, and a determined effort must be made to rectify anaemia before term is reached.

The patients have a low haemoglobin concentration and a low red cell count, with a low colour index and mean corpuscular haemoglobin concentration. In severe cases there is polychromasia, a low mean corpuscular volume and a low serum iron level. In practice not all these observations are made routinely, and in many cases the diagnosis is made by observing a satisfactory response to treatment with iron. But if there is not a quick response, or if the haemoglobin level is less than 9 g/100 ml, then a complete blood count is required.

In patients from tropical countries iron deficiency anaemia during pregnancy may result from worm infestation, and this may need investigation and treatment.

Treatment.   There is usually time to treat the patient with oral iron. It is essential to make sure that adequate doses of an active preparation are being swallowed. The ordinary doses may be doubled but nothing is gained by increasing the dose still further. There is a limit to the amount of iron that can be absorbed, and with larger doses gastro-intestinal symptoms may occur.

Patients who do not respond, and in whom full investigation has not shown any other type of anaemia nor any condition such as chronic pyelonephritis, may be treated with parenteral iron.

Parenteral iron may also be used if pregnancy is advanced and time is short, but if the patient is very near to term blood transfusion will be the only way to raise the haemoglobin level quickly enough. In cases of very severe anaemia, such as may be seen in tropical countries, there is a risk of overloading the circulation by transfusion, and either packed cells must be given slowly, or an exchange transfusion performed. As a general rule no patient should be allowed to go into labour with a haemoglobin level below 10 g/100 ml.

Parenteral iron may be given by a deep intramuscular injection of an iron-dextran compound (Imferon) or an iron-sorbitol compound (Jectofer). Each of these contains the equivalent of 50 mg of iron per ml, and the patient is given a daily injection of 2 ml until a satisfactory response is obtained. Iron-dextran (but *not* iron-sorbitol) may also be given by 'total dose' intravenous infusion, and this method may be useful for women with severe iron deficiency anaemia who are unlikely to attend for a series of injections. The patient is admitted to hospital for 6 hours and 1 litre of normal saline containing the calculated dose of iron-dextran is administered by slow intravenous drip. It is assumed that 250 mg of iron are required to raise the haemoglobin level by 1 g/100 ml, and the dose is calculated accordingly. Anaphylactic reactions to intravenous iron occasionally occur, so the initial drip rate should be very slow and the infusion closely supervised.

Megaloblastic anaemia

For normal maturation of red cells in the bone marrow folic acid is required. If there is a deficiency of folic acid the marrow becomes full of megaloblasts, and the number of mature red cells in the peripheral blood is reduced. The blood will contain macrocytic cells and occasional nucleated red cells (although the latter are rarely found in the blood during megaloblastic anaemia of pregnancy).

Folic acid is essential for the synthesis of nucleic acid. During pregnancy, because of the increased fetal demand and inadequate absorption from the diet, anaemia due to folic acid deficiency may occur. It is relatively rare in this country, but much more common in some tropical countries. It occurs most commonly in multigravidae, in whom it may recur in successive pregnancies, and it is relatively more common in twin pregnancies.

The anaemia may develop rapidly in late pregnancy, and is often severe with a haemoglobin concentration of less than 9 g/100 ml. The diagnosis should be considered in any case of severe anaemia during late pregnancy, and also in any case in which there is no response to the administration of adequate doses of iron.

The clinical and haematological pictures are often confused because folic acid deficiency is accompanied by iron deficiency. Thus the macrocytes which are found in the peripheral blood in non-pregnant women with folic acid deficiency are rarely seen in pregnant women. Confirmation of the diagnosis is made by measuring the serum folate level or examining bone marrow obtained by sternal puncture, but it is often simpler to apply a simple therapeutic test by giving folic acid 20 mg orally daily, when there will be a rapid rise in the haemoglobin level in genuine cases.

Most obstetricians give folic acid prophylactically during pregnancy in doses of 0.5 mg daily in combined pills with iron. The fear that administration of folic acid might mask the diagnosis of Addisonian anaemia is unfounded, as this disease is not likely to be found in women of childbearing age.

Tropical megaloblastic anaemia.   Megaloblastic anaemia is a common complication of pregnancy in some tropical countries. These cases also appear to be due to folic acid deficiency, but they are complicated by additional dietary deficiencies of protein or iron, or by blood destruction by malaria or haemoglobinopathies, or by blood loss from hook worm infestation.

Haemoglobinopathies

The normal haemoglobin molecule of the adult (HbA) has four polypeptide side chains, two alpha and two beta chains, so that the molecule can be designated $\alpha_2\beta_2$. In the normal adult about 2 per cent of the haemoglobin is of a different type (HbA$_2$) in which two of the polypeptide chains have a different amino acid sequence (δ), so that the designation of the molecule is $\alpha_2\delta_2$.

During intrauterine life fetal haemoglobin (HbF) is found, with two different polypeptide chains from HbA, represented as $\alpha_2\gamma_2$. Fetal haemoglobin is more resistant to denaturation with alkali than adult haemoglobin, and this is the basis of the Kleihauer test (see p. 448). At term the blood contains 70 per cent HbF, but this starts to disappear after delivery so that by the time the infant is a year old only traces remain. However, if there is any disorder in which formation of HbA is impaired, such as the hereditary haemoglobinopathies described in the rest of this section, large amounts of HbF are found.

Abnormal haemoglobins.　Over 100 variants of the haemoglobin molecule have been found. These have been given various designations, sometimes letters of the alphabet and sometimes with reference to places of discovery. There are two main types of abnormal haemoglobins which are encountered in pregnant women.

In the first there are alterations of the amino acid structure of the polypeptide chains. The glutamic acid of HbA is replaced by valine in HbS and by lysine in HbC. Haemoglobin S is related to sickle cell disease and trait. In the second type the amnio acid sequences are normal but production of the α or β chains is impaired, causing thalassaemia.

Most of the abnormal haemoglobins are inherited by Mendelian laws. The clinical manifestations depend on (1) the types of haemoglobin present and (2) their relative proportions, which in turn largely depend on whether the inheritance is homo- or heterozygous.

As the haemoglobins carry different electrical charges they can be distinguished by electrophoresis.

Haemoglobin S.　*Sickle cell disease* is usually fatal in childhood and therefore rare in pregnant women. It occurs almost entirely in Negroes who originated from central Africa. In sickle cell disease the trait is inherited from both parents, so that the phenotype may be designated SS (homozygous). The importance of this haemoglobin is that whenever the oxygen tension in any part of the body falls the red cells assume a sickle shape and 'sludge' together, obstructing the circulation. Infarcts of various organs occur. There may be crises with severe abdominal pain or pain in the long bones. Haemolysis of the abnormal cells occurs and causes anaemia. There may be enlargement of the liver and spleen, and ulceration of the legs. Death may occur from thrombosis in a vital organ, or from pulmonary embolism. If a woman survives to become pregnant severe crises may occur, and thrombosis of placental blood vessels may cause fetal death.

Sickle cell trait is common and usually harmless. Many Negroes inherit HbS from only one parent, so that less than half of their haemoglobin is of this type. The phenotype may be designated AS (where A stands for normal adult haemoglobin). There is often some HbF present. In this heterozygous state, which can be recognized by electrophoresis, the concentration of HbS is usually too low for serious sickling to occur in the tissues. However, patients with sickle cell trait seem to be liable to pyelonephritis in pregnancy.

Haemoglobin C. This abnormal haemoglobin is also found in Negroes. Heterozygous inheritance (AC) is harmless, but with homozygous inheritance (CC) haemolytic anaemia may occur. HbC is of more importance when it is combined with inheritance of HbS (see below).

Thalassaemia. Thalassaemia was so named because it was first thought to be restricted to Mediterranean peoples, but in fact it occurs more widely, especially in the near and far East. It is caused by defective formation of either the α or the β chains. Both types may be of homo- or heterozygous inheritance, the former being termed thalassaemia major and the latter thalassaemia minor.

β thalassaemia minor is the variety which is most likely to concern the obstetrician. Only one β chain is affected and there is only mild hypochromic anaemia, with occasional splenomegaly. There is a raised level of HbA_2 and often of HbF. It is important to realize that the anaemia is not due to iron deficiency; it is useless to prescribe iron, and prolonged iron administration could cause haemosiderosis. β thalassaemia is more serious if it is combined with inheritance of S or C haemoglobin (see below).

α thalassaemia minor is of little obstetric importance.

Patients with α thalassaemia major are unlikely to survive beyond childhood, and β thalassaemia major causes fetal death from hydrops fetalis.

Mixed haemoglobinopathies. Mixed forms of disease are common. The effects produced depend on the chains involved. If both abnormal genes affect the same chains the effects are serious. In SC disease both β chains are abnormal and no HbA can be found; the patient is therefore as badly off as with homozygous SS disease. Similarly β thalassaemia with HbS or HbC results in severe anaemia. On the other hand combinations of S or C inheritance with α thalassaemia do not do this.

Management of haemoglobinopathies during pregnancy. With such complex problems and numerous combinations, some of which are very rare, the obstetrician will obviously need to seek expert guidance in diagnosis and treatment.

With the advent of large immigrant communities, Britain, in common with many other Western countries, now has many women attending antenatal clinics who may have haemoglobinopathies, and in some of these the effect of pregnancy may be serious. All women coming from countries where these disorders are common, such as Africa, the West Indies, Mediterranean countries and Asia, should have a blood electrophoresis examination at their first antenatal attendance.

Sickle-cell disease. Treatment with iron should be avoided as these patients have a high serum iron concentration and a low iron-binding capacity, so that administered iron may be deposited in the reticulo-endothelial system with haemosiderosis. Folic acid 15 mg daily should be given. In crises adequate oxygenation and hydration must be ensured, and heparin is given if bone pain or pulmonary thrombosis or embolism develops. Infections are vigorously treated with antibiotics and sodium bicarbonate is given to correct acidosis. It is particularly important to avoid hypoxia or circulatory depression if an anaesthetic is required for operative delivery.

Very severe anaemia, with haemoglobin levels of 5 g/100 ml or less, may develop in late pregnancy, and exchange transfusion may be required before labour. In less severe cases a cautious transfusion with packed cells may be given.

Sickle-cell trait.   So long as adequate amounts of HbA are present there is unlikely to be anything more than mild anaemia during pregnancy, but there is an increased susceptibility to urinary tract infection.

Thalassaemia.   Heterozygotic thalassaemia minor is unlikely to require special treatment during pregnancy.

Mixed haemoglobinopathies.   Combinations such as SC disease may cause severe anaemia and occasional crises during pregnancy, and would then require the same treatment as for SS disease.

Antenatal diagnosis of fetal haemoglobinopathy.   By fetoscopy it is now possible to obtain a sample of fetal blood at about 16 weeks, and it may be possible to determine whether the fetus has inherited a serious haemoglobinopathy such as sickle cell disease, and selective termination is then possible. Fetoscopy carries the risk of abortion and loss of a normal fetus, but in cases with a high risk of inherited disease many parents would accept this in order to avoid the possibility of birth of an affected child.

Heart disease in pregnancy

Although most patients with heart disease will go through pregnancy and labour successfully when their management has been conducted efficiently, that there is an added risk is shown by the fact that heart disease is the commonest 'associated disease' to cause maternal death.

Cardiovascular changes during pregnancy

There is a steady increase in blood volume from about 8 weeks until about 35 weeks, when the volume is some 30 per cent greater than the non-pregnant volume. In the last 5 weeks of pregnancy the volume falls slowly and to a variable extent until delivery. After delivery there is a return to non-pregnant levels over 4 to 6 weeks.

The cardiac output follows the changes in blood volume, rising from an average of 5.5 litres per minute in the non-pregnant woman to an average of 7 litres per minute at 34 weeks. This output is maintained until term, and reaches a further peak at times during the second stage of labour.

There is another transient rise as the uterus retracts down during the third stage, and after that the output falls concurrently with the decrease in blood volume.

There must obviously be an additional flow of the same degree in the pulmonary circuit as in the general circulation. The increased flow is largely distributed through the uterus, breasts and kidneys, but there is also some dilatation of peripheral skin capillaries. The maternal side of the placental circulation resembles an arterio-venous shunt, and it takes up an increasing part of the cardiac output in the last trimester of pregnancy.

Aetiology of heart disease in pregnancy

Rheumatic heart disease remains the commonest cause of heart disease during pregnancy although it is now becoming less common. Mitral stenosis is the commonest lesion found, and there may also be mitral regurgitation or aortic regurgitation; aortic stenosis is rarely seen.

Congenital heart disease now accounts for more than 30 per cent of cases. On the whole those patients who survive to the age of childbearing are those without cyanosis or gross disability, including cases of patent interatrial or interventricular septal defect, patent ductus arteriosus, aortic coarctation or pulmonary stenosis. Other cases of congenital heart disease are rare in pregnancy, although the successful results of modern cardiac surgery bring more survivors to adult life.

Bacterial endocarditis may occur as a complication of rheumatic valvular disease or of congenital lesions, and as a rare result of streptococcal puerperal infection.

Cardiac failure is a rare complication of severe and relatively acute *hypertension* (e.g. during eclampsia), but is hardly ever seen in cases of chronic essential hypertension during pregnancy. Coronary thrombosis is very rare during pregnancy.

Puerperal cardiomyopathy. This term refers to rare cases of myocardial failure of unknown aetiology occurring in late pregnancy or the puerperium, and sometimes recurring in successive pregnancies. There is tachycardia, gallop rhythm and reversible cardiac dilatation, but the exact pathology is uncertain, and it is doubtful if it is a single clear-cut clinical entity.

Diagnosis

The heart should always be examined carefully at the first antenatal visit. The diagnosis of cardiac disease during pregnancy is sometimes difficult. Dyspnoea of slight degree and oedema of the ankles may occur in normal pregnancy. A soft systolic murmur without any other evidence of cardiac disease may have no significance, but any diastolic murmur or any harsh systolic murmur always suggests organic disease. It is often difficult to assess the size of the heart during pregnancy, and radiological studies (with the fetus screened off) may be necessary. Rotation of the axis of the heart occurs during pregnancy, which gives a false impression of enlargement and also may cause changes in the electrocardiograph.

Cyanosis, fibrillation or unequivocal evidence of pulmonary congestion, such as haemoptysis or moist râles, are always serious signs of organic disease.

Prognosis

Although the lesions present in particular cases are obviously important, especially in cases of congenital heart disease, the functional capacity of the myocardium is the most significant factor in prognosis, and for this reason it was formerly the practice to classify cases of heart disease in pregnancy thus:

Grade I. No dyspnoea or limitation of activity.

Grade II. Dyspnoea, with some limitation of activity.

Grade III. Severe dyspnoea with limitation of even ordinary activity, but comfortable at rest.

Grade IV. Dysponea even at rest, or history of cardiac failure.

However cardiologists now seldom use this classification and prefer to assess the severity of heart disease during pregnancy on objective evidence obtained by clinical, electrocardiographic and echocardiographic examination, supplemented by radiological studies, taking care to protect the fetus from radiation.

Deterioration of even mild cases may sometimes occur during pregnancy, and respiratory infection will increase the danger. Careful assessment of all women with cardiac lesions should be made in early pregnancy by an experienced cardiologist, and he should continue to see them at intervals during pregnancy and the puerperium. The ideal plan is for such an assessment to be made before the pregnancy begins.

Management

The majority of patients with cardiac disease who become pregnant have only minor disability and will not require special treatment although, as indicated above, they should all be supervised during pregnancy by a cardiologist working closely with the obstetrician. Depending on the severity of the case, good antenatal care will include:

(a) Adequate rest at home (10 hours at night and 2 hours horizontal rest in the afternoon) with provision of help at home and transport to and from the hospital.

(b) Avoidance of respiratory infection—shunning people with obvious colds and crowded places of entertainment—and immediate treatment of any respiratory infection.

(c) Any dental sepsis should be treated, and if extractions are required penicillin should be given before and afterwards to reduce the risk of bacterial endocarditis.

(d) Prevention and treatment of anaemia.

(e) Admission to hospital for rest at any time if the cardiac condition seems to be deteriorating. For the more severe cases 2 or 3 weeks rest in hospital prior to labour is desirable.

(f) Digitalis may be needed for cases with arrhythmia or cardiac failure. Diuretics such as frusemide or chlorothiazide may be of help if there is fluid retention.

(g) Special problems arise with patients who have had a valvular prosthesis inserted and for whom anticoagulant treatment is essential. Oral anticoagulants are continued during pregnancy but, as these drugs reach the fetus and might cause intracranial or other haemorrhage during delivery, a change to heparin, which does not cross the placenta, is made before labour. With anticoagulant drugs the risk of uterine haemorrhage is small as myometrial contraction will effectively control blood loss.

Cardiac surgery. In early pregnancy a decision may need to be made whether cardiac surgery is indicated or, if the lesion is unsuitable for operation, about termination of pregnancy. Open-heart surgery cannot be performed during pregnancy but simpler procedures such as valvotomy can be carried out. Most patients, even those with quite severe disease, can tolerate pregnancy, so that termination is rarely essential. However, the longer term effects of bringing up the child need to be considered in deciding whether termination is to be advised in a particular case.

Cases of coarctation of the aorta run a slight risk of developing a dissecting aneurysm, but this risk does not justify Caesarean section nor operation on the aorta during pregnancy.

Heart failure. Acute pulmonary oedema is most frequently seen in patients with tight constriction of the mitral valve; congestive failure is usually encountered in patients with gross cardiac enlargement, some of whom may be fibrillating. These patients need to be nursed in a propped-up position. Salt and fluid intake are restricted. Digitalis is indicated for congestive heart failure and especially if there is fibrillation. In acute pulmonary oedema morphine and oxygen are given, and venesection may be needed. Labour should never be induced in haste because the heart is in failure; in most cases improvement can be obtained before delivery.

Mode of delivery. Easy vaginal delivery should be the aim, and fortunately this often occurs. In the first stage analgesic drugs should be given in adequate doses, because tachycardia due to pain may be the starting point of failure. Intravenous infusions are best avoided, but if essential must be used with care not to overload the circulation. The second stage should be short, and if this is proving not to be the case then prolonged expulsive effort is avoided by forceps delivery or vacuum extraction under pudendal block with, if necessary, nitrous oxide and oxygen given with care. If a general anaesthetic becomes necessary the services of an experienced anaesthetist should be secured, and every effort made to avoid hypoxia. Epidural anaesthesia should not be used except for very mild cases because of the risk of hypotension.

The sudden increase in blood volume caused by uterine contraction after delivery of the placenta may occasionally precipitate acute pulmonary oedema or heart failure and it is wisest not to use ergometrine or Syntocinon in the third stage unless postpartum haemorrhage occurs.

The indications for Caesarean section are the same as for a patient with a normal heart, and it should not be undertaken except for an obstetric reason.

Postnatal care.   Even after a normal vaginal delivery heart failure can occur in the puerperium. The patient must have additional rest at this time, and may need a longer than average stay in hospital. In all but the mildest cases a course of penicillin should be given for the first 14 days post partum to guard against bacterial endocarditis. The patient should be encouraged to feed her baby unless there is very severe heart disease.

Family planning and cardiac disease.   Women with cardiac disease should limit their families to one or two children because the strain of pregnancy and labour are only the beginning of the additional physical and mental strain involved in the care of children. Except in mild cases the contraceptive pill is best avoided because of the risk of thrombo-embolism. The progesterone-only pill, the intrauterine device or the diaphragm are alternative methods of contraception for patients with severe cardiac disease. Termination of pregnancy may need to be considered if unplanned pregnancy occurs. Sterilization is a useful procedure once a patient has completed her family. It is best postponed for two or three months after delivery, when it can be performed through a small incision or by laparoscopy, although for the latter the anaesthetic must be carefully given.

Hypertension and renal disease

See pp. 200–211.

Pulmonary tuberculosis and pregnancy

The incidence of pulmonary tuberculosis during pregnancy is now so low in the United Kingdom that routine radiological examination of the chest in antenatal patients has been given up, but in communities with a significant incidence of the disease this investigation should be carried out, care being taken to shield the uterus from the x-rays.

Pregnancy does not adversely affect the course and prognosis of the disease, provided that the usual treatment is carried out. Termination is not necessary except in occasional advanced cases. The fetus is practically never infected *in utero*. Chemotherapy is the essential part of treatment, but streptomycin should be avoided if possible because long-continued treatment with it may affect the fetal VIIIth nerve. The risk of this is small, so that streptomycin may be used if for any reason it is considered to be an essential part of the mother's treatment. Apart from this pregnancy and labour are managed in the normal way.

The aim of treatment is to make the mother sputum-negative by the time the baby is born. If this is achieved the baby can be left with the mother in the ordinary way, and vaccinated with BCG. If the sputum is still positive at the time of delivery the baby will have to be separated completely from the mother until the BCG vaccination has built up resistance to the disease; this will take at least six weeks. If the mother is sputum negative there is no objection to breast feeding.

Long-term follow-up of these patients is important to ensure that the prescribed course of treatment is completed and that recurrence does not occur. Every effort must be made to improve the patient's diet and living conditions. Family planning advice is given so that further pregnancy is avoided for at least one year after completion of treatment.

Other respiratory diseases during pregnancy

Pneumonia. Lobar pneumonia is very uncommon with pregnancy today, but bronchopneumonia may complicate upper respiratory tract infections and viral pneumonia may occur. Vigorous treatment for bacterial infections with broad-spectrum antibiotics is essential. If the patient becomes seriously ill with high fever, abortion, premature labour or intrauterine fetal death may occur.

Asthma. Most cases are unaffected by pregnancy, but cases of emotional origin may be worse if pregnancy is resented, or better if it is welcomed. If cortisone is the only treatment which gives relief there is no contraindication, but it should not be used in the first 12 weeks because of a possible teratogenic effect. Inhalations of sympathomimetic or antihistamine preparations may be used.

Emphysema, bronchitis and bronchiectasis. During pregnancy the vital capacity is not reduced but pulmonary ventilation is increased, and patients with rigid rib cages may have severe dyspnoea. An antibiotic such as ampicillin 250 mg twice daily may be given regularly during the winter months to prevent superadded infection. If there is severe dyspnoea assistance with forceps or the vacuum extractor in the second stage of labour may be required.

Sarcoidosis.   This disorder appears to improve during pregnancy, but is likely to relapse afterwards.

Carbohydrate metabolism in pregnancy

Glycosuria

Glycosuria often occurs during pregnancy as a result of a lowered renal threshold. The glomerular filtration of glucose is so much increased that incomplete reabsorption takes place in the tubules. The usual upper limit of glucose excretion during pregnancy is 140 mg/24 hours, but this is often exceeded and may reach 1 g/24 hours. The amount of glycosuria varies both from day to day and during each day. An early morning specimen of urine, excreted when the blood sugar level is low, is less likely to show glycosuria than a specimen collected after a meal. However, in pregnancy the situation is complicated because there is only a tenuous relationship between blood glucose levels and glycosuria as demonstrated by the glucose oxidase test strip (Clinistix). These strips appear to be less sensitive during pregnancy because of the presence of substances such as ascorbic acid in the urine which interfere with the reaction.

Glycosuria by itself does not have any significance, but it needs to be distinguished from glycosuria due to diabetes mellitus. Glycosuria found before the 16th week or occurring on two or more occasions in late pregnancy should be investigated by means of a standard 50 g oral glucose tolerance test. In cases of glycosuria in pregnancy it is uncommon to discover diabetes except when there are other indicators of diabetes, especially a close family history of the disease, or a history of the birth of a baby weighing 4.5 kg or more.

Glucose tolerance in pregnancy

During pregnancy the fasting levels of blood glucose are lower than in non-pregnant women by an average of 0.5 mmol/l. The peak levels of blood glucose after meals are higher, especially in late pregnancy. The tendency to post-prandial hyperglycaemia occurs in spite of increased insulin production, so that there is in effect a decreased sensitivity to insulin. To maintain glucose homeostasis the pregnant woman must produce more insulin. Most women are able to respond to this demand, but a few are unable to do so and develop diabetes. The diabetogenic effect of pregnancy is increased by repeated pregnancies and by obesity. The need for increased production of insulin during pregnancy is seen in insulin-dependent diabetics, whose insulin dosage often has to be increased three-fold as pregnancy advances.

Glucose and insulin relationships in mother and fetus

Glucose crosses the placenta freely; insulin does not. Hyperglycaemia in the mother is reflected by hyperglycaemia in the fetus. If there is persistent maternal hyperglycaemia in late pregnancy, as in diabetes, the fetal pancreas responds by producing an excess of insulin which cannot cross back into the maternal circulation and may therefore cause fetal hypoglycaemia.

Diabetes mellitus in pregnancy

Most cases of pregnancy complicating diabetes are seen in women who are already diabetic at the start of the pregnancy. Most of these patients will already have been treated with insulin, but some of the older women with maturity-onset diabetes will have been treated with diet alone, or with diet and oral hypoglycaemic agents.

The term *chemical diabetes* is applied when a woman has diabetes by the usual standards of glucose testing, but is symptom free. *Latent gestational diabetes* is the term used when a patient develops diabetes during pregnancy but reverts to normal after the pregnancy. A *potential diabetic* has an increased tendency to develop the disease during pregnancy, recognized by having had a heavy baby previously (4.5 kg or more) or by having a family history of diabetes in a parent or sibling.

Effect of pregnancy on diabetes. As noted above, the insulin requirement almost invariably needs to be increased during pregnancy to maintain control, and ketosis is more apt to occur because of the increased loss of glucose in the urine. Patients who are ordinarily treated by diet alone may need insulin during pregnancy.

Effect of diabetes on pregnancy. Unrecognized or badly treated diabetes leads to complications in both mother and baby.

Maternal complications include urinary tract infection, candidiasis of the vulva and vagina, pre-eclampsia and hydramnios.

Fetal and neonatal complications include an increased incidence of congenital abnormalities, intra-uterine death in late pregnancy or death soon after birth from hypoglycaemia, and respiratory distress syndrome in the newborn. The infant is characteristically large (with enlargement of all the organs) and plethoric from polycythaemia, which gives rise to an increased incidence of neonatal jaundice. The risk of birth trauma is greater because of the large size of the fetus. The combined effect of all these factors is an increased perinatal mortality.

Management. The incidence of the complications listed above and the perinatal mortality rate can be greatly reduced by very careful control of maternal diabetes at every stage of pregnancy. In the case of an established diabetic an assessment of her condition should ideally be made *before* the pregnancy occurs. Some diabetics with severe nephropathy or retinopathy may need to be advised against pregnancy; the perinatal mortality is especially high in cases with these complications. Good control of the diabetes during the months preceding conception and during the first trimester should reduce the incidence of congenital abnormality, which is now the most important single cause of perinatal loss.

It has been suggested that a variant of haemoglobin A, known as Hb A$_1$ which is produced by slow glycosylation of Hb A during the life of the red cell may be a useful indicator of preceding average blood glucose levels. A level of Hb A$_1$ above the normal proportion of 3–4 per cent of the total amount of haemoglobin suggests that there has been an abnormally high average level of blood glucose during the preceding two to three months. Diabetic women who have a high level of Hb A$_1$ (more than 10 per cent) in early pregnancy may have an increased tendency to fetal abnormality. When the level is high in late pregnancy the fetus is more likely to be overweight. If the Hb A$_1$ index is high pregnancy should be postponed until better control of the diabetes had been achieved.

Close co-operation between obstetrician and diabetic physician throughout pregnancy is essential if a satisfactory outcome is to be achieved. The need to increase the insulin dosage progressively as pregnancy advances, to adjust the diet and to monitor blood glucose levels means that these women are best treated in specialized units with the ability to admit the patient at any time when control is less than perfect. For the intelligent and well-motivated patient control of blood glucose levels can be improved by employment of Dextrostix and a glucose monitor which she uses in her own home two or three times a week. Patients are commonly admitted to hospital at about 34 weeks gestation, and then kept under constant supervision until delivery.

Obstetric management. Apart from routine antenatal care, an early ultrasonic scan of the fetus should be made to establish maturity and exlude gross fetal abnormality. Thereafter fetal growth can be followed by repeated ultrasonic examinations. In late pregnancy daily observation by the mother of fetal movements and, when possible, frequent cardio-tocographic studies and ultrasonic observations of fetal breathing movements should help to prevent the unexpected late intrauterine deaths that used to occur in cases of badly controlled diabetes. Placental function tests may also be performed in cases with any suspicion of insufficiency (see p. 57).

Premature delivery to avoid late intrauterine fetal death has been a standard procedure for many years, but may be less necessary when very good control of the maternal diabetes has been maintained. However, at present for most patients induction of labour or planned Caesarean section at 38 weeks is probably wise, provided that the lecithin-sphingomyelin ratio in a sample of liquor amnii is satisfactory (see p. 369). Vaginal delivery should always be the aim, but obstetric complications and the difficulty of controlling diabetes throughout a long labour lead to a relatively high Caesarean section rate. During labour diabetic control is best maintained by the administration of glucose and insulin intravenously at a controlled rate by means of an infusion pump. Continuous fetal heart monitoring and fetal blood sampling (p. 352) are employed to detect fetal distress.

As soon as the baby is delivered it should be handed over to an expert in neonatal care. Ensuring that the lecithin-sphingomyelin ratio in the liquor is normal before delivery has reduced the incidence of fatal respiratory distress syndrome almost to nothing, and early feeding counteracts any tendency to neonatal hypoglycaemia. If the infant's haematocrit (packed cell volume) is greater than 70 per cent then 10 per cent of the estimated blood volume is removed by venesection and replaced by an equal volume of serum.

There is no contraindication to breast feeding, and the majority of diabetic mothers feed their babies successfully.

Family planning. For diabetics this is an essential part of postnatal care. Most of the patients will be content with two or three children and once the family is complete sterilization is the most satisfactory long-term solution. For short-term family planning there is no contraindication to the use of the oral contraceptive pill or to the intrauterine device.

Acute specific fevers

Although pregnancy does not alter the course of most specific fevers the fetal results may be serious. With high fever and toxic effects either miscarriage or premature labour may occur. Some organisms reach the fetus, including those of rubella, smallpox, vaccinia, chickenpox, typhoid fever, toxoplasmosis, Coxsackie virus disease and cytomegalic inclusion disease.

Rubella. The importance of rubella as a cause of congenital abnormality was first recognized by Gregg in 1941. Maternal viraemia results in direct infection of the fetus via the placenta. Fetal infection is as likely to occur with a subclinical infection as with severe infection of the mother. The result of fetal infection varies greatly, including fetal death, birth of a fetus with active rubella, congenital malformation, and in some cases no apparent damage. In some epidemics the incidence of damage has been 50 per cent in the 1st month, 30 per cent in the second month and 15 per cent in the third month; with rare cases of damage after this. The congenital defects produced vary according to the stage of pregnancy. Infection during the first and second months may produce congenital cataract or cardiac valvular lesions; during the third month deafness may result. Follow-up studies have shown that deafness and visual or neurological defects may not be recognized until late in childhood. One study showed that 23 per cent of children exposed to rubella *in utero* who were apparently normal at birth showed defects by the age of 2.

The clinical diagnosis of rubella-like illness is difficult, and a diagnosis of rubella is only correct in about 20 per cent of cases. It is therefore necessary to carry out immunological investigations whenever possible. The best test is the haemagglutination inhibition test, which depends on the fact that serum containing antibody inhibits the agglutination of day-old chick erythrocytes by the virus. Haemagglutination inhibition antibodies appear soon after the rash and reach peak titres in 6 to 12 days. Absence of antibody immediately after exposure to infection indicates susceptibility and its presence indicates previous infection and immunity. Patients who present within two weeks of exposure and who have a rapid rise in antibody titres in blood samples taken one or two weeks apart are showing signs of infection.

An effective vaccine is now available against rubella, consisting of living but attenuated virus. It is sad that numerous children still suffer damage from this virus, although prevention of fetal rubella is possible. Since 1970 rubella vaccination has been offered to all girls aged 11 to 14 in the United Kingdom, but unfortunately it is still only accepted on their behalf by 70 per cent of parents. Vaccination is also offered to all women who are seronegative and are at special risk of exposure to rubella, such as nurses and teachers. Much is now being done by health authorities to try to increase the acceptance rate of vaccination. No dangerous complications of the vaccination have been reported, but living virus is used and if the recipient became pregnant soon after its administration the fetus might be affected. Adult women must be warned of this and instructed to use contraception for three months.

Pregnant women must be advised to avoid contact with any known case of rubella. In antenatal clinics every patient should have her antibody status determined at her first visit. This indicates those women who are immune because of previous infection, which may be useful information if any exposure occurs. The women who are susceptible should be vaccinated as soon as the pregnancy is over. Termination of pregnancy is justifiable if a patient has certain evidence of infection in the first trimester.

Measles. Measles is reported to have affected the fetus *in utero*, but has not been proved to cause fetal abnormalities.

Typhoid fever. Before the introduction of antibiotics typhoid fever was a serious complication of pregnancy in that abortion, stillbirth or premature labour occurred in many cases. The bacilli have been demonstrated in the organs of the fetus.

Smallpox. The prognosis of smallpox during pregnancy is more serious than in the non-pregnant woman, the confluent and haemorrhagic types being commoner. Abortion, stillbirth or premature labour may occur, and children have been born with the eruption.

Vaccination during pregnancy may rarely cause fetal infection and death. The risk is very small, but vaccination should not be performed during pregnancy unless the mother has been in contact, or has a strong possibility of coming in contact, with smallpox.

Chickenpox. There is no evidence that this infection causes congenital abnormalities, but the child may be born covered with the rash.

Scarlet fever. This disease is caused by the haemolytic streptococcus which may also cause puerperal fever, and a scarlatiniform rash can occur in cases of puerperal streptococcal infection. If the disease occurs during pregnancy abortion may occur, but there is no evidence that the fetus is infected.

Poliomyelitis. Susceptibility to this disease may be increased during pregnancy, but the point is disputed. During the initial pyrexial illness or during severe hypoxia fetal death may occur, but the virus does not cause fetal abnormalities, and paralysis of the newborn is exceedingly rare. During labour special care is only required if respiration is impeded, and then forceps delivery is better than Caesarean section. Immunization against poliomyelitis can safely be carried out during pregnancy.

Chorea. So-called chorea gravidarum is Sydenham's (rheumatic) chorea occurring during pregnancy. If a patient who has recently had chorea becomes pregnant a recrudescence of the symptoms is common. Recovery is the rule and termination of pregnancy is not required.

Malaria. During pregnancy severe exacerbation of latent malaria may occur, and disease which is already active may be made worse. Abortion, premature labour and low birth weight frequently occur, especially in cases of malignant tertian malaria. The suppressive drug pyrimethamine (Daraprim) 25 mg weekly should be given to all pregnant women in malarious areas. If infection occurs the same treatment is given as to the non-pregnant.

Influenza. A severe attack of influenza may have the same effect on pregnancy as any other severe fever in causing abortion or intrauterine fetal death. With infection in the first trimester the incidence of congenital abnormality, particularly neural tube defects, may be slightly increased.

Toxoplasmosis. This is an uncommon disease caused by a small protozoon *Toxoplasma gondii*. In England the incidence of congenital toxoplasmosis is 1 in 5000 to 10 000 pregnancies; the disease is more common on the continent of Europe. The mother may only have a transient febrile illness, but the disease is transmitted to the fetus, in which it causes encephalomyelitis and choroidoretinitis. The effect on the fetus is greatest when infection occurs in the second trimester. Most infants die, but those that survive for a time may have blindness, mental defects, hydrocephalus and calcification of the cerebral lesions. Diagnosis is difficult but a complement fixation test is available. Fortunately one attack gives immunity, and subsequent children are normal.

Cytomegalic inclusion disease. The group of cytomegalic viruses (CMV) are found in many animals, and in the Western hemisphere most humans show antibodies to them after the age of 35. In the East the infection is acquired in early life and most children have antibodies. Although it requires very close contact to transfer the virus, an infected individual carries it permanently and is capable of passing on the virus. The clinical picture is extremely variable and often resembles that of glandular fever. Even if the effects in the mother are mild or subclinical the fetus may be badly affected. The majority of babies born after CMV infection during pregnancy progress normally, but those who are affected show abnormalities of the central nervous system, with a high incidence of mental retardation and deafness. Diagnosis is made by a complement fixation test. There is no effective treatment or prevention.

Diseases of the alimentary tract

Dental caries.   Decayed teeth and gingivitis are often observed during pregnancy or after delivery. The popular saying is 'For every child a tooth', and the popular belief is that the caries is caused by calcium deficiency. Since the enamel is not vascularized decalcification is not possible, but if dentine has already been exposed then decay may progress more rapidly. Dental inspection and treatment should be carried on in pregnancy. Fillings or extractions should be performed under local anaesthesia if possible, and if a general anaesthetic is required 'gas' in a dental chair is more dangerous in pregnancy than at other times. A proper anaesthetic with every precaution taken against hypoxia should be given.

Ptyalism is excessive salivation. Patients sometimes think that they are producing more saliva during pregnancy, but there is no evidence that this is so. In early pregnancy a nauseated patient may fail to swallow her saliva and keep spitting it out. Reassurance is all that is needed.

Heartburn.   During pregnancy the cardiac sphincter is relaxed and acid regurgitation may occur. Sometimes troublesome heartburn is due to a hiatus hernia. Relief may be obtained with alkalies in either tablet or liquid form. The symptoms are often worse if the patient lies flat or bends over.

Peptic ulcer.   Symptoms nearly always improve during pregnancy, probably because the gastric acidity falls and there is an increased secretion of mucus. Perforation or haematemesis are very rare during pregnancy.

Appendicitis.   Appendicitis is not common during pregnancy. The danger is enchanced because it is sometimes difficult to make an early diagnosis and there may be widespread peritonitis. Abortion may also occur.

Abdominal pain on the right side during pregnancy may be due to pyelonephritis, extrauterine gestation, torsion of an ovarian cyst, red degeneration of a fibromyoma, biliary or renal colic, or appendicitis. A small right-sided concealed accidental haemorrhage may also simulate appendicitis. The most frequent error is to confuse pyelonephritis with appendicits; in every case the urine must be carefully examined.

The symptoms of appendicitis are little altered during pregnancy, but the site of the pain and of maximum tenderness may be higher than usual because the caecum and appendix are displaced upwards.

Appendicectomy should be performed in spite of the pregnancy. A muscle splitting incision should be made at the site of maximum tenderness and every effort made to avoid handling the uterus. Antibiotic cover is advised, and drugs such as isoxsuprine or ritodine (p. 345) may be given to reduce the risk of premature labour.

Intestinal obstruction. The commonest cause of intestinal obstruction during pregnancy is a band resulting from adhesions following a previous operation; the obstruction occurs because of altered positions of the viscera brought about by the growth of the uterus. Other causes of obstruction during pregnancy are strangulated internal or external hernia, volvulus, intussusception and mesenteric thrombosis. Neoplasms of the bowel are rare.

The especial danger of intestinal obstruction during pregnancy is the delay that often elapses before the diagnosis is made, the symptoms so often being attributed to the pregnancy. The classical symptoms of pain, vomiting and constipation will be present, but the physical sign of distention is masked by the pregnant uterus. A scar on the abdomen of a patient whose chief complaint is vomiting should always suggest the possibility of intestinal obstruction. Pyelonephritis, appendicitis, hyperemesis gravidarum, ureteric calculus and torsion of the pedicle of an ovarian cyst would all need to be considered in making the diagnosis.

When the diagnosis has been made laparotomy is performed without delay. Intravenous infusion of saline and gastric suction are started before the operation. Laparatomy for the relief of obstruction can be a difficult operation even without pregnancy, and if the bulk of the uterus interferes seriously it may have to be emptied by Caesarean section before the operation for relief of obstruction can proceed.

Hernia and pregnancy. As a general rule herniae are not made worse by, and do not affect the course of, pregnancy. The growing uterus usually pushes the bowel away from the orifices of inguinal and femoral herniae, and eventually blocks access to them. Rarely these types of herniae first appear during pregnancy, but fluctant swellings which appear in the groin during pregnancy are usually found to be varicoceles.

In the case of umbilical hernia if intestine is adherent to the sac it may rarely be dragged upon by the growing uterus to cause intestinal obstruction.

Ulcerative colitis. This disease is sometimes worse during pregnancy and is sometimes first diagnosed at that time. Women with active colitis should not become pregnant, but once the acute symptoms have subsided they may accept the risk of reactivation. The usual treatment, including steroids and prednisolone retention enemata may be used during pregnancy.

Liver disease in pregnancy

Acute infective hepatitis.   Pregnant women may suffer from both types of hepatitis, Type A which is caused by a virus excreted in the faeces by a patient with the disease, and Type B which is due to a virus spread by transfusion of infected blood or plasma or by injection with contaminated needles. The virus responsible for Type B can be identified by an antigen on its surface (Australia antigen).

Both types of hepatitis usually follow a similar course during pregnancy to that in non-pregnant women, and spontaneous recovery is to be expected. In a small number of cases, and more commonly in developing countries, liver damage is so severe that death occurs. Hepatitis during pregnancy does not cause fetal abnormalities, but abortion may occur or intrauterine death in late pregnancy. At least half of babies born to mothers who have had Type B hepatitis during pregnancy will show hepatitis B antigen in their blood, and a proportion of them develop hepatic lesions.

Medical and nursing staff may be infected with Type B virus contained in blood from a patient via any small cut or abrasion, or from contact with a Type B case, and these patients are best placed in a specialized liver unit.

Toxic hepatitis caused by chemical agents.   Hepatic necrosis may occur a few days after prolonged or repeated administration of fluothane (Halothane) anaesthesia during pregnancy, and its use should be avoided at that time. Hepatic necrosis may also be caused by chloroform, and in rare instances by other substances including trichlorethylene and chlorpromazine compounds.

Eclampsia.   Hepatic lesions of a specific type may occur (p. 195).

Acute hepatic failure during pregnancy ('Obstetric acute yellow atrophy'). This is a rare condition which occurs in late pregnancy. Acute fatty degeneration of centrilobar liver cells causes the rapid onset of vomiting, upper abdominal pain and jaundice. Most cases progress to coma and death in a few days. The cause is unknown, and there is no effective treatment, although a few cases have survived after early delivery. This condition does not seem to be the same as the acute hepatic necrosis which rarely follows acute viral hepatitis.

Recurrent cholestatic jaundice of pregnancy.   Very slight jaundice may occur as a result of oestrogen-induced cholestasis. This causes pruritus, and biochemical examination shows slightly raised levels of bilirubin, alkaline phosphatase and transferase in the serum. Women who are affected are unduly sensitive to oestrogens and develop this condition in every pregnancy and if they take oral contraceptives. No treatment is required and complete recovery occurs after the pregnancy or on stopping the oral contraceptive.

Other causes of jaundice in pregnancy. All the other causes of jaundice in non-pregnant women may occur during pregnancy and give difficulties in diagnosis. Examples are obstructive jaundice from gallstones, haemolytic jaundice from mismatched transfusion and jaundice from infection with haemolytic organisms.

Venereal diseases in pregnancy

Gonorrhoea. The disease may be contracted before pregnancy, at the time of conception, or during pregnancy. Uncomplicated gonorrhoea does not diminish the chance of conception, but gonococcal infection of the Fallopian tubes is likely to cause sterility.

The symptoms and signs of gonorrhoea are not modified by pregnancy. Women with gonorrhoea are often symptom-free. When vaginal discharge is present it may be due to associated trichomonal or candidial vaginitis, both of which are more likely to be more severe and persistent in pregnant than in non-pregnant women.

Gonorrhoea is unlikely to affect the pregnancy, although in a few cases the infection has spread to the uterine cavity and Fallopian tubes after delivery. During labour the baby's eyes are in danger of being infected, and the discovery of conjunctivitis is occasionally the first reason for suspecting the disease.

Careful investigation of any abnormal urethral or vaginal discharge during pregnancy is essential. Swabs for microscopical examination and bacterial culture are taken directly from the urethra and cervix with the aid of a speculum. If it is not possible to plate the swabs onto warm blood agar plates immediately they are placed in Stuart's medium for transport to the laboratory.

Treatment. A single injection of 2.4 g of procaine penicillin is usually sufficient; this may be combined with probenecid 1 g. If the patient is allergic to penicillin or the organism is resistant there is a wide choice of effective antibiotics, but tetracycline should not be used during pregnancy. Cure must be established by repeated bacteriological tests and efforts must be made to treat the partners of patients. Serological tests for possible concurrent syphilis are made both before and after penicillin treatment.

Gonococcal conjunctivitis of the newborn. In this country prophylactic instillation of drops of 1 per cent silver nitrate solution into the eyes of the newborn infant has been given up because of the chemical conjunctivitis it caused, and because antibiotic treatment is now effective if infection should occur. In every case of neonatal conjunctivitis swabs must be taken for microscopy and bacterial culture. Penicillin or chloramphenicol eye drops are used 6-hourly until the report is received (see p. 506).

Syphilis. The importance of syphilis in pregnancy is that the causative organism, *Treponema pallidum*, crosses the placenta and invades the fetus. Fetal infection is most likely when the mother is in the primary or secondary stage of the disease. Severe fetal infection will cause intra-uterine death, followed by late abortion or premature delivery. With less severe infection the fetus may be born alive with congenital syphilis. The baby may be light-for-dates and show enlargement of the liver and spleen, purpura, thrombocytopenia and anaemia. At birth there may be bullous lesions on the skin (syphilitic pemphigus). After three or four weeks a widespread maculo-papular rash may appear over the trunk and often the palms and soles, with 'mucous patches' in the mouth and 'condylomata' around the anus. There may be nasal infection and osteochondritis of long bones. Choroiditis may occur.

Sometimes there are no signs at the time of birth, but manifestations appear later in childhood.

Diagnosis. All pregnant women must have a screening blood test for syphilis in early pregnancy. The Kahn and Wassermann tests also give a positive reaction in cases of yaws, and more specific tests such as the TPI (treponema pallidum immobilization) test or the FTA (fluorescent treponemal antibody) test are needed to confirm a suspicion of maternal syphilis. These tests are also performed on the newborn child if there is any possibility of congenital infection.

Treatment. If treatment is given early in pregnancy the fetal infection will be cured. Treatment in late pregnancy may precipitate a Herxheimer reaction, causing fetal death. This may be prevented by giving the mother prednisolone 5 mg three times daily for 4 days before starting antibiotic treatment. Benzylpenicillin 2.4 g is injected intramuscularly and repeated after two weeks. In penicillin sensitive patients erythromycin 500 mg three times daily for 21 days is an alternative treatment.

Neonatal infection. The baby should be barrier nursed because any cutaneous or mucosal lesions are infectious. Procaine penicillin 200 000 units is injected intramuscularly dialy for 15 days, and the clinical and serological response is observed.

Yaws. Occasionally a positive test for syphilis will be found in a patient from central America, the West Indies or Africa who is in fact suffering from yaws. This endemic disease is acquired in youth from skin contact, and is caused by an organism closely related to *Treponema pallidum*. Yaws is a mild disease in temperate climates and does not harm the fetus. However, in view of the diagnostic difficulties it is usually wise to treat all sero-positive patients as if they have syphilis.

Herpes genitalis. Herpetic lesions of the vulva and vagina are caused by sexually transmitted infection with type 2 herpes virus. If the disease is acquired by the mother during pregnancy there is a strong probability of abortion in early pregnancy or of infection of the fetus in late pregnancy.

The fetal infection may occur as an ascending infection when the membranes rupture or during birth, but the high incidence of abortion and of premature birth suggests that transplacental infection may also occur. Infected babies have widespread lesions in the central nervous system, the eyes, the skin and the mouth, with a high mortality and much morbidity in survivors. If the diagnosis is made during pregnancy and the membranes are intact delivery should be by Caesarean section.

Neurological diseases during pregnancy

Epilepsy. Epilepsy has no significant effect on pregnancy, even in patients in whom the fits are difficult to control. There is no tendency to abortion or premature labour. The effect of pregnancy on epilepsy is extremely variable, and there is just as good a chance of the disease being improved as there is for it to be made temporarily worse. Drug treatment is continued during pregnancy. Ideally sodium valproate should be substituted for phenytoin before the woman becomes pregnant, because there is a slight risk of a teratogenic effect with the latter (see p. 64).

In women with pre-eclampsia it is possible that a grand mal epileptic fit could be mistaken for an eclamptic fit. The two types of fit cannot be distinguished, and if a patient with hypertension or proteinuria has a fit, even if she is an epileptic, it is safest to assume that she has developed eclampsia and to treat her accordingly.

Myasthenia gravis. Pregnancy has a variable effect on this disease. The dosage of neostigmine may need to be altered, but pregnancy and labour are usually uneventful. Uterine action is unaffected but forceps delivery or vacuum extraction may be required because of weak voluntary effort. For this local analgesia should be used if possible, as these patients are unduly sensitive to general anaesthesia. Postpartum exacerbation of the disease is common and should be watched for. The newborn infant may be temporarily affected and hypotonic and motionless after birth. The myasthenia of the baby passes off after about ten days, and treatment is only necessary if there is difficulty in breathing, sucking or swallowing.

Multiple sclerosis. The present-day view is that pregnancy has no effect on this disease and that any changes which occur during pregnancy would have taken place in any case. Spinal and caudal analgesia should be avoided at delivery. The question of termination of pregnancy sometimes arises because of the family problems of an incapacitated woman.

Subarachnoid haemorrhage. Rupture of an intracranial aneurysm may occur during pregnancy, or a patient may become pregnant who has previously had this accident. Unless the haemorrhage occurred within six weeks of delivery, or there is hypertension, assisted vaginal delivery is preferable to Caesarean section.

Cerebral thrombophlebitis.   Thrombosis of cerebral veins or dural sinuses may occur during pregnancy or the puerperium. A few cases are associated with pelvic infection, but often the cause is obscure. There may be general signs such as headache, fits and coma, often with fever and vomiting; or there may be focal neurological signs such as hemiplegia or aphasia. Anticoagulant drugs are given, and recovery may occur.

Acroparaesthesia (carpal tunnel syndrome).   See p. 63.

Cramp in pregnancy.   See p. 62.

Endocrine disorders in pregnancy

Addison's disease.   Addison's disease rarely complicates pregnancy. It presents the same features during pregnancy as in the non-pregnant state. Addisonian crises may occur at any time, but most often during early pregnancy when vomiting may accentuate any electrolytic disturbance, during the stress of labour, or during the early puerperium. The patient's replacement dosage of cortisone and fludrocortisone is continued during pregnancy, and will often need to be increased if abnormal loss of sodium occurs. Frequent estimations of serum electrolytes are necessary to ensure adequate replacement therapy. To cover the stress of labour hydrocortisone 200 mg is injected intramuscularly at the onset, and 100 mg every six hours until delivery. Anaesthetics must be administered cautiously.

Acute adrenal failure.   Rarely, as a result of septicaemia, haemorrhagic shock or amniotic embolism, haemorrhages in the adrenal glands cause acute adrenal insufficiency, so that the patient does not respond to normal resuscitative measures. If this occurs hydrocortisone is given intravenously in high dosage.

Administration of corticosteroids during pregnancy.   Women who have been receiving treatment with corticosteroids for any conditions before becoming pregnant may occasionally collapse under mild stress during pregnancy or labour, and this possibility should be remembered when any patient shows unexpected response to stress. The slow recovery of adrenal function after adminstration of corticosteroids means that any patient who has had such treatment during the twelve months preceding her pregnancy should be given hydrocortisone, as described above, during labour.

Although there is a very slight risk of corticosteroids given during pregnancy causing cleft lip or palate in the fetus, experience suggests that the risk can be ignored with doses of the order of 100 mg of cortisone or 20 mg of prednisolone daily.

Phaechromocytoma.   This is a very rare but exceedingly dangerous complication of pregnancy which is due to a tumour of the adrenal medulla that produces an excess of noradrenaline and adrenaline. Any stress or painful stimulus, or any mechanical disturbance of the tumour, causes the release of these substances and paroxysmal hypertension and tachycardia, during which cardiac failure may occur. In the attack there is pallor, sweating, headache and sometimes vomiting. Attacks may occur during pregnancy and simulate pre-eclampsia, but also occur during labour or soon after delivery. Anaesthesia and operations are especially liable to precipitate an attack, and a number of patients have died of so-called shock, the tumour only being found at postmortem examination. It is the paroxysmal nature of the attacks which should arouse suspicion. It is not usually possible to palpate the small tumour, but the urinary excretion of catechol amines and of vanillyl mandelic acid is increased.

If the diagnosis is made during pregnancy it is best to deliver the patient by Caesarean section when the fetus is sufficiently mature. Any hypertensive crisis is controlled by giving phentolamine intravenously. The tumour is removed later.

Disorders of the thyroid gland. The thyroid gland becomes larger and more vascular during pregnancy as a result of increased secretion of thyroid stimulating hormone by the anterior pituitary gland. The level of protein-bound thyroxine is raised, but the free thyroxine level (T_4) is normal. The basal metabolic rate is increased by up to 20 per cent, partly as a result of increased oxygen consumption by the uterus and feto-placental tissues.

Non-toxic enlargement of the thyroid gland. Simple colloid goitres, such as occur in districts where iodine is deficient, enlarge in pregnancy and if such a tumour is retrosternal it may press on the trachea. Surgical treatment can be carried out if necessary during pregnancy, but thyroxine should be given post-operatively to guard against hypothyroidism. In Hashimoto's disease the firm enlargement can be reduced without the need for surgery by administration of thyroxine.

Hyperthyroidism. Mild hyperthyroidism is not uncommon during pregnancy. If the overactivity of the gland is caused by an abnormal long-acting thyroid stimulator this will cross the placenta and cause neonatal hyperthyroidism. This subsides within three weeks.

Because of the raised basal metabolic rate and the enlargement of the thyroid gland which normally occur during pregnancy the diagnosis of mild hyperthyroidism may be difficult, and careful clinical assessment and assay of T_4 will be needed.

The treatment most commonly employed during pregnancy is with antithyroid drugs such as carbimazole and thiouracil. As these drugs cross the placenta there is a risk of fetal hypothyroidism. The risk can be avoided by keeping the mother euthyroid and by giving a small dose of T_4 such as 0.2 mg daily during the last trimester. This will cross the placenta and reach the fetus. Breast feeding is contraindicated as antithyroid drugs are excreted in the milk.

Hypothyroidism. Severe hypothyroidism causes infertility. Pregnancy may occur in mild cases, but there is an increased risk of abortion. Treated cases of myxoedema who become pregnant require an increased dose of T_4.

Diseases of the skin during pregnancy

Physiological changes are described on pp. 38, 39. Almost any of the multitudinous diseases of the skin can occur during pregnancy, and conditions specifically related to pregnancy are rare. These include:

Pruritis.   Generalized pruritus may occur with cholestatic jaundice (p. 232) and a complaint of abdominal pruritus is not uncommon. Treatment is not very effective, but warm alkaline baths or the application of calamine lotion are often tried.

Pruritus vulvae may occur with infection by candida, which is common in diabetics, or in any case in which there is vaginal discharge.

Prurigo gestationis.   This condition was first described by Besnier, and consists of a papular eruption on the abdomen, thighs and buttocks, on the dorsal surfaces of the hands and feet. The lesions are small, discrete and very irritating. They resolve after delivery. Calamine lotion or phenol lotion (1 per cent) may be helpful, or oral antihistamines such as chlorpheniramine tablets (Piriton) 4 mg four times daily.

Herpes gestationis.   This rare disease may recur in successive pregnancies. Severe pruritis is followed by the development of red erythematous patches on the abdomen and legs. These give way to rings of vesicles which appear in crops, and sometimes coalesce to form bullae which may become pustular or haemorrhagic. The patient is ill with fever, rigors and vomiting, and there is a striking eosinophilia. The clinical picture is similar to that of dermatitis herpetiformis.

Recovery is the rule, although there have been a few fatal cases. If the patient becomes severely ill abortion or intrauterine fetal death may occur. There is no specific treatment but corticosteroids may control the lesions and systemic antibiotics are required for infection.

Malignant disease during pregnancy

Malignant disease is uncommon in association with pregnancy, and apart from choriocarcinoma is never caused by it. When malignant disease is diagnosed during pregnancy the treatment of the disease becomes the first consideration. In only a few cases is surgical treatment or radiotherapy possible without affecting the fetus; in many cases the pregnancy must be brought to an end. In early pregnancy termination may be advised; in the second half of pregnancy a difficult choice sometimes has to be made between postponing early delivery in the interests of the fetus or of delivering a premature baby to allow treatment of the malignant disease to start. The patient's wishes and the nature of the disease will have to be taken into account.

Carcinoma of the cervix (p. 248) and carcinoma of the breast are the two lesions in which early treatment is especially important during pregnancy, although whether pregnancy has any adverse effect in these conditions is doubtful.

Mental illness and childbirth

See pp. 438 – 445.

22

Abnormalities of the pelvic organs complicating pregnancy, labour and the puerperium

Retroversion of the uterus

Pregnancy often occurs in a retroverted uterus and is nearly always uneventful. In the great majority of cases the uterus rises up normally into the abdomen at about the 12th week. In only a small minority of cases the uterus remains retroverted, and as it grows it comes to fill the pelvic cavity completely. The cervix is directed forwards, and even slightly upwards (see fig. 22.1). The uterus is then said to be *incarcerated*. As the bladder base is attached to the supravaginal cervix the base of the bladder is distorted and the urethra is elongated. Retention of urine follows and the bladder becomes distended.

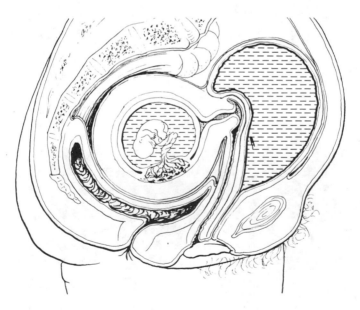

Fig. 22.1 Retroversion of the pregnant uterus.

240

The acute retention is extremely painful, and if it is not relieved by catheterization overflow incontinence will eventually occur with frequent escape of small volumes of urine. If the condition is still left unrelieved cystitis develops, and in the past cases of necrosis of the bladder mucosa have occurred.

Diagnosis

If difficulty in micturition occurs between the 12th and 16th weeks of pregnancy the possibility of incarceration of a retroverted uterus must always be considered. On abdominal examination the distended bladder will be felt; it may contain as much as 3 litres of urine, and must not be mistaken for the pregnant uterus. On vaginal examination the posterior vaginal wall is found to be pushed forward by a smooth elastic swelling which occupies the hollow of the sacrum. On seeking the cervix it is found to be high up behind the symphysis pubis and directed forwards and slightly upwards; this shows that the swelling in the pelvis is the uterus.

This condition might be confused with a pelvic haematocele with retention of urine (p. 143), but in the latter the uterus is displaced forwards and the cervix is directed backwards, and there is a history of severe pain in early pregnancy.

Another uncommon condition which might give rise to similar symptoms is pregnancy with a fibromyoma in the posterior wall of the uterus. If the tumour is soft and the cervix is displaced forwards diagnosis may be very difficult. However, passage of a catheter would relieve the retention, and the tumour would then still be treated expectantly and would not require surgical treatment in early pregnancy.

Treatment

If a patient is found to have a pregnancy in a retroverted uterus before the 12th week there is no need to interfere as the uterus will probably right itself and rise up into the abdomen as it enlarges. The patient should only be kept under observation.

In the few cases in which retention occurs a catheter is immediately passed and the bladder is drained continuously; in acute retention there is no danger in emptying the bladder quickly. As the bladder empties the uterus nearly always rises up into the anteverted position and into the abdomen.

Only in extremely rare cases in which spontaneous correction of the position of the uterus does not follow catheterization will correction by manipulation under anaesthesia be required.

Abnormal anteversion; pendulous abdomen

In multiparae with very atonic abdominal muscles, or very rarely in primigravidae with spinal deformity or gross pelvic contraction, the fundus uteri may fall right forwards. The uterus is abnormally anteverted in the pendulous abdomen. During pregnancy a belt or corset will be needed, and labour should be conducted with the patient on her back until the head has engaged in the pelvic inlet. Assistance with forceps or the vacuum extractor may be required because of the laxity of the abdominal muscles.

Sacculation of the pregnant uterus

This very rare condition may result from disproportionate expansion of either the anterior or posterior uterine walls. If a retroverted uterus becomes incarcerated and abortion does not occur the anterior wall may bulge into the abdominal cavity. Posterior sacculation has followed the obsolete operation of ventrofixation, in which the anterior surface of the uterus is attached to the abdominal wall.

Prolapse of the pregnant uterus

Pregnancy may occur in a partially prolapsed uterus. In such cases as the uterus grows it eventually becomes too large to sink through the pelvic brim and usually, although not invariably, the cervix is then drawn up and no longer descends. Minor degrees of prolapse only require support with a ring pessary until the uterus has grown well up into the abdomen.

Pregnancy in a completely prolapsed uterus is very rare. As a rule the cervix becomes retracted when labour begins, but on rare instances it remains protruding through the vulva, becomes oedematous, and may fail to dilate. Any infection of the cervix should be treated by application of an antiseptic such as chlorhexidine to reduce the risk of puerperal sepsis, but the most important point is to keep the patient in bed for some days before labour, with the cervix within the vagina to allow the oedema to subside.

It is usual to defer operations for prolapse until the patient has completed her family. If, however, she becomes pregnant again after a repair has been carried out some obstetricians would always advise delivery by Caesarean section; but others recommend vaginal delivery with a wide episiotomy. If the cervix has been amputated it usually dilates more quickly than usual, but occasionally because of scarring it either tears or fails to dilate. In such a case Caesarean section is carried out.

It would be generally agreed that in a case where there was stress incontinence before the repair, and in which this complaint has been cured, Caesarean section should be advised.

All these cases should be delivered in hospital.

Congenital abnormalities of the uterus and vagina

The more gross uterine abnormalities are often accompanied by infertility, but lesser degrees of malformation do not prevent pregnancy occurring.

A woman with a double uterus may become pregnant in one or both sides. The risk of abortion or premature labour is increased, but labour is often normal. If pregnancy occurs in one uterus it is possible for the other one, which undergoes both myometrial and decidual hypertrophy, to obstruct the descent of the presenting part into the pelvis, and Caesarean section may be necessary. The non-pregnant uterus is sometimes mistaken for a pelvic tumour such as an ovarian cyst.

With a bicornuate or septate uterus there may be a malpresentation such as a transverse lie or a breech presentation, and this would be likely to recur in successive pregnancies. Such uterine abnormalities may also cause repeated abortion.

A vaginal septum may be present with or without a double uterus. Sometimes there is no obstruction to delivery, but in many cases the septum has to be excised or divided during labour.

Uterine fibromyomata

The incidence of uterine fibromyomata during pregnancy is about 5 per 1000 in white women, but is much higher in Negro women.

Effects of pregnancy on fibromyomata

During pregnancy the tumours may undergo several pathological changes:

1. **Increase in size and softening.** There is hypertrophy of the muscle fibres of the tumour as in the rest of the myometrium, and there is also increased vascularity and oedema, so that it becomes larger and softer, and may also be flattened out.

2. **Necrobiosis (red degeneration).** This change is seldom seen in fibromyomata except during pregnancy. Rapid degeneration and partial necrosis of the tumour occurs, associated with thrombosis of efferent veins from the capsule of the tumour. Its cut surface has a reddish-purple colour, and the softened tumour has a faint odour like that of stale fish.

The patient experiences pain at the site, and the fibromyoma becomes very tender. There is usually pyrexia, and sometimes vomiting. Fortunately in most cases the symptoms and signs subside spontaneously in a few days without treatment.

3. **Torsion of the pedicle** of a pedunculated subserous tumour is a rare accident, but is more common during pregnancy than at other times.

Effects of fibromyomata on pregnancy, labour and the puerperium

Pregnancy.   Miscarriage is sometimes associated with fibromyomata, although it is difficult to be sure that any particular miscarriage is due to this cause. In theory it is most likely to occur with a submucous tumour.

Labour.   Fibromyomata occur most commonly in the body of the uterus, and such tumours are drawn up out of the pelvis as the uterus enlarges, so that they do not obstruct labour. Cervical fibromyomata which remain in the pelvis prevent the head from engaging, may cause malpresentations, and will obstruct labour.

The third stage of labour may be complicated by postpartum haemorrhage, especially with submucous tumours, and particularly if the placental attachment is over the tumour.

Puerperium.   A submucous fibromyoma may become infected during labour, and separation of a necrotic tumour may cause late postpartum haemorrhage. After delivery fibromyomata regress as part of the general process of involution of the uterus, but they do not totally disappear.

Diagnosis

Fibromyomata which are projecting are easily felt in the wall of the pregnant uterus, and are distinguished from fetal parts by their fixed position. They become more evident when the uterus contracts, whereas fetal parts become less obvious. They may be very difficult to detect when they have become softened and flattened in the uterine wall; however such tumours are very unlikely to interfere seriously with labour.

If a woman who is known to have a fibromyomatous uterus becomes pregnant the signs of pregnancy are sometimes masked, or confusion may arise about the expected date of delivery because the uterus is larger than expected for the period of amenorrhoea. The tumours may make the swelling feel unlike the normal pregnant uterus in shape or consistency, or make it difficult to feel fetal parts. Confusion will be increased if there is amenorrhoea from some cause other than pregnancy, such as the menopause. Conversely bleeding from threatened abortion may be attributed to menstrual bleeding if the signs of pregnancy are obscured.

In cases of doubt an immunological test for pregnancy is performed, and ultrasonic examination may be very helpful, showing the presence in the uterus of a gestation sac containing a fetus, and later the fetal heart movements will be detected.

Treatment

Pregnancy. Most women with fibromyomata pass through pregnancy without difficulty. Any threat to miscarry calls for rest.

If necrobiosis (red degeneration) occurs the symptoms may be severe enough to require admission to hospital, but they almost always subside within a week or so without any treatment other than rest in bed and analgesic drugs. Myomectomy is unnecessary and carries a high risk of abortion and also of severe haemorrhage during the operation.

Torsion of a pedunculated subserous fibromyoma causes severe pain and vomiting and calls for laparotomy and removal of the tumour. Two rare conditions with which torsion of a fibromyoma may be confused are torsion of the pregnant uterus itself, and intraperitoneal haemorrhage from a ruptured vein on the surface of a fibromyoma.

Labour. All pregnant women with fibromyomata should be delivered in hospital. Towards the end of pregnancy, at about the 36th week, the important decision as to the method of delivery will have to be made; first,

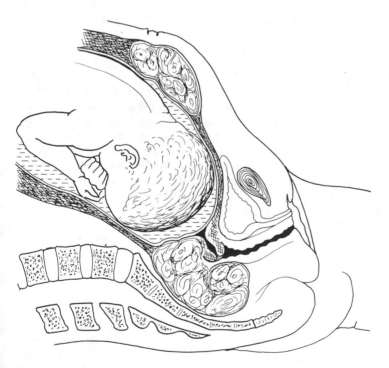

Fig. 22.2 Fibromyomata complicating pregnancy. The tumour in the anterior wall of the uterus has been drawn up out of the pelvis as the lower segment was formed, but the tumour arising from the cervix remains in the pelvis and will obstruct labour.

whether it is to be vaginal or abdominal; and, secondly, if abdominal, whether hysterectomy or myomectomy should be combined with the Caesarean operation.

If a fibromyoma is situated in the pelvis and offers obstruction to vaginal delivery Caesarean section is imperative and should be performed before term. Such cases are uncommon because most fibromyomata grow from the upper uterine segment and rise into the abodmen during pregnancy, or occasionally even in the early stage of labour.

In the other cases, which form the large majority, individual decisions have to be made, and the age and parity have an important bearing. Often the pregnancy is the first at an age when the prospects of future childbearing are diminishing, and there may have been previous infertility. Natural delivery would be chosen for a patient with a small fibromyoma situated in the upper uterine segment, whereas in the case of a patient with a large number of tumours Caesarean section with hysterectomy might be advised. The larger the number and the greater the size of the tumours, the stronger is the indication for abdominal delivery. Failure of the head to engage before the onset of labour in a primigravida, or a malpresentation, would weight the scales heavily in favour of Caesarean section.

If the decision is reached to perform Caesarean section should the fibromyomata be dealt with at the same operation, and if so by myomectomy or hysterectomy? Caesarean section with myomectomy is to be avoided because of the danger of haemorrhage from the cavities left after enucleation of the tumours. Even after careful obliteration with mattress sutures haemorrhage often continues from the stitch holes and suture lines. Myomectomy after Caesarean section is only advisable in the case of pedunculated tumours or when the fibromyomata are small or few in number (when Caesarean section is of dubious necessity). In those cases in which Caesarean section has been decided upon but which are unsuitable for myomectomy there are only two alternatives: either to leave the tumours to be dealt with later, or to remove the uterus with the tumours. If the patient has the family she wants, and when there are numerous tumours, hysterectomy will be advised. If myomectomy is proposed it is best to defer this until involution is complete after an interval of three months.

Ovarian tumours

Ovarian tumours are not commonly associated with pregnancy, the incidence being less than 1 in 1000 cases. Any type of ovarian tumour may be found, but simple serous cysts and benign teratomatous cysts are most often found. The most important fact to bear in mind is that it is impossible to exclude the possibility that an ovarian tumour or cyst may be malignant. About 10 per cent of tumours in patients under 30 are malignant, and this proportion rises in older patients.

Torsion of the pedicle of an ovarian tumour occurs more often during pregnancy than at other times, and it may also occur during the puerperium. Rupture of a cyst or intracystic haemorrhage may also occur, but not more commonly during pregnancy than at other times. Injury and necrosis may occur from pressure on a cyst during labour, and infection and suppuration may follow.

Usually pregnancy is undisturbed by the tumour unless torsion or some other complication occurs. Labour is unaffected unless the tumour lies in the pelvic cavity; in that case obstruction is probable. This is relatively more common than with fibromyomata because the latter usually rise up into the abdomen before labour begins.

Diagnosis

In the early months of pregnancy the uterus is easily distinguished by bimanual examination from the rounded and usually mobile ovarian tumour lying behind it in the recto-vaginal pouch. A useful sign when it can be obtained is the periodical contraction of the pregnant uterus.

The chief condition which has to be distinguished from an intrapelvic ovarian cyst associated with pregnancy is retroversion of the gravid uterus. Contrary to expectation an ovarian cyst is not displaced to one side but lies in the midline behind the uterus. It is cystic and tense, and a groove may be felt between the cervix, which is directed downwards and backwards, and the cyst. A retroverted gravid uterus is also felt centrally in the recto-vaginal pouch, but the body of the uterus is soft, and the cervix is directed forwards.

A twisted ovarian cyst with an early uterine pregnancy might be mistaken for a tubal pregnancy, but the correct treatment is laparotomy for both conditions. An ovarian tumour that cannot be recognized as a separate structure from the uterus might lead to an erroneous diagnosis of a fibromyoma, a bicornuate uterus or, because the uterus appears to be unduly enlarged, twin pregnancy or hydramnios.

In the last month of pregnancy an ovarian tumour is sometimes discovered in the pelvis when an examination is made to investigate non-engagement of the fetal head, although the tumour should have been found at the examination at the time of booking.

In all cases of doubtful diagnosis useful information can be obtained from ultrasonic examination or from careful examination under anaesthesia.

Treatment

An ovarian tumour discovered during pregnancy should be removed as soon as it is diagnosed (except during the first 12 weeks) because of the possibility that it may be malignant. Moreover it is subject to the risks of torsion of the pedicle, rupture and intracystic haemorrhage. It is wise to wait until after the 12th week before operating, as there is a risk of mis-carriage if the corpus luteum has to be removed with the ovary before the placenta has taken up its hormonal function. If the tumour proves to be innocent every effort is made to conserve ovarian tissue; the cyst or tumour is enucleated from the rest of the ovary.

If the diagnosis is not made until late in pregnancy, and the ovarian tumour is not in the pelvic cavity, natural delivery is awaited and the tumour is removed in the early puerperium. If the tumour is in the pelvis, even if it is cystic, it is likely to obstruct delivery and Caesarean section with removal of the tumour is necessary.

Carcinoma of the cervix uteri

Carcinoma in situ

During pregnancy carcinoma *in situ* (pre-invasive carcinoma) is found more often than invasive cancer of the cervix, as might be expected because patients who ultimately develop invasive cancer may have carcinoma *in situ* for many years beforehand.

It is the usual practice to take a cervical smear from patients at the time of their first visit to the antenatal clinic. If abnormal cells are found the cer-vix is carefully examined with a speculum. Any area of suspicious appear-ance is examined by simple biopsy; often nothing suspicious is seen and then the patient is followed for the rest of pregnancy by repeated speculum examination and smears.

If a biopsy during pregnancy shows invasive cancer the treatment described below is applied forwith, but if only carcinoma *in situ* is found the pregnancy is allowed to continue, and if after delivery malignant cells are still present in the smear a complete cone biopsy is carried out. Cone biopsy during pregnancy may cause abortion, and the vascular cervix bleeds very freely. It is therefore postponed until after delivery when possi-ble, but it will occasionally be justified during pregnancy if cells that are regarded as coming from an invasive cancer are repeatedly found. In most cases it is safer to defer the biopsy until after delivery, when the ultimate treatment is determined by the extent of the carcinoma *in situ* and the age and parity of the patient. (See *Gynaecology by Ten Teachers*).

If any patient has not had a cervical smear examination during preg-nancy this must be done in the postnatal clinic.

Invasive carcinoma

Invasive cancer of the cervix is a rare complication of pregnancy because the disease most often arises in the later years of menstrual life, when pregnancy is less likely to occur. Apart from early diagnosis by cervical smear, when there may be no symptoms, the disease is first discovered because of slight bleeding from the cervix, sometimes after coitus or examination. It quickly progresses in the same way as in the non-pregnant woman, with free bleeding and purulent discharge from a friable or ulcerated lesion on the cervix. When there is any doubt about the nature of such a lesion biopsy is essential.

If the growth is endocervical intermittent bleeding will be the only sign at first, and delay in diagnosis may occur because this is attributed to threatened abortion or antepartum haemorrhage.

Treatment. Opinions differ about the best method of treatment. For growths in an early stage many surgeons recommend immediate Wertheim's hysterectomy. In the early weeks this can be performed without emptying the uterus, but later on hysterotomy or Caesarean section would be the first step of the operation.

Other authorities prefer to treat such early cases by intrauterine insertion of caesium or radium, but the uterus would first have to be emptied by suction cannula, hysterotomy or Caesarean section according to the stage of the pregnancy. Another possible course is to give external irradiation first; abortion of a dead fetus would follow and then the caesium could be inserted.

In more advanced cases the uterus is emptied by hysterotomy or Caesarean section so that caesium can be inserted and teleradiation given. In advanced cases vaginal delivery carries the dangers of severe haemorrhage, tearing of the lower segment and puerperal sepsis. Delay in treatment in the fetal interest would only be justified in a very advanced case in which the maternal prognosis was already very bad.

23

The fetus at risk in late pregnancy; intrauterine fetal death

During pregnancy and labour the fetus may be at risk of damage or death from many causes. However it has become the custom to talk of the fetus at risk in the more limited sense of at risk from acute or chronic placental insufficiency. Acute placental failure may result from accidental antepartum haemorrhage after placental function had previously seemed quite normal, or it may come at the end of a phase of gradually declining placental efficiency. In the latter case acute failure may become manifest during labour when the uterine contractions interfere with blood flow. This failure we commonly call fetal distress. It is discussed in Chapter 33, p. 351.

The importance of acute anoxia which may cause sudden fetal death during labour has been appreciated for a long time. Awareness of the long-term damage which may result from chronic intrauterine malnutrition and leads to the birth of a light-for-dates baby is more recent.

Placental insufficiency during pregnancy

During pregnancy the fetus depends on the placenta and the umbilical vessels for transport of oxygen and nutrients from the maternal blood, and for excretion of carbon dioxide and the products of metabolism. Because of the constancy of the mother's internal environment the composition of the blood reaching the placenta is unlikely to vary much except in desperate conditions of maternal circulatory failure or asphyxia, or in cases of gross metabolic disturbance such as severe diabetes or renal disease. Even if the maternal nutrition is poor the maternal blood will show little alteration, and this explains the fact that a normal sized child may be born in such circumstances, and that the fetus of a mother with poor iron reserves is not anaemic as long as her serum iron concentration is maintained. Fetal ill-health therefore seldom arises because of alteration in the biochemical quality of the maternal blood—the ability of the placenta to act as an organ of transfer is the important consideration.

Restriction of the maternal blood flow through the placental site—sometimes seen in patients with arterial disease for example—can have a serious effect upon fetal growth and development. Placental tissue may be lost by the separation from the uterine wall that occurs when abortion threatens or when there is a small accidental haemorrhage. Spasm or thrombosis of small decidual vessels may also have the same effect. In a few patients who give birth to babies who have obviously suffered from chronic placental insufficiency the placenta is small for no apparent reason.

If pregnancy is prolonged beyond term the placenta sometimes becomes inadequate for the needs of the large and still growing fetus. Significant structural changes in the placenta are seldom found in such cases. There may be calcification of the decidual plate, but the intervillous circulation is not impaired by this. Although intrauterine death before the onset of labour is rare in cases of postmaturity, fetal distress may occur during labour.

Intrauterine death may occur in cases of diabetes but the cause of this is uncertain (see p. 225). The fetus is often very large, but so is the placenta, and placental failure is not an adequate explanation.

In cases of haemolytic disease the placenta is large and oedematous, with persistence of Langhans' layer of cytotrophoblast in the villi, but the fetus probably dies from cardiac failure caused by the severe haemolytic anaemia rather than from placental insufficiency.

Tests of placental function

It is obvious that there is much still to be discovered about placental function, but the practical need for the obstetrician is to obtain some warning of placental insufficiency, so that the fetus at risk of intrauterine death may be delivered before this occurs. Conversely, such a test might be reassuring, and prevent the unnecessary hazard of premature delivery. Unfortunately there is no absolutely reliable test for placental function. Clinical judgment must still be used. Indeed clinical assessment of the patient is usually the basis for requesting the more sophisticated physical or biochemical tests of function that we now use so commonly.

Three important clinical indicators of placental function are the pattern of maternal weight gain, and the growth of the uterus and fetus.

The maternal weight should normally increase by about 0.5 kg weekly after the first trimester, provided that the patient is not dieting or vomiting, and has no other disorder causing malnutrition. The components of this weight gain include the fetus, placenta, liquor, uterus, breasts and the fat store. In addition there is the increase in blood volume and extracellular fluid. These very diverse components are all dependent directly on placental function, or indirectly on it by way of the hormones it produces. Thus failure to gain weight adequately should be regarded as an indication to carry out some other placental function tests.

Uterine growth is not always easy to assess, and the variation between observers may be considerable. Nevertheless simple measurements of the height of the fundus above the symphysis pubis have more to recommend them than the common practice of assessing fundal height in relation to the umbilicus or xiphisternum. The fundal height should increase by about 1 cm weekly from the 16th week of pregnancy, and with an average sized fetus remains about 3 cm less than the number of weeks of gestation. Measurements of abdominal girth are much less satisfactory indicators of uterine growth. In the case of both measurements the variability is lessened appreciably if the same person sees the patient at each antenatal visit. If the uterus seems to be growing slowly this is another reason to perform other placental function tests.

Fetal growth.   The most reliable measurements of the fetus are obtained with ultrasound. Serial measurements of the biparietal diameter of the fetal head are comparatively easy to obtain with the relatively simple apparatus that is now becoming widely available. It should be remembered that the head of the fetus is a privileged area in so far as the greatest part of the cardiac output with the most highly oxygenated blood is diverted there. It is therefore the last part of the fetus to suffer from malnutrition. If earlier signs of poor growth are to be sought it is better to measure the girth of the fetus at the point of entry of the umbilical cord and to relate this to the size of the head. This technique calls for more sophisticated apparatus and a great degree of expertise on the part of the operator.

Fetal activity.   The most important indicator of placental function is the wellbeing of the fetus. A valuable sign of a healthy fetus is vigorous activity. The mother may be able to give some indication of this by keeping a 'kick count'. She can be asked to note how frequently the baby moves in a given period, perhaps 30 minutes. Alternatively she can be asked to note how long it takes for the baby to move ten times. A more sophisticated way of assessing fetal activity is to produce a continuous record of the fetal heart rate over a period of 30 minutes or more. This can be done with an abdominal lead and an electronic ratemeter. A change in rate with fetal activity, together with variability in the interval between beats (p. 355) is associated with fetal health. A further refinement is to record with a tocograph the spontaneous contractions of the uterus, or in some instances oxytocin induced contractions, and to relate the heart rate changes to the stress of the uterine activity. A change in heart rate is normal with a uterine contraction, but with a healthy fetus the change is reversed immediately the contraction passes off.

Placental function tests.   Attempts have been made to judge the functional activity of the placenta by measuring one or more of its hormone or enzyme products in maternal blood or urine. Blood levels of oestrogens and progesterone vary with placental function, but diurnal variations and variations due to activity and posture are so great that they are unreliable indicators of fetal wellbeing. The excretion in the maternal urine of oestrogens (particularly oestriol, see p. 57) during a 24-hour period gives a more consistent indication of placental function. The normal range of values for excretion is considerable, and isolated observations are of little value, but repeated observations may show an obvious trend.

Other tests which are less frequently employed include serum levels of placental lactogen (HPL) and of heat-stable alkaline phosphatase.

Postmaturity

Postmaturity means the prolongation of pregnancy beyond its normal duration. It is important because surveys of perinatal deaths have shown that after term the risk of intrauterine death increases, and also the stillbirth rate. However, there is no agreement on the normal limits of pregnancy. The difficulty in making any definition is that the precise date of conception in any particular pregnancy is unknown, and even with regular menstrual cycles of normal length the date of ovulation is only approximately known. In women with irregular or prolonged cycles calculations based on the date of the last menstrual period are bound to be inaccurate.

Apart from the uncertainty about the date of ovulation, it is improbable that all fetuses will mature in precisely the same number of days. The cause of the onset of labour at term is unknown (p. 67).

Diagnosis. General statistical statements based on large numbers of cases can easily be made, showing that delivery takes place during the 42nd week in about 25 per cent of cases, during the 43rd week in about 12 per cent, and during the 44th week in about 3 per cent; but in any particular pregnancy the diagnosis of postmaturity is often uncertain.

In cases in which the date of the last menstrual period is absolutely certain, and in which the previous menstrual cycles were of normal length, the diagnosis of maturity can reasonably be based on this. If the menstrual history is uncertain an attempt can be made to assess maturity by scrutiny of the antenatal records to discover whether the size of the uterus was determined by bimanual examination at an early visit by an experienced obstetrician. Between the 8th and the 14th weeks an accurate assessment of the uterine size can generally be made. Ultrasonic measurements of the crown-rump length of the fetus up to about the 14th week, and of the biparietal diameter of the fetal head up to about the 28th week, give reliable indication of the duration of gestation. The date at which the mother first felt fetal movements may be of interest, but as this can range from 16 to 22 weeks depending on her previous obstetric experience and her obesity this is hardly reliable enough evidence on which to base any important decision.

Other tests for the assessment of maturity include radiological examination of fetal ossific centres, and chemical and cytological examination of liquor amnii. These tests are mentioned on p. 53 but they are now infrequently used.

Clinical significance. The delayed onset of labour might in theory have two disadvantages: (1) The placental function may become inadequate after term as the uterine blood flow diminishes and degenerative changes progress, with a large fetus that is still growing. (2) There may be mechanical difficulties during labour because of the increased size of the fetus, and perhaps the uterus which is slow to begin labour may also prove to be inefficient during labour.

The risk of the fetus dying in the uterus from anoxia before the onset of labour has probably been exaggerated, although this does occasionally occur. However, there is good evidence that the risk of fetal distress and fetal death during labour is greater in postmature than in normal cases. In part this is due to more difficult labour because of the larger size of the fetus and incoordinate uterine action. The skull of the postmature fetus is more ossified, so that moulding is less easy.

The risk of anoxia in postmature cases is increased if there is also hypertension, and perhaps in the case of an elderly primigravida.

Medico-legal significance.   Postmaturity may be of medico-legal importance, as a husband may question the paternity of a child born more than 44 weeks after he left his wife. In law each case is decided on the medical evidence, and there is no legal definition or set upper limit for the normal duration of pregnancy. In one astonishing decision a child born 346 days after the last cohabitation was judged to be legitimate, but in another case a child born after 360 days was adjudged illegitimate on appeal.

Management.   Postmaturity is often a cause of worry, and sometimes of expense and inconvenience, to the mother. Pressure is often put upon the obstetrician to induce labour. While this is often justifiable in cases in which the menstrual history is certain, in other cases there is a risk that the fetus may, after induction, prove to be premature rather than postmature. The clinical evidence must be carefully reviewed before deciding to induce labour.

Since patients and their relatives tend to worry when the date given to them as the expected date of delivery has been passed, it is most desirable that every patient should be told that the calculated date is only an approximation, and that normal labour often starts a week or more later.

Each case of suspected postmaturity should be dealt with according to its special circumstances. There is no justification for making a rule that all cases must be induced at some stated week of pregnancy; the risks of indiscriminate induction might well exceed those of postmaturity. There will be more anxiety in the case of elderly primigravidae, or patients with hypertension. Induction might well be recommended if the fetus is evidently large, and for patients' in whom there is a risk of disproportion if the fetus continues to grow. There can be little justification for induction until the patient is at least two weeks overdue except in cases with hypertension or some other reason to suspect placental insufficiency.

Some obstetricians have advised that amnioscopy should be performed on alternate days in these patients. The tubular amnioscope is passed through the cervix to inspect the liquor through the intact transparent membranes. If the liquor is stained with meconium this is certainly evidence of fetal distress; but in most of the postmature cases that develop fetal distress the liquor is clear beforehand, and this investigation is therefore not recommended.

Labour may be induced in cases of postmaturity by amniotomy in the usual way, followed if necessary by an oxytocin infusion. Very careful monitoring of the progress of the labour and of the condition of the fetus are required. If there is evidence of fetal hypoxia during the first stage of labour, preferably confirmed by examination of a sample of fetal blood, Caesarean section may be necessary. In the second stage clinical signs of fetal distress would call for forceps delivery without delay.

Intrauterine death of the fetus

In addition to cases in which the fetus dies during delivery as the result of asphyxia or difficult labour, others are seen in which it dies *in utero* before labour starts. This is usually followed by expulsion of the fetus from the uterus within a few days. However, in exceptional cases the dead fetus is not expelled from the uterus at once, but is retained for several weeks.

Causes

In some cases the cause of death is obvious; but in others it is obscure, because autolysis of the tissues of the fetus and placenta occurs, and as a result postmortem findings are difficult to interpret. The causes of intrauterine fetal death may be classified under the following headings:

1. *Pre-eclampsia, essential hypertension and chronic renal disease.* Fetal anoxia is produced by reduction in the maternal blood supply to the placenta because of spasm, and sometimes thrombosis, of the maternal vessels. Added to this there may be separation of the placenta by accidental haemorrhage or extensive clotting of maternal blood around the chorionic villi.

2. *Diabetes mellitus.* If maternal diabetes is poorly controlled fetal death *in utero* often occurs (p. 225).

3. *Postmaturity.* This is an uncommon cause of fetal death before labour (see above).

4. *Accidental antepartum haemorrhage.* See p. 157.

5. *Cord accidents.* True knots in the cord or constriction of the cord round a limb are very rare causes of fetal death.

6. *Haemolytic disease.* Death of a hydropic fetus usually occurs (p. 449).

7. *Unexplained placental insufficiency.* Apart from the cases of preeclampsia, hypertension and renal disease already mentioned, in a few patients unexplained placental insufficiency occurs in successive pregnancies. The fetus does not grow at the normal rate and intrauterine death may occur. The placenta is found to be small but appears to be normal in other

respects. In the absence of any explanation for some of the cases the only advice which can be offered is to rest in bed during most of the pregnancy, with the hope that this will increase the uterine blood flow. Delivery before the time at which previous deaths occurred is wise, either by induction of labour or Caesarean section. Placental function tests may give some guidance in deciding when to advise delivery.

8. *Fetal malformation.* With gross malformation intrauterine death sometimes occurs.

9. *Infective diseases.*   Any disease that causes high fever and toxaemia may cause fetal death.

Untreated syphilis will often lead to fetal death, and rare fetal infection with smallpox, herpes virus or other viruses may cause death. Severe rubella is sometimes fatal to the fetus.

Pathological anatomy

The fetus is usually born in a macerated condition, that is to say its skin is peeling and stained reddish-brown by absorption of blood pigments. The whole body is softened and toneless; the cranial bones are loosened and easily moveable on one another. The liquor amnii and the fluid in all the serous cavities contain blood pigments. Maceration occurs rapidly, and may be advanced within 24 hours of fetal death. It is not accompanied by an offensive odour.

Symptoms and diagnosis

The patients may notice that the fetal movements have not been present for several days, and the breasts may diminish in size. In cases of hypertension the blood pressure sometimes falls. The following signs may be found:

After the 24th week the fetal heart sounds can usually be heard with a stethoscope; failure to hear them on careful auscultation will be strong presumptive evidence of fetal death. Ultrasonic apparatus can detect fetal blood flow as early as the 8th week of pregnancy, and a careful and repeated search for evidence of fetal life should be made with this.

The uterus may be found to be smaller than the duration of pregnancy would warrant. A more accurate sign is to note how much alteration takes place in the size of the uterus during a period of observation. For this the bladder must be empty and the level of the fundus accurately noted. The patient is examined week by week. If uterine enlargement is not observed in four weeks this strongly suggests that the fetus is dead. In some cases the uterus not only ceases to grow but gets smaller because of absorption of the liquor amnii.

Sometimes secretion of colostrum from the breasts occurs a few days after the death of the fetus.

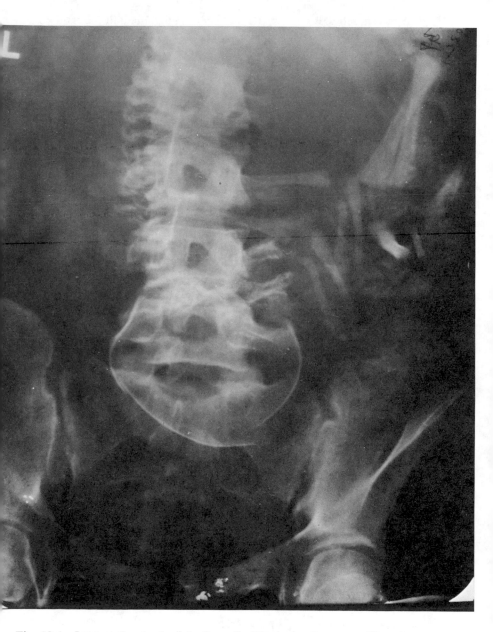

Fig. 23.1 Intra-uterine death of the fetus. Spalding's sign is present. There is marked overlapping of the bones of the vault of the skull.

A radiograph will show overlapping and disalignment of the skull bones (Spalding's sign) and occasionally the presence of gas in the fetal heart and great vessels (Roberts' sign). Spalding's sign is not usually present until a week after fetal death, but gas formation may be seen after only two days. Immunological tests for pregnancy are usually negative within a week after the death of the fetus, but sometimes a weakly positive test persists for a time, presumably because some chorionic tissue is still active. The excretion of oestriol in the mother's urine falls sharply.

It will be seen that fetal death is difficult to diagnose from a single examination of the patient, and it may be necessary to watch the patient for a time before deciding that the fetus is dead. Very little importance should be attached to the patient's statements about fetal movements; false hope will lead to confusion of intestinal with fetal movement.

Management

In the majority of cases labour soon follows death of the fetus, but in a few cases labour does not occur for several weeks. In these cases there is no urgent call for interference, unless the complication of hypofibrinogenaemia occurs (p. 431). If the patient becomes greatly distressed when she knows that the fetus is dead the labour can be induced, but amniotomy is unwise because of the risk of anaerobic uterine infection from growth of bacteria in the dead placental and fetal tissues if labour does not follow quickly.

Oxytocin infusion will often bring about evacuation of the uterus, but prostaglandins are more effective. When given intravenously they often have unpleasant side effects from stimulation of the intestine, but these can be avoided by the use of vaginal pessaries. It is also possible to induce labour by the intra-amniotic injection of a hypertonic solution of urea (p. 374).

24

Dystocia (introduction)

Before reading the next four chapters the student may find it helpful to have a brief general survey of the causes of dystocia, which means difficult or prolonged labour. Dystocia has many causes, but these can be divided into three main categories:

1. Obstruction to delivery caused by a fetal malposition or malpresentation, or rarely a fetal malformation such as hydrocephaly.

2. Obstruction to delivery caused by an abnormality of the birth canal such as a contracted pelvis, or by a tumour lying in the pelvic cavity.

3. Weak or incoordinate action of the uterus.

Maternal and fetal factors may be combined. For example, with disproportion between the size of the head and the pelvis it is the relative and not the absolute size of the structures which matters. Again, in attempting to overcome mechanical obstruction the uterine action may become abnormal.

Not all causes of dystocia are absolute; with strong uterine action minor degrees of disproportion can be overcome, and spontaneous correction of some malpositions of the fetal head may occur.

Some causes of dystocia (for example weak uterine action) may act throughout all the stages of labour, whereas others only cause difficulty in the second stage (for example persistent occipito-posterior position of the occiput).

In the following chapters the general scheme set out above is followed. Fetal causes of delay are described in Chapter 25 on Malpresentations. Abnormalities of the birth canal are described in Chapter 26 on Disproportion (with pelvic tumours in Chapter 38). Abnormal uterine action is discussed in Chapter 27. The disastrous effects of unrelieved obstruction during labour are described in Chapter 28.

25

Fetal malposition and malpresentation, and fetal abnormalities which cause dystocia

Occipito-posterior positions of the vertex

The mechanism of labour in occipito-posterior positions of the vertex has already been described in Chapter 10 (pp. 97 – 99). In most cases in which the occiput lies posteriorly at the onset of labour normal vaginal delivery occurs. With good flexion of the head the occiput, being the first part of the head to meet the pelvic floor, usually undergoes long rotation forward through three-eighths of a circle and is thus directed to the space below the pubic arch. In about one-fifth of the cases this does not occur and the malposition persists. A short backward rotation of one-eighth of a circle may then take place which results in the occiput being directed so as to lie in the hollow of the sacrum. This may occur because the head is poorly flexed, so that the first part of the fetal head to meet the pelvic floor is the sinciput, and this part of the head then rotates forward.

The direction of rotation of the fetal skull may also be influenced by the shape of the cavity and outlet of the pelvis. In the android type of pelvis (p. 297) there is narrowing of the pelvic cavity from side to side, and the size of the cavity tends to diminish in the lower straits. The angle of the pubic arch is less acute and the ischial spines project more into the birth canal. There therefore tends to be less room in the anterior part of the pelvis and a posterior position of the occiput may persist even with good flexion of the head.

With an occipito-posterior position the head is pushed downwards and forwards against the back of the symphysis pubis rather than directly downwards onto the cervix. Thus some of the effectiveness of the uterine contractions is lost and cervical dilatation tends to be slow. The cervix may be compressed between the head and the pubis, so that progressive oedema of the anterior lip of the cervix occurs.

Diagnosis

Diagnosis during pregnancy is of no importance except that the occipito-posterior position must be recognized as a cause of non-engagement of the head before the onset of labour. During labour a lack of flexion of the head may be suspected if there is early rupture of the membranes, and there is a possibility of prolapse of the umbilical cord if this occurs.

Abdominal examination. During the intervals between uterine contractions slight flattening of the lower abdomen may be observed, and the limbs, being in front, are easily felt. It may be difficult to define the back or to hear the fetal heart. This should be listened for well to the side of the abdomen and towards the mother's back, but it may sometimes be best heard in the midline when the sounds are heard through the chest wall of the fetus. The head usually descends through the pelvic brim as labour proceeds, but descent may be slow because with poor flexion a wider diameter presents. It must not be forgotten that failure to descend can also be caused by contraction of the brim.

Vaginal examination. Early in labour it may be difficult to reach the presenting part, and the bag of membranes may bulge in an elongated manner and rupture early. When the head has entered the pelvic cavity the most striking feature is the ease with which the anterior fontanelle can be felt. This fontanelle is directed forwards and to the left in the right occipito-posterior position, and forwards and to the right with a left occipito-posterior position. The anterior fontanelle is more easily felt because the head is less well flexed, and also because it lies well forward when the head is in the occipito-posterior position. An attempt should be

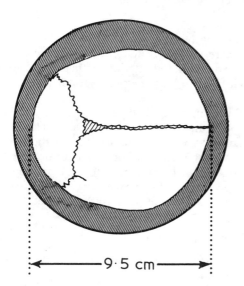

Fig. 25.1 Vaginal palpation of head in right occipito-lateral position. The circle represents the pelvic cavity with a diameter of 11 cm. The head is well flexed and only the posterior fontanelle is felt.

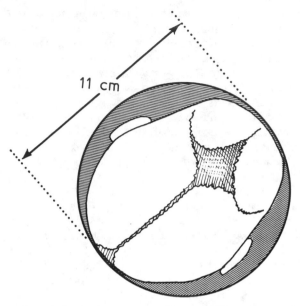

11 cm

Fig. 25.2 Vaginal palpation of head in right occipito-posterior position. The head is poorly flexed so that the anterior fontanelle presents.

made to assess the degree of flexion of the head, as the well-flexed head is more likely to rotate. If only the anterior fontanelle can be felt the head is poorly flexed; it is less poorly flexed if both the anterior and posterior fontanelles can be felt; and it is well flexed if only the posterior fontanelle is felt. (Figs. 25.1, 25.2.)

Although the diagnosis should be made early in labour, it not infrequently happens that the position is unrecognized until there is delay in the second stage of labour. Diagnosis by vaginal examination may then be difficult owing to the formation of a caput succedaneum over the presenting part. Before forceps delivery, when it is essential to have accurate knowledge of the direction of the occiput, the fingers may be passed higher to feel for the free margin of an ear, which will point to the occiput.

The course of labour in occipito-posterior positions

In about 70 per cent of cases spontaneous rotation of the occiput to the anterior position occurs, and in about another 10 per cent of cases the occiput undergoes short rotation so that delivery in the occipito-posterior position (face-to-pubes) can occur. In the remainder assisted rotation will be required.

During labour the uterine contractions may be ineffective, and it has been suggested that the poorly flexed head fails to provide the reflex stimulation of the lower segment that is produced by the more pointed vertex with full flexion. A long first stage is likely to be followed by a long second stage, for the woman is tired and the uterus may be less capable of further strong contractions.

Moulding of the head. When the fetal head descends through the birth canal and flexion of the head is poor the skull will be compressed in the occipito-frontal diameter (Fig. 25.3) If the alteration in shape is

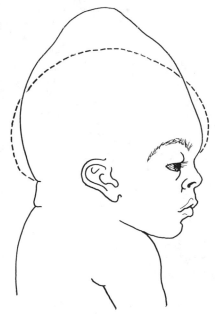

Fig. 25.3 Moulding of head and formation of caput succedaneum in persistent occipito-posterior position.

extreme the structures of the skull may not adapt well to the relatively sudden change. Great compression along the occipito-frontal diameter causes tension in the posterior vertical part of the falx cerebri. This elevates the tentorium cerebelli, which may ultimately tear at its free margin. The upward dislocation of the tentorium may result in rupture of the great cerebral vein (vein of Galen) or a tributary, and fetal damage or death from intracranial haemorrhage.

Management of labour

First stage of labour.   The first stage is managed as in a normal case. Nothing can be done to correct the malposition or to influence the rotation of the head at this stage.

The frequency, duration and strength of the uterine contractions, the dilatation of the cervix, and the fetal heart rate are observed in the ordinary way, and preferably recorded on a partogram (p. 116). If progressive cervical dilatation does not occur the effect of augmenting the uterine action with a Syntocinon drip by the method described on p. 316 may be tried. If this does not result in better progress in a few hours Caesarean section is performed. Caesarean section will also be required if fetal distress occurs.

Second stage of labour.   A mistaken diagnosis of full dilation of the cervix is not uncommon in these cases, when the patient complains of rectal discomfort and a desire to bear down. Vaginal examination is essential to establish that the second stage has been reached. The degree of flexion of the head and its position are determined by palpation of the fontanelles. Continued deflexion, a large caput succedaneum or marked over-riding of the skull bones suggest that spontaneous rotation may not occur.

In most cases, provided that the uterine contractions are strong and the patient is able to make good expulsive efforts the occiput rotates forward and spontaneous delivery takes place. In other cases the baby may be delivered face-to-pubes without any difficulty, although there is a greater risk of a perineal tear.

The indications for interference in these cases are:

1. Failure of the presenting part to descend.
2. Fetal distress.
3. Maternal distress.

An accurate diagnosis of the exact position of the head is essential. No condemnation can be strong enough for the haphazard application of forceps, made in the hope that strong traction will overcome most difficulties in the second stage.

Arrest of the head which is caused by a persistent occipito-posterior position of the occiput occurs during the second stage of labour and in the pelvic cavity. Except in very rare cases of contraction of the outlet of the pelvis vaginal delivery is possible after correction of the malposition. (Arrest at the pelvic brim is not caused by a posterior position of the occiput, even if this is present, but by disproportion, for which Caesarean section is indicated).

Because the head in the occipito-anterior position presents a smaller and more favourable diameter, the first step in assisting delivery is rotation of the fetal head. This can be performed:

(a) manually,
(b) with Kielland's forceps,

(c) and may occur during traction with the vacuum extractor if the cup is applied to the occipital part of the vertex.

(a) Manual rotation. Unless an epidural anaesthetic has already been given, a pudendal block or general anaesthesia will be required. After careful diagnostic examination the head is rotated with the hand in the appropriate direction. Thus if the fetus is in the right occipito-posterior position the head is rotated so that the occiput travels round the right wall of the pelvis until the occiput is directly anterior. The opposite direction of rotation is followed for a left occipito-posterior position. The shoulder girdle of the fetus should be rotated at the same time as the fetal head. If this is not done the head will tend to slip back after rotation into an oblique or transverse diameter of the pelvis. Rotation of the shoulder girdle may be achieved by pressure through the abdominal wall with an external hand (Fig. 25.4).

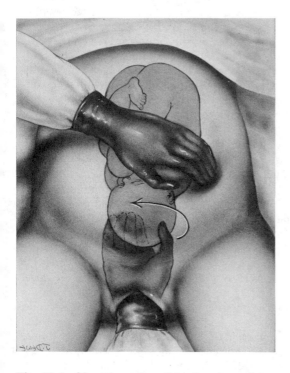

Fig. 25.4 Manual rotation of the fetus in occipito-posterior position. The right hand passes between the pelvic wall and the fetal head and is about to rotate the head. The left hand placed on the abdomen will assist this rotation by pressure on the shoulder.

It is undesirable to displace the head upward if this can be avoided, as it will make subsequent application of the forceps more difficult. It is often possible to achieve rotation with the use of the half hand; this means that rotation is effected by tangential pressure on the side of the head with the fingers, without grasping the head. After rotation to the occipito-anterior position has been achieved the fingers are kept in place to hold the head in position until the obstetric forceps are applied to complete the delivery.

Difficulties arise if manual rotation is unsuccessful and the operator does not realise this, or if the forceps are applied to the head in any other position than with the sagittal suture in the antero-posterior diameter of the pelvis. The forceps will then not lock properly and the handles will not lie together. Squeezing the handles will only compress the head and may cause fetal injury, and when traction is applied the blades may slip off and cause maternal injury as well.

(b) Kielland's forceps. This instrument is of relatively light construction and is designed so that it can be used for rotation of the fetal head, in addition to traction. The pelvic curve of the shank has been greatly reduced, and the lock allows one shank to slide upwards or downwards on the other (see Fig. 35.2). In experienced hands the instrument is safe and most satisfactory, but it is potentially dangerous in the hands of anyone not trained in its use. The technique of application of Kielland's forceps differs from that for ordinary forceps in that the instrument is applied with reference to the fetal head in whatever position it lies, and not in relation to the pelvis. These forceps are used to rotate the head until the occiput lies anteriorly before traction is applied. Details of the method of use are given on p. 388. If the instrument is incorrectly used damage to both maternal tissues and the fetal head may occur.

(c) Vacuum extraction. If the extractor is applied as near to the occipital end of the vertex as possible and traction is applied forward rotation of the head often occurs. For the method of application see p. 392.

Arrest at the pelvic outlet. If it is found that arrest has occurred when the head is so low in the pelvic cavity that with each contraction of the uterus the fetal scalp is easily visible it is probable that further progress is being prevented by the muscles of the pelvic floor. To reach this level the head will already have undergone a considerable degree of moulding into the shape described for the persistent posterior position of the occiput (p. 263). It may be found easier to perform an episiotomy and assist the delivery of the baby in the unrotated occipito-posterior position. The large occipito-frontal diameter, albeit shortened by moulding, will have to pass through the pelvic floor and therefore the episiotomy should be adequate. Traction with the obstetric forceps must be careful and only moderate force should be used. The instrument was not designed to fit the head in this position and may slip off. However, only moderate traction is necessary to complete the delivery of a fetal head which is arrested by the perineal muscles at this low level. The vacuum extractor can be used instead of the forceps.

If there is any difficulty in extraction this is due to some cause other than the resistance of the pelvic floor and perineum. On rare occasions severe outlet contraction with narrowing of the subpubic arch may cause arrest of the head. This ought to have been diagnosed at an examination of the patient during pregnancy or at least at some earlier stage of labour, when a decision might have been made to deliver the patient by Caesarean section. At this late stage the best plan is to attempt delivery with the obstetric forceps. Such a 'trial of forceps delivery' should only be conducted in the operating theatre with all preparations made for Caesarean section. Under general anaesthesia an accurate application of the forceps is obtained. Traction must be very cautious and failure to effect delivery must be treated by immediate Caesarean section.

Deep transverse arrest of the head

This term denotes arrest in labour when the fetal head has descended to the level of the ischial spines and the sagittal suture lies in the transverse diameter of the pelvis. The occiput is on one side of the pelvis and the sinciput on the other; the head is badly flexed. The condition is only diagnosed during the second stage of labour. Unlike the persistent occipitoposterior position in which birth of the baby occurs face-to-pubes, if the head is firmly fixed in the transverse position obstructed labour will occur.

The occiput may have been obliquely posterior at the onset of labour and only partly rotated forward, or it may have descended from an initial transverse position.

In an android pelvis the anterior surface of the sacrum may be straight, and the ischial spines may be prominent because the side walls of the pelvis are convergent. The head fails to descend to the pelvic floor, where rotation of the head normally occurs.

Diagnosis. The diagnosis rests on vaginal examination made during the second stage of labour because the progress of labour has ceased. The head will be found to be arrested at the level of the ischial spines, with the sagittal suture lying in the transverse diameter of the pelvis. Both fontanelles are usually palpable.

Management. The head must be rotated so that the occiput is brought to the front and then, and only then, are forceps applied. Rotation may be done manually or with Kielland's forceps. Exactly the same procedure is followed, and exactly the same precautions are taken, as have already been described for rotation of the head from the occipito-posterior position.

Very rarely indeed all attempts at rotation fail because the head is impacted in the pelvic cavity, and the fetus may be dead. If it is alive Caesarean section is performed, but otherwise the safest procedure is to perform craniotomy (p. 404). A slight reduction in the size of the fetal head usually allows it to be extracted with the forceps without difficulty.

Face presentation

Face presentation, in which the head is fully extended, occurs about once in 300 labours, and is slightly more frequent in multiparae than in primigravidae. It may be primary or secondary. *Primary face presentation* means that the fetus presents by the face before labour begins; *secondary*

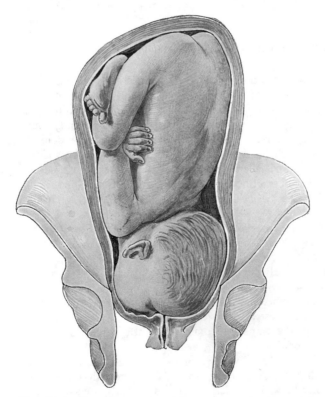

Fig. 25.5 Face presentation. Right mento-posterior position. The face from the chin to the bregma presents, the submento-bregmatic diameter occupying the right oblique diameter of the pelvic inlet. The back faces forward and to the left, but is extended instead of flexed as in a vertex presentation, so that the breech is more prominent and more easily palpated.

face presentation means that the head becomes fully extended during labour.

Causes

The commonest type of case is one in which a normal fetus actively holds its head extended, and even after delivery the infant may keep its head in an attitude of exaggerated extension for some days. In spite of this the head can be flexed on to the chest, showing that there is no increase in extensor tone.

Fetal deformities such as anencephaly, iniencephaly or congenital tumours of the neck may also cause this malpresentation.

A rare theoretical cause of secondary extension is a flat pelvis, when the wider biparietal diameter of the head cannot pass the pelvic brim. Once the head is deflexed, as may also occur with an occipito-posterior position, uterine contractions may increase the extension and thus cause a face or brow presentation.

Mechanisms

The chin is the denominator and four positions are conventionally described, analogous to the corresponding positions of the vertex from which they may be said to arise namely (1) right mento-posterior, (2) left mento-

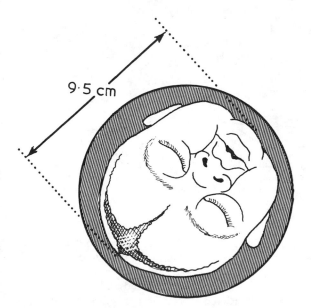

Fig. 25.6 Vaginal examination in left mento-anterior position. The circle represents the pelvic cavity with a diameter of 11 cm.

posterior, (3) left mento-anterior and (4) right mento-anterior. The mento-anterior positions are relatively more frequent.

In a mento-anterior position the head engages and descends with increasing extension, so that the submento-bregmatic diameter (9.5 cm) comes through the cervix. When the chin reaches the pelvic floor it undergoes internal rotation through one-eighth of a circle, and the submental region comes to lie under the subpubic arch. The head is then born by a movement of flexion, the submento-vertical diameter (11 cm) distending the vulva. Restitution occurs and is followed by external rotation as in vertex presentations.

In a mento-posterior position a similar mechanism occurs, except that the chin has to undergo internal rotation through three-eighths of a circle (Fig. 25.7).

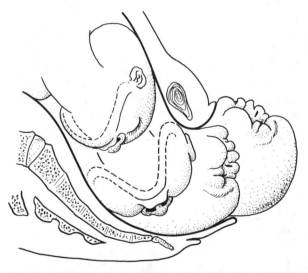

Fig. 25.7 To show mechanism of labour with a face presentation. The head descends with increasing extension. The chin reaches the pelvic floor and undergoes forward rotation. The head is born by flexion.

Backward short rotation of the chin sometimes occurs, but a fetus in such a persistent mento-posterior position cannot be delivered unless it is very small. This is because the head is already fully extended, and further extension to deliver the head is impossible. The head and thorax become impacted in the pelvis, and obstructed labour occurs unless assistance is given.

Moulding. In a face presentation the submento-vertical diameter of the head is compressed, causing elongation of the occipito-frontal diameter (Fig. 25.8). This shape of the head is called dolichocephaly.

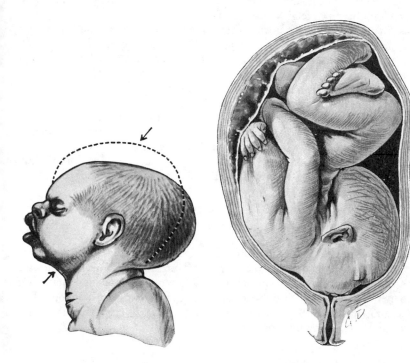

Fig. 25.8 Moulding in face presentation. The arrows indicate the direction of the pressure which shortens the diameter between the submento-vertical and submento-bregmatic diameters. The splitting of the skin in the front of the neck and the swelling of the face are also shown.

Fig. 25.9 Face presentation. To show findings on abdominal examination. In mento-posterior positions, the marked prominence of the occiput will be found on the same side as the back. Above this an interval may be detected before the back is felt running up into the unduly prominent breech.

In mento-anterior positions the small parts are very distinctly felt owing to the way they are thrust forward towards the abdominal wall. On auscultation the heart sounds may be heard most plainly on the same side as the small parts are felt.

Diagnosis

Abdominal examination. With a mento-posterior position the cephalic prominence is very easily felt and appears to overlap the symphysis; it is felt on the same side as the back, from which it is separated by a deep sulcus. The podalic pole is unduly prominent. It may be difficult to locate and hear the fetal heart sounds.

With a mento-anterior position the cephalic prominence is again felt on the same side as the back, but the latter, being posterior, is difficult to feel, and the prominent chest may be mistaken for it. The fetal heart is easily heard over the chest, and small parts may be felt on the same side. Radiological examination will settle the diagnosis.

Vaginal examination.   Early in labour it may be difficult to reach the presenting part. As the face fits less well than the vertex the membranes may rupture early. When the presenting part has engaged in the brim and can be felt, the supra-orbital ridges, the bridge of the nose and the alveolar margins within the mouth are recognized. Care must be taken not to injure the eyes when palpating the face. If the face is oedematous it can be mistaken for the breech.

Prognosis

Many face presentations are delivered naturally without difficulty. Face presentations are less favourable than vertex presentations because the face is a less efficient dilator of the cervix, and because spontaneous rotation of the mento-posterior positions occurs late in the second stage of labour. The emerging diameter, the submento-vertical (11 cm), is larger than that with a normal vertex presentation.

Management of labour

The patient is kept in bed during the first stage, and a vaginal examination is made as soon as the membranes rupture to exclude prolapse of the cord. An epidural block or infiltration of the perineum with local anaesthetic and an episiotomy are advisable in primigravidae if there is any delay when the face reaches the pelvic floor. With a mento-anterior position spontaneous delivery is to be expected. If there is delay in the second stage from inadequate expulsive forces there is no difficulty in applying the forceps.

With a mento-posterior position time should be allowed for spontaneous rotation, which will only occur late in the second stage. If spontaneous rotation does not occur manual rotation of the head to the mento-anterior position is attempted under pudendal block or general anaesthesia, and after rotation delivery is completed with the forceps. The expert may prefer to use Kielland's forceps, with which the chin is rotated forwards while traction is applied.

Caesarean section is only necessary when there is some complication, such as a contracted pelvis or prolapse of the cord, or when the presenting part fails to descend. In a neglected case in which impaction has occurred, with obstructed labour and fetal death, the head can be perforated through the orbit to facilitate delivery.

The face is always somewhat swollen and discoloured after a face delivery, and the parents should be warned that it may be temporarily unsightly, but that complete recovery is to be expected.

Brow presentation

The causes of a primary brow presentation include those of a primary face presentation, but in some cases the reason for partial extension of the head

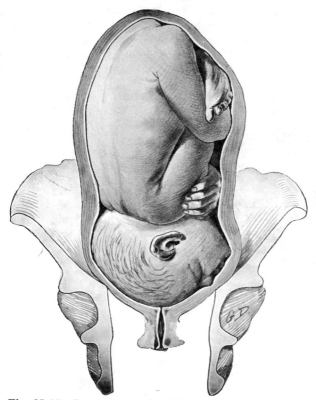

Fig. 25.10 Brow presentation. The head is above the brim and not engaged. The mento-vertical diameter of the head is trying to engage in the transverse diameter at the brim.

is not evident. All face presentations must pass through the stage of partial extension.

Two types of secondary extension occur, one at the level of the pelvic brim and the other at a lower level in the pelvis. Descent of the wider biparietal diameter of the head may be impossible if the pelvic brim is contracted, and the narrower anterior part of the head may descend a little into the pelvis, so that the head becomes partially extended.

Similarly in some cases of occipito-posterior position the wider occipital end of the head may lie in the sacro-cotyloid bay of the pelvis where it is held up, while the sinciput descends and extension of the head occurs in the cavity of the pelvis. This can only occur with a relatively small fetus.

A persistent brow presentation is fortunately rare. If a head of normal size lies with its longest diameter of 13 cm across the brim of a normal pelvis it cannot engage (Fig. 25.11). With a fetus of average size obstructed labour would result and there is no mechanism to describe. However, when the fetal head is small in proportion to the pelvis it may be driven down into the pelvic cavity and actually be born as a brow presentation.

With a brow presentation the head becomes very much moulded, with compression of the mento-vertical diameter and lengthening of the occipito-frontal diameter.

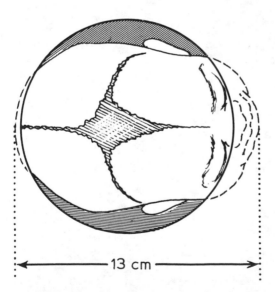

Fig. 25.11 Vaginal examination with brow presentation. The circle represents the pelvic cavity with a diameter of 1Γcm. The mento-vertical diameter of 13 cm is too large to permit engagement of the head.

Diagnosis

In cases in which extension of the head occurs early in labour the diagnosis may be difficult. On abdominal examination the head is above the brim, with some overlap, and the cephalic prominence is on the same side as the back. This malpresentation should always be suspected when non-engagement of the head is noted early in labour, particularly in the case of a patient who has had previous easy deliveries.

As a rule the membranes rupture early in labour, and there is some risk of prolapse of the cord. On vaginal examination, except in the case of extension of a head lying in the occipito-posterior position in the pelvic cavity, the presenting part will be high. The examining finger encounters the forehead, with the orbital ridges in front and the anterior fontanelle behind.

Management

In a few cases a brow presentation is discovered by x-ray examination performed to investigate a high head in the antenatal period. If there is no evidence of disproportion or any other abnormality nothing should be done, as in most cases the head will flex when labour starts, and spontaneous delivery will occur.

If the head is discovered to be partially extended in early labour and there is no evidence of severe disproportion a short trial of labour is permitted, and this may result in further extension of the head to a face presentation and engagement of the pelvic brim. If the head fails to engage or if there is evidence of disproportion Caesarean section is performed.

If the head has entered the pelvic cavity in an occipito-posterior position and undergone further extension there will be a brow presentation with the chin directed anteriorly. The cervix becomes fully dilated but the head is arrested. If the head is now rotated anteriorly so that the occiput becomes anterior flexion of the head occurs and vaginal delivery with forceps is usually easy. Rotation may be peformed manually or with Kielland's forceps.

Breech presentation

Breech presentation occurs in about 3 per cent of labours, but breech presentation is found more commonly than this before term. It is found in about 25 per cent of pregnancies at the 30th week, and so the incidence is higher in premature births. Spontaneous version occurs in all but a small number of cases by the 36th week.

There are two main varieties of breech presentation. In the commonest variety, especially in primigravidae, both hips are fully flexed but the

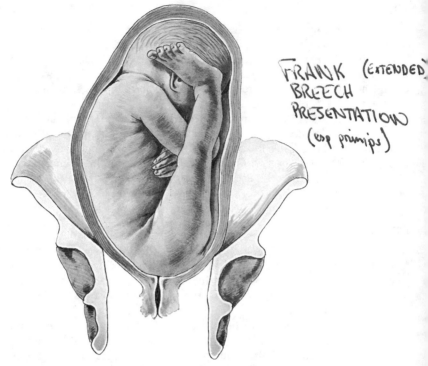

FRANK (EXTENDED) BREECH PRESENTATION (esp primips)

Fig. 25.12   Frank breech presentation with extension of the legs.

knees are extended (Fig. 25.12). This is called an *extended or frank breech*. If the legs are fully flexed at both hips and knees (Fig. 25.13) the term *flexed or complete breech* is applied.

In the course of obstetric manipulations one leg of a breech may be drawn down through the cervix while the other leg remains extended at the knee and flexed at the hip, when the term *half breech* is sometimes used.

With the breech with extended legs (frank breech) the buttocks accurately fit the lower segment and cervix and prolapse of the cord is an uncommon complication, whereas it may sometimes occur with a flexed breech.

Causation

In most instances breech presentation occurs by chance and there is no other underlying abnormality. Before the 30th week of pregnancy the uterine cavity is more or less spherical and the long axis of the fetus may lie in any direction. In late pregnancy the cavity is ovoid, with the fundus

Causes   1. Polyhydramnios
2. Multiparae ē lax muscles
3. Twins
4. Placenta praevia
5. CPD
6. Pelvic tumours

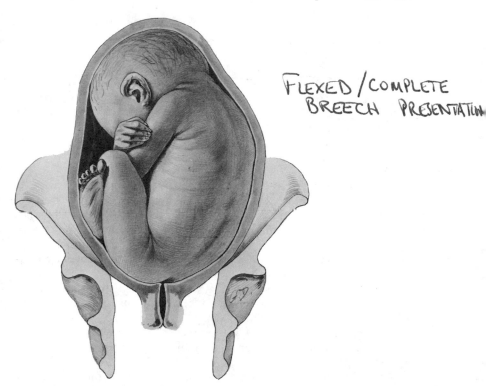

FLEXED / COMPLETE
BREECH PRESENTATION

Fig. 25.13 Complete breech presentation with flexion of the legs.

wider than the lower pole. Fetal movements normally turn the fetus until the flexed legs occupy the more spacious upper part of the cavity and the head fits into the narrower lower part. If kicking movements are ineffective because the legs are extended, or the frank breech becomes engaged in the pelvic brim, then a breech presentation will persist. Further fetal growth makes the free space in the uterus relatively less, so that spontaneous version becomes less possible as term is approached. Extension of the legs is probably the most common reason for persistent breech presentation.

If there is an excess of liquor free fetal movement may continue, and a breech presentation at term may occur by chance. For the same reason malpresentations are more common in multiparae with lax uterine and abdominal musculature.

With twin pregnancy either fetus may prevent the head of the other from engaging, and will also prevent free movement in the uterus, so that malpresentations are common.

1. Hydrocephalus
8 Bicornuate uterus.
EXTENSION OF LEGS

In a small proportion of cases some underlying abnormality will be discovered which prevents the head from entering the pelvis, and in some of these cases a breech presentation may occur. Such abnormalities include placenta praevia, contraction of the pelvic brim, and pelvic tumours. In the same way breech presentation may occur in cases of hydrocephalus. In rare cases in which pregnancy occurs in one horn of a double uterus breech presentation may occur because the horn tends to be narrow with the wider pole below.

Diagnosis

(a) During pregnancy. During pregnancy the diagnosis is made by abdominal examination. The fetal head is felt as a hard, spherical and easily movable object in the fundal region of the uterus. The patient may have noticed discomfort in this region. Admittedly the breech of a mature fetus may feel firm, but it is never so hard nor so movable as the head. If a considerable amount of liquor is present the head can be balloted from side to side between the two hands.

The fetal heart sounds are heard at a higher level than in the case of a cephalic presentation; at term the point of maximal intensity is at the level of or slightly above the umbilicus.

If the diagnosis is uncertain in late pregnancy vaginal examination may resolve it, but if doubt still remains a radiological or ultrasonic examination should be made.

(b) During labour. After rupture of the membranes additional information can be obtained by vaginal examination. In the case of a flexed breech a foot may present and the projection of the heel will distinguish it from a hand. With an extended breech the rounded buttocks superficially resemble a fetal head, but the hardness of bone is absent, and the anus and sacrum should be identifiable, and the scrotum in a male.

Mechanism of labour

Four positions of the breech are conventionally described: (1) Left sacro-anterior, (2) right sacro-anterior, (3) right sacro-posterior and (4) left sacro-posterior. However, in most cases the bitrochanteric diameter (10 cm) engages in the transverse diameter of the pelvic brim, with the back to the front. During labour the breech descends into the pelvic cavity and then internal rotation brings the bitrochanteric diameter into the antero-posterior diameter of the pelvic outlet. The breech is born by lateral flexion of the trunk, the anterior buttock appearing first. This movement of lateral flexion is determined by the curve of the birth canal, and more flexion is necessary with a rigid perineum. At one time it was thought that if the legs of the fetus were extended they splinted the trunk and prevented

4 positions
1. Left sacro anterior
2. Right sacro anterior
3. Left sacro ~~anterior~~ posterior
4. Right sacro ~~ante~~ posterior

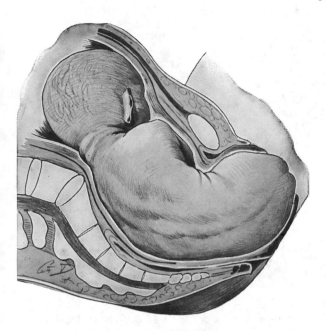

Fig. 25.14 Lateral flexion of the body during delivery of the breech. The anterior (right) buttock is under the pubic arch, and the posterior (left) is escaping over the perineum. The child's sacrum looks directly to the mother's right side, and the body is flexed round the symphysis. The shoulders are entering the pelvis in the oblique diameter so that there is also a slight twist on the body.

lateral flexion. This is not the case, and the frank breech usually descends easily. Its conical shape makes it a better dilator of the cervix than the rounded head.

The rest of the trunk is born by further descent, together with the arms which normally remain flexed in front of it. The anterior shoulder emerges first under the pubic arch and is quickly followed by the other. The flexed head engages in the transverse diameter of the pelvic brim. Forward rotation of the back occurs as the head descends into the pelvic cavity and then undergoes internal rotation, with the occiput coming to lie behind the symphysis pubis. The neck rests against the pubic arch as the head is born by the face sweeping over the perineum (fig. 25.15). Posterior rotation of the occiput occurs infrequently, and then the head is born face-to-pubes. This mechanism is less favourable as the larger occipito-frontal diameter of the head distends the vulva.

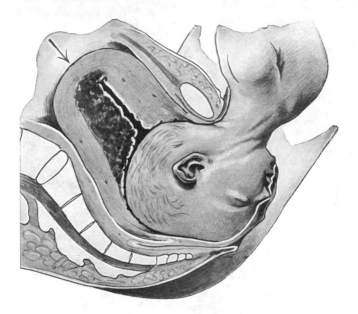

Fig. 25.15   Birth of the aftercoming head. The nape of the neck is under the symphysis, the chin is escaping over the perineum. In delivery the child's body is supported by holding the ankles. The arrow indicates the direction of maternal expulsive efforts. Sudden expulsion of the head may be prevented by gentle pressure on the brow.

Prognosis

The fetal mortality is higher in breech than in vertex delivery, even if complications such as contracted pelvis, placenta praevia, fetal abnormality or prematurity are excluded. In cases of complicated breech presentation, particularly those in which the fetus is premature, the fetal mortality may be as high as 20 per cent. In mature uncomplicated cases it is between 2 and 5 per cent. The increased mortality in mature uncomplicated cases is caused by (1) intracranial injury and (2) anoxia.

(1) Intracranial injury.   The risk of a tentorial tear and intracranial haemorrhage is greater with an aftercoming head. Less time is available for moulding, and rapid compression of a badly flexed head is particularly likely to produce this injury. Intracranial injury accounts for more than half the perinatal mortality in breech delivery.

Breech birth is particularly dangerous in the presence of even slight disproportion between the size of the pelvis and the head. Pelvic contraction should be diagnosed at antenatal examinations. If in a primigravida a breech presentation persists every effort should be made to prove that the pelvis is normal in shape and size, including taking a lateral x-ray view of the pelvis, before the onset of labour. In multiparae, even if the previous confinements have been normal and easy, there cannot be complete freedom from anxiety about breech delivery; the perinatal mortality rates for breech delivery are very similar in multiparae and primigravidae. A large fetus will cause difficulty as readily as a slightly contracted pelvis, and the fetus tends to increase in size with increasing parity.

(2) Fetal anoxia. Interference with the placental circulation may occur from compression of the umbilical cord by the aftercoming head during delivery, and also from uterine retraction which may separate the placenta before birth of the head. Delay in the delivery of the head for more than 10 minutes after the body has been born is very likely to endanger the baby's life from asphyxia. Even if the delay is not as long as this there is some risk to the fetus from premature inspiration with the aftercoming head undelivered, when mucus may be inhaled into the air passages and obstruct them after delivery.

Fetal asphyxia may also be caused by prolapse of the umbilical cord. This is rare with a frank breech, but more likely with a flexed breech.

Management

Because of the increased risk of a breech presentation every case must be under the management of someone with good obstetric experience, and all such cases must be delivered in hospital unless the presentation can be changed in the antenatal period by external version.

External cephalic version. External version means changing the fetal presentation by manual pressure through the mother's abdominal wall. It is desirable to correct a breech presentation by version so long as the operation does not itself increase the risk to the fetus. Version should not be attempted if there is:

1. Gross pelvic contraction, when Caesarean section is necessary. There is no purpose in attempting version in such a case, but in a case of doubtful disproportion version may be useful so that a trial labour can subsequently be conducted with the vertex presenting.
2. Placenta praevia or other cause of antepartum haemorrhage, because of the risk of causing further placental separation. Some consider that there is also a risk of antepartum haemorrhage in cases of hypertension and in patients who have previously threatened to miscarry.
3. A classical Caesarean or hysterotomy scar in the uterus.
4. Twin pregnancy, when version is prevented by the second twin.

There is also some risk of causing the passage of a few fetal red cells into the maternal circulation, and this might be important if the mother was rhesus negative and her husband rhesus positive.

External version should not be attempted before the 34th week, because in a large proportion of cases spontaneous cephalic version will occur. On

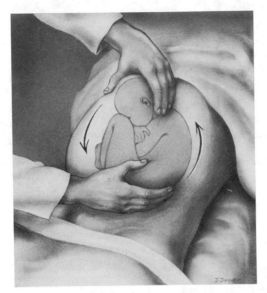

Fig. 25.16 External cephalic version. The breech has been disengaged from the pelvic inlet. Version is performed in the direction which increases flexion.

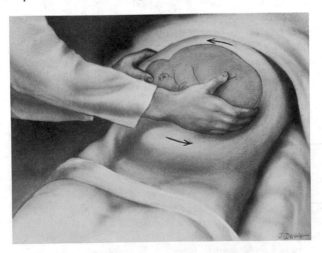

Fig. 25.17 External cephalic version, continued.

the other hand, after the 38th week version is unlikely to succeed because of the size of the fetus and the relative decrease in the volume of liquor. Factors which make version difficult are abdominal fat, failure of the patient to relax her abdominal muscles, uterine irritability, deep engagement of the breech and extension of the legs.

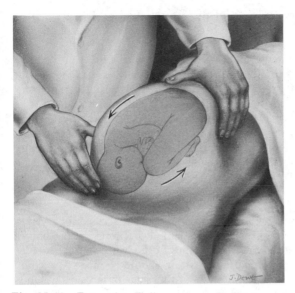

Fig. 25.18 External cephalic version completed.

Before version is attempted the exact position of the fetus must be determined by palpation, and the fetal heart auscultated. Relaxation of the abdominal muscles may be easier if the patient bends her knees slightly, and it is sometimes helpful to slope the head of the bed downwards for a time before attempting version as this may disengage the breech. The first step is to disengage the breech from the pelvic brim; if this cannot be done no further attempt at version should be made. The breech is pushed upward with the fingers of both hands, then pressed upward and laterally with one hand while the other hand presses on the head, displacing it in the direction which will increase flexion (Fig. 25.16). Only if the long axis of the fetus can be brought across the long axis of the uterus will version succeed. Steady pressure is more likely to be effective than jerky movements. After any attempt at version, successful or otherwise, the fetal heart rate should be counted.

If version failed it used to be common practice to give an anaesthetic in the hope of relaxing the abdominal muscles and the uterus. The only anaesthetic agents now in common use that will relax the uterus (as distinct from the abdominal muscles) are ether, cyclopropane and fluothane (Halothane). The last is often preferred although it carries some risk of hepatic necrosis. Anaesthesia for version has the great disadvantage that increased force is liable to be used on the uncomplaining patient, with a risk of placental separation or premature labour. Some obstetricians still use anaesthesia for selected cases, but the majority do not use it. If an anaesthetic is given, and version fails, a thorough assessment of the pelvis is possible, so that a decision about the best method of delivery can be made. Immediately after version the head is high and not engaged, and this should not be taken as evidence of disproportion.

Before discussing the management of vaginal breech delivery it must be asked whether, in view of the fetal risk, Caesarean section should not always be preferred. In experienced hands the fetal risk of breech delivery may not greatly exceed that of cephalic delivery, and the maternal risk is increased by section. Yet because unexpected fetal deaths occur with vaginal breech delivery there is today an increasing use of Caesarean section, both electively before labour and during labour if any difficulty arises. We return to this topic on p. 289.

Management of vaginal breech delivery

The conduct of the first stage of labour is exactly as described for a vertex presentation. Early rupture of the membranes may occur, as the presenting part, particularly of a flexed breech, may not fit the brim well. As soon as the membranes rupture a vaginal examination should be made to exclude prolapse of the umbilical cord. Throughout this stage of labour a watch is kept, as always, for failure of progress or any evidence of maternal or fetal distress.

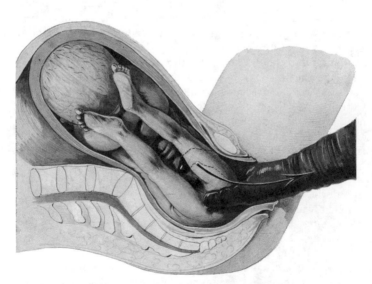

Fig. 25.19   Traction of the anterior groin in a sacro-lateral position of the breech with extended legs. The breech has descended deeply into the pelvis so traction with a finger in the groin completes the delivery usually after an episiotomy has been performed.

In the second stage a vaginal examination must always be made to confirm full dilatation before the patient is allowed to bear down. Spontaneous descent of the breech onto the pelvic floor usually occurs, whether the legs are extended or not. When the breech reaches the pelvic floor the patient should be placed in the lithotomy position. Episiotomy is performed as a routine so that the intact perineum will not provide any obstacle to the delivery of the breech, and to facilitate the ultimate delivery of the fetal head. Epidural analgesia is excellent for these cases, but if it is not used then a pudendal block or local infiltration is necessary for the episiotomy.

In the case of a flexed breech the feet and legs present and as they appear they are eased out. If the legs are extended the anterior buttock first becomes visible. The minimum of assistance is given by digital traction in the anterior groin (Fig. 25.19) and by traction in the posterior groin as the breech is born. Traction should only be made when the uterus is contracting. Delivery of the breech will nearly always occur by this method.

Arrest of descent of the breech. It is uncommon for the breech to be arrested before it has descended into the pelvic cavity. This event demands immediate examination to determine the cause, which is usually contraction of the pelvis or an unduly large fetus. The difficulty might be overcome by breech extraction, but in nearly every instance, except for the delivery of a second twin when the birth canal is fully dilated, Caesarean section is preferable. Breech extraction of a large fetus, or delivery through an incompletely dilated cervix, gives disastrous results.

For breech extraction (as might be performed for a second twin), the patient is anaesthetized and her bladder is emptied. The whole hand is inserted and the breech is pushed up to the level of the pelvic brim. The anterior leg is brought down through the cervix first, by pressing into the popliteal space and abducting the thigh. This will flex the knee, and the foot can be grasped and brought down. The posterior leg is then brought down in the same way. Unless each leg is first flexed, pulling on the knee may fracture the femur. Delivery can now proceed, only applying traction to the legs if there is not spontaneous progress.

Delivery of the trunk and head. As soon as the umbilicus is born pulsation of the cord can be observed. Compression of the cord by the side walls of the birth canal may sometimes cause spasm of the umbilical vessels and obliterate the fetal pulse, but the fetal heart sounds can still be heard through the abdominal wall. Absence of pulsations during delivery is not an immediate indication for haste; too rapid extraction of the fetus may cause death from intracranial haemorrhage.

A finger should be inserted into the vagina to make certain that the arms are lying folded on the chest. As delivery of the shoulders proceeds the baby's body is allowed to hang down to exert slight traction in the direction of the pelvic axis. As soon as the head has descended onto the pelvic floor and the nape of the neck can be seen below the pubic arch, the baby's legs are held just above the ankles, and by exerting slight traction its body

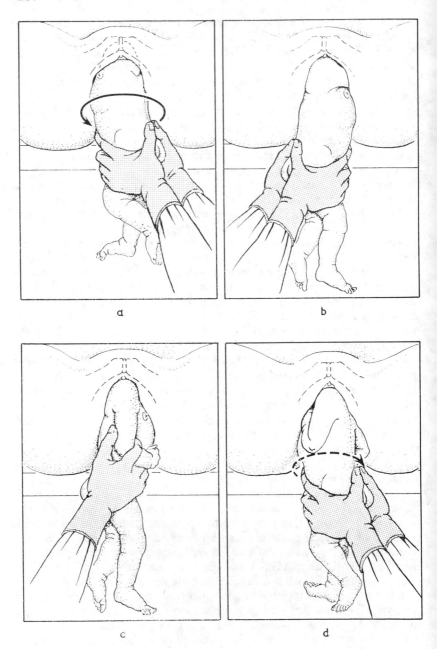

Fig. 25.20   Løvset's manoeuvre.

is lifted to the horizontal position. The face will then appear at the vulva and, as the baby can now breathe, the head can be delivered slowly and carefully. Lifting the baby's body upwards before the head has passed completely through the brim will not assist delivery, and may injure the cervical spine. In many units forceps are used routinely for the delivery of the head as described below.

Extension of the arms. Spontaneous delivery may not occur if the arms are extended. This should be suspected if descent of the fetus is not continuous after delivery of the thorax, and if the arms cannot be felt in the pelvic cavity. This complication must be dealt with at once by Løvset's manoeuvre. This depends on the facts that as a result of the curvature of the birth canal the posterior shoulder must be at a lower level than the anterior shoulder, and that the subpubic arch is the shallowest part of the pelvis. By downward traction the anterior shoulder is brought to lie behind the symphysis pubis so that the inferior angle of the scapula can be seen (Fig. 25.20). When this is done the posterior shoulder will lie below the promontory of the sacrum and below the pelvic brim. The pelvic girdle and thighs are then firmly held with both hands and the fetus is turned through 180° with the back upwards, while moderate traction is maintained. By this means the posterior arm is brought to the front and inevitably appears under the pubic arch. The arm may be delivered spontaneously; otherwise it is easily hooked out with a finger. The other shoulder, which previously lay anteriorly and above the brim of the pelvis, now lies in the hollow of the sacrum. The fetus, therefore, is rotated through 180° in the opposite direction, the fetal back again being kept upwards. The remaining arm will appear under the pubic arch and can easily be delivered.

Difficulty with the aftercoming head. After the birth of the shoulders the flexed head normally enters the pelvis in the transverse diameter of the brim. As descent occurs the head undergoes internal rotation so that the occiput comes to lie behind the symphysis pubis. The neck rests under the pubic arch and normally the head is born by a movement of flexion. In most cases the head is brought into the pelvis by allowing the fetal trunk to hang downwards for not more than one minute. Any failure of descent or difficulty in the delivery of the head calls for immediate assistance. The body of the baby having been born, the placental circulation is impaired by retraction of the uterus and pressure on the cord, and respiratory efforts will certainly be made. If the birth is not completed within the next few minutes death from asphyxia is likely. The obstetric forceps must be available for immediate use at every breech delivery whenever the descent of the head is arrested. The body of the baby is lifted well forward by an assistant and the blades are applied beneath it. The fingers of the right hand steer the left blade of the forceps to the left side of the pelvis, and then the right blade is applied. Only moderate traction

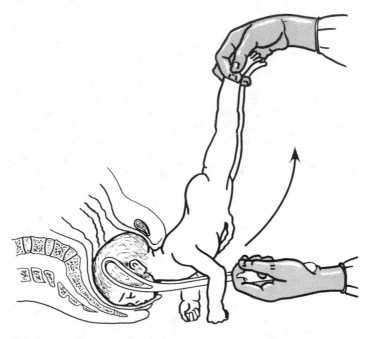

Fig. 25.21   Delivery of the aftercoming head with forceps.

should be required to complete delivery as episiotomy has already been performed.

Very rarely the fetal head cannot be made to enter the pelvic brim. This means that an error of judgment has been made and pelvic contraction has been overlooked (or very rarely that hydrocephalus is present). Apart from the fact that the head may be lying transversely, flexion will almost certainly be poor, and the application of forceps at this level would be difficult and dangerous. The best hope of saving a desperate situation is to pass one hand up in front of the fetal thorax, where one finger presses on the jaw to produce flexion. The other hand is passed along the back until the index and middle fingers can curve over the shoulders to exert traction (Fig. 25.22). The head is drawn down by traction on the shoulders, and if necessary rotated until the neck lies under the pubic arch. Delivery may then be completed with forceps as already described. This sort of traction may cause injury to the cervical spine or to the brachial plexus.

Difficulty at the pelvic outlet may occur if it is contracted, or if the occiput has rotated posteriorly. Delivery is achieved with forceps. If the occiput lies posteriorly and cannot be rotated the forceps are applied in front of the baby's body, which is supported by an assistant.

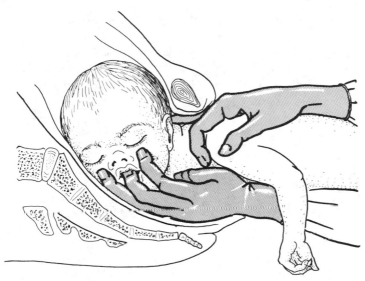

Fig. 25.22 Jaw and shoulder traction applied to a fetus with the head at the level of the pelvic brim. Forceps could not be applied at this level.

The place of Caesarean section for breech delivery

It is evident from the preceding description of breech delivery that damage to the fetus may occur even though it is born alive. Morbidity is difficult to measure, but follow-up studies of infants after breech delivery show an increased incidence of physical and mental retardation. This fact is appreciated by many women, and with their knowledge of the increased mortality, prompts them to request delivery by Caesarean section. Some obstetricians would agree, and regard breech presentation as an indication for elective Caesarean section, and they point out that even if labour is allowed to start many cases will require section for delay or fetal distress.

Even if this view is not wholly accepted it is generally agreed that any additional complication during pregnancy, or anything untoward in the patient's history, is an indication for section. Caesarean section would be advised for any primigravida over 35 years of age, and for any woman who has previously been infertile or has had stillbirths.

Pelvic contraction, even if it is only slight, is an indication for section, including any case with a true conjugate of less than 10 cm. An android pelvis is particularly unfavourable.

Caesarean section would also be performed in cases associated with placenta praevia, and in cases of prolapse of the cord before full dilatation of the cervix.

Transverse and oblique lie (shoulder presentation)

The fetus may lie with its long axis transverse or oblique in the uterus, when the point of the shoulder is usually the presenting part. After rupture of the membranes an arm may prolapse. Shoulder presentations occur about once in 500 labours.

Cause

The commonest cause of an oblique lie is multiparity associated with a lax uterus and abdominal wall. It is not infrequently found on antenatal examination before 36 weeks and it is therefore more common in cases in which labour starts prematurely. An oblique lie may be found with hydramnios or multiple pregnancy, and may be caused by anything which prevents engagement of the fetal head, such as contracted pelvis, placenta praevia or a pelvic tumour. If a transverse lie occurs in a primigravida or recurs in successive pregnancies the possibility that it is due to a uterine malformation (arcuate or subseptate uterus) must be considered.

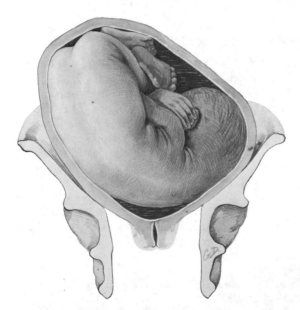

Fig. 25.23 Shoulder presentation: dorso-anterior position. The head is in the left iliac fossa, the back lies anteriorly and obliquely, and the breech is on the right above the right iliac fossa.

Positions

The fetus may lie with the head in either iliac fossa, with the back sloping obliquely across the pelvic brim, while the breech usually occupies a somewhat higher position than the head, on the opposite side of the abdomen. Only two positions are described, dorso-anterior and dorso-posterior, the former being the more common.

Diagnosis

On abdominal examination the uterus appears asymmetrical, and is broader than usual with the fundus lower than expected for the duration of pregnancy. On palpation the hard round head is felt in one iliac fossa, with

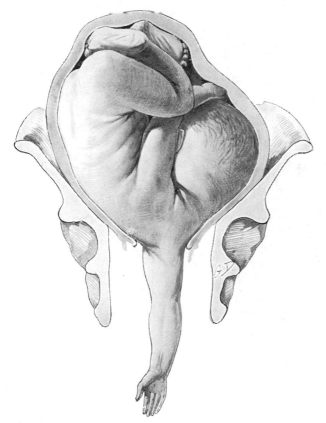

Fig. 25.24 Shoulder presentation with prolapse of arm. The shoulder and arm, forming the apex of the wedge, are driven into the brim; the head and neck on the one side and the trunk on the other form the sides of the wedge.

the softer breech on the opposite side. No presenting part is felt over the brim. In the centre of the abdomen the back will be felt in dorso-anterior positions, and small parts in dorso-posterior positions. The fetal heart sounds are usually heard just below the umbilicus (Fig. 25.23).

On vaginal examination at the beginning of labour the presenting part is too high to be felt. During labour the membranes usually rupture early. When the cervix becomes dilated an arm or a loop of cord may prolapse. Diagnosis of a shoulder presentation depends on recognition of the acromion process, scapula and adjacent ribs. A prolapsed arm must be distinguished from a leg; the elbow is sharper than the knee, and absence of a heel and abduction of the thumb will distinguish a hand from a foot.

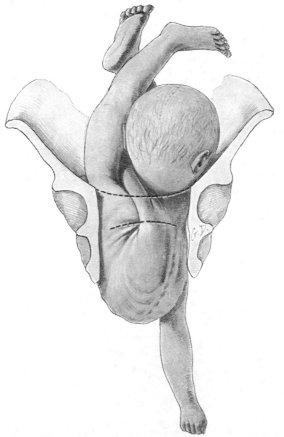

Fig. 25.25   Spontaneous evolution. The body is squeezed past the head by extreme flexion; the ribs distend the perineum, whilst the breech occupies the sacral hollow.

Course of labour

A fetus lying obliquely cannot be born naturally unless it is macerated or very premature. There is no true mechanism of labour, and an untreated case will end in obstructed labour and fetal death.

Spontaneous rectification to a vertex or more rarely a breech presentation may sometimes occur in early labour, but cannot do so after prolapse of an arm. Spontaneous delivery may rarely occur with a macerated or very premature infant when the body is delivered doubled up (Fig. 25.25).

Prognosis

Neglected or unrecognized shoulder presentations are extremely serious, since all the risks of obstructed labour are present, including rupture of the uterus. In the case of the fetus, death is usual from interference with the placental circulation or prolapse of the cord. A few cases will be associated with placenta praevia, contracted pelvis or pelvic tumour.

Treatment

During pregnancy. During pregnancy an oblique lie should be corrected by external version to a vertex presentation. In a multigravida with a lax uterus the malpresentation often recurs, and for such an *unstable lie* repeated version may be necessary. After the 38th week the patient is admitted to hospital, so that external cephalic version may be performed and a Syntocinon infusion started. When the uterus starts to contract regularly the correction of the malpresentation is checked, and if the head is over the pelvic brim the membranes are ruptured. To reduce the risk of prolapse of the cord the patient should be kept in bed until labour is well established with the head in the pelvis.

If an oblique lie is secondary to a contracted pelvis, placenta praevia or pelvic tumour Caesarean section will be required.

During early labour. If an oblique lie is discovered early in labour it may still be corrected by external version if the membranes are intact. Once the lie has been corrected the membranes should be ruptured and the uterine contractions will usually maintain a longitudinal lie. If an oblique or transverse lie persists in labour Caesarean section is performed, being safer than the dangerous operation of internal podalic version, in which a leg of the fetus is pulled down and it is then delivered as a breech.

Late in labour when the shoulder has become impacted. In neglected cases when the uterus is tonically retracted any form of version is extremely dangerous, owing to the very great risk of rupturing the thinned out lower uterine segment. If the fetus is alive, which is seldom the case, Caesarean section may be considered. If the fetus is dead the usual procedure is decapitation (see p. 408). After division of the neck of the fetus the trunk can be delivered by traction on the prolapsed arm and head with forceps.

Compound presentations

Prolapse of a limb with a vertex presentation is known as a compound presentation. Commonly it is a hand which comes down, very rarely a foot. Prolapse of an arm occurs when the head does not fit the brim well. If the head is not low in the pelvic cavity the arm often goes back as the head descends, and active treatment is not required. If the head is lower in the pelvis and its progress is arrested the arm should be replaced under anaesthesia. Delivery is completed with forceps if the cervix is fully dilated.

When a foot presents with the head it may be pushed up under anaesthesia, or it may be better to pull on the foot and push up the head, turning the fetus into a breech presentation.

Fetal malformations that cause difficulty in labour

These are mentioned in this chapter to complete the discussion of fetal causes of dystocia.

Hydrocephaly.   This may be discovered during pregnancy if the head is noticed to be unduly large, or during the course of investigation of suspected disproportion. Radiological examination will make the diagnosis. During labour the wide separation of the cranial bones at the sutures may be recognized on vaginal examination. As the head cannot enter the pelvis a breech presentation may occur.

Obstruction during labour is treated by perforation of the head (see p. 404).

Iniencephaly.   In this abnormality the head is hyperextended and the tissues over the occiput and sacrum are fused. It is recognized radiographically. Induction before the 32nd week may avoid the need for Caesarean section.

Anencephaly.   In some cases of anencephaly difficulty in delivery of the shoulders may occur, because they have not been preceded by a head of normal size. There should be no hesitation in performing cleidotomy and applying strong traction in the axilla.

Conjoined twins.   Conjunction of twins may be suspected during pregnancy if ultrasonic or radiological examination shows that the twins constantly maintain the same relative positions, especially if they are facing one another. In other cases the diagnosis is made during twin labour when

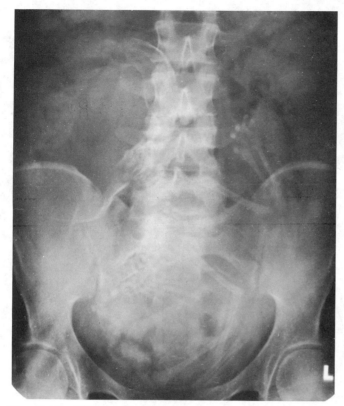

Fig. 25.26   X-Ray shows typical appearance of hydrocephalus. Note wide separation of bones of the vault of the skull; also the large size of the fetal head in comparison with other fetal bones.

there is delay and a hand is passed into the uterus to determine the cause. Surprisingly, vaginal delivery has not infrequently been reported when the twins have been small and the junction between them has been fairly pliable, but in most cases Caesarean section is unavoidable, and is preferable to embryotomy.

26

Pelvic abnormalities and cephalo-pelvic disproportion

Pelvic abnormalities

The size of the female pelvis is of primary importance; if it is large enough there will be no difficulty in the passage of the fetal head through it. The shape of the pelvis is of secondary importance, and only has a bearing on the mechanism of labour and the ease of delivery if the pelvic dimensions are small in relation to those of the head passing through it.

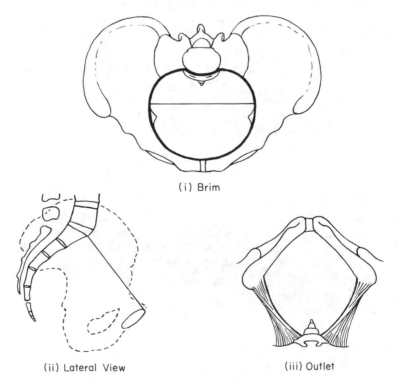

(i) Brim

(ii) Lateral View

(iii) Outlet

Fig. 26.1   The gynaecoid pelvis.

Certain terms are used to describe variations in the shape of the pelvis which were discovered by anatomical and radiological studies. Very few pelves fit the criteria exactly, and any pelvis may be a mixture of the types about to be described.

1. The *gynaecoid pelvis* conforms to the accepted female type in that the brim is rounded, with the widest transverse diameter slightly behind its centre (Fig. 26.1). The subpubic arch is rounded, with an angle of at least 90 degrees.

2. The *android pelvis* has many of the characteristics of the male pelvis. The brim is heart-shaped, so that the widest transverse diameter is much nearer to the sacrum than it is in the gynaecoid pelvis (Fig. 26.2). The side walls tend to converge, and the subpubic arch is generally narrow, with an angle of 70 degrees or less. Both the antero-posterior and transverse diameters of the outlet tend to be reduced. This type of pelvis is funnel-shaped, with diameters which decrease from above downwards, and disproportion thus becomes worse as labour proceeds.

3. The *anthropoid pelvis*. The antero-posterior diameter of the brim exceeds the transverse diameter (Fig. 26.3). The pelvis tends to be deep

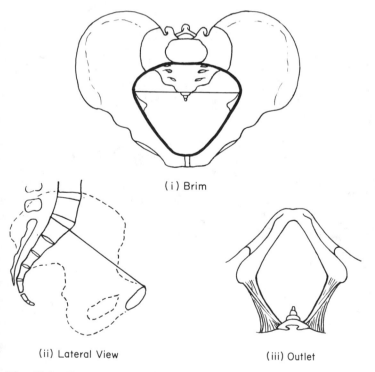

(i) Brim

(ii) Lateral View

(iii) Outlet

Fig. 26.2 The android pelvis.

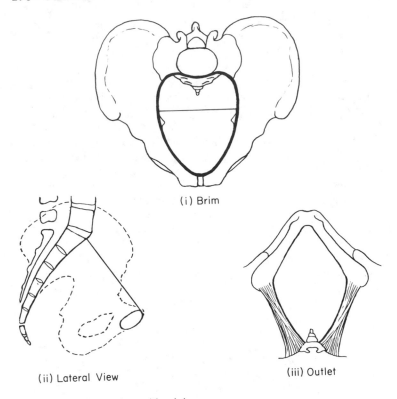

(i) Brim

(ii) Lateral View

(iii) Outlet

Fig. 26.3 The anthropoid pelvis.

and the sacrum often has six segments instead of five; this is known as a high assimilation pelvis. Very often the sacrum and the axis of the pelvis cavity are less curved than in the gynaecoid pelvis, and the subpubic arch may be a little narrow, but the sacro-sciatic notches are wide and the antero-posterior diameter of the outlet is large, so there is no difficulty.

4. The *platypelloid pelvis* is described as the simple (non-rachitic) flat pelvis. The brim is elliptical with a wide transverse diameter (Fig. 26.4). The subpubic arch is wide and rounded.

It is emphasized that, except in the case of the android pelvis, these variations in shape have little effect on the normal mechanism of labour unless there is considerable reduction in the size of the pelvis. The android pelvis is the least favourable because of the tendency to contraction of the outlet. The anthropoid pelvis favours engagement of the head in the antero-posterior diameter of the brim, and if it is in the occipito-posterior position it may fail to undergo internal rotation, but it is usually delivered face-to-pubes without difficulty.

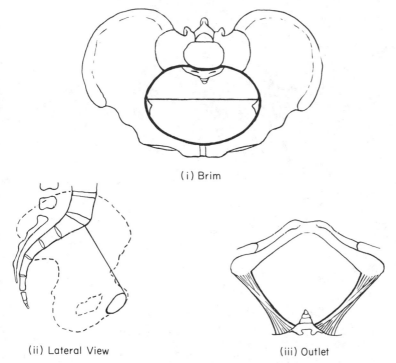

(i) Brim

(ii) Lateral View

(iii) Outlet

Fig. 26.4 The platypelloid pelvis.

Abnormalities of the pelvis

Abnormalities of the pelvis may be classified into 3 groups:
1. Those caused by developmental abnormalities of the pelvis.
2. Those caused by disease or injury of the pelvic bones.
3. Those caused by abnormalities of the spine, hip joints or lower limbs.

Developmental abnormalities of the pelvic bones. Developmental variations in shape have already been described, and the android pelvis is the only one of these that commonly affects labour adversely. However, even a round gynaecoid pelvis may be small in size, and is then called a *generally contracted pelvis*.

The presence of a 6th segment in the sacrum which may be found with an anthropoid pelvis has given rise to the term *high assimilation pelvis*, but this is not of great significance.

Very rarely malformation of the pelvis may result from defective development of one side of the sacrum, which is fused with the ilium. This is known as the *oblique pelvis of Naegele*, and if bilateral as the *transversely contracted pelvis of Robert* (see Figs. 26.5, 26.6).

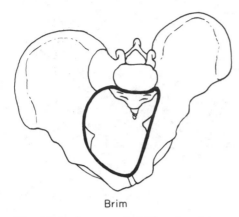

Brim

Fig. 26.5　Asymmetrical Naegele pelvis.

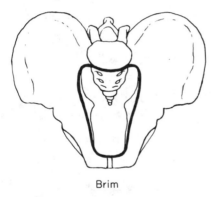

Brim

Fig. 26.6　Transversely contracted, Robert's pelvis.

Disease or injury of the pelvic bones.　The most important abnormality in this group is rickets, which causes softening of the bones in early childhood, with flattening of the pelvic brim (Fig. 26.7). Fortunately rickets is becoming uncommon in this country. A similar disease, osteomalacia, which may occur in adults, can cause very severe distortion of the pelvis; it is almost unknown in Britain, but may still occur in Africa and Asia.

Pelvic deformity may be caused by malunited fractures, or by new growths arising from the pelvic bones.

Abnormalities of the spine, hip joints and lower limbs.　The shape and inclination of the pelvis may be affected by kyphosis of the spine or spondylolisthesis (Figs. 26.8, 26.9).

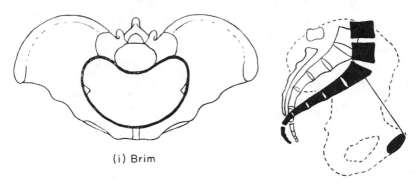

(i) Brim

(ii) Lateral View
(Showing forward displacement
of the sacral promontory)

Fig. 26.7 Rachitic pelvis.

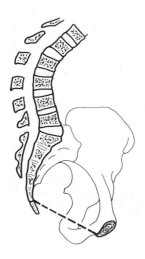

Fig. 26.8 Kyphosis with forward rotation of the lower part of the sacrum and reduction of the antero-posterior diameter of the pelvic outlet.

Disease of a hip joint, particularly congenital dislocation, and abnormalities of the lower limbs which alter the distribution of weight and tilt the pelvis, may cause an oblique distortion of the pelvis. This is unlikely to occur unless the disease was present before the completion of bone growth at about 17 years. As scoliosis is usually present such a pelvis has been described as a scoliotic pelvis, although the pelvic deformity is not caused by the scoliosis.

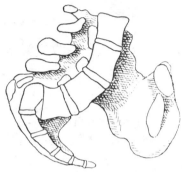

Fig. 26.9   Spondylolisthetic pelvis.

Labour in the presence of pelvic abnormality

The course of labour in a woman with an abnormal pelvis will depend to some degree on the type of abnormality but far more on the degree of disproportion. When the size of the fetal head exceeds the size of the pelvis even after moulding has taken place normal vaginal delivery will clearly be impossible. If, however, there is not absolute disproportion vaginal delivery may occur if the uterine contractions are sufficiently strong to overcome the relatively increased resistance.

In practice the type of deformity is less important than the size of the pelvis relative to that of the head. The management of labour will depend on this relationship and on the strength of the uterine contractions. The mechanism of the passage of the head through the pelvis will differ according to the shape of the pelvis, but in general there is a tendency with most pelvic abnormalities for the fore-pelvis to be small, thus increasing the risk of persistent occipito-posterior positions or deep transverse arrest. If vaginal delivery has to be assisted with forceps, delivery of the fetus in the occipito-posterior position (face-to-pubes) may be preferable to rotation to the anterior position if the transverse diameters of the pelvis are reduced, as in a small android or anthropoid pelvis.

Cephalo-pelvic disproportion

Disproportion between the size of the fetal head and that of the maternal pelvis will cause difficult labour and danger to the fetus. The size of the head at term is genetically related to the size of the maternal pelvis—small women tend to have small babies—so that in the absence of pelvic deformity the majority of labours proceed without mechanical difficulty. However, the obstetrician must always be on the lookout for possible disproportion, both in the antenatal clinic and during labour.

In cases of disproportion it is usually found that the pelvic inlet presents the most difficulty. If the widest diameter of the head will pass through the inlet it will usually pass through the pelvic cavity and outlet. Occasionally the pelvis is to some degree funnel-shaped with a narrower outlet than inlet, but even in this case the head will often pass because by the time it has reached the outlet its diameters have been reduced by moulding. In every case of disproportion the efficiency of the uterine contractions plays a major part in determining whether vaginal delivery will occur.

The diagnosis of disproportion

The diagnosis of disproportion is made on the basis of the previous obstetric history, digital vaginal examination of the pelvis and an assessment of the degree of descent of the head through the pelvic inlet in late pregnancy. In the past many patients also had radiological pelvimetry, but recently in developed countries it has been found that it is comparatively rare for a patient to have a pelvis too small to allow the passage of a normal sized fetus, provided that there are good uterine contractions. This, together with an increasing reluctance to subject the fetus to x-rays, has led to a change in emphasis in the diagnosis and management of disproportion.

The following are the steps in the antenatal diagnosis of disproportion:

Past obstetric history. A distinction is made between primigravidae and multigravidae. In a multigravida the pelvis has been tested up to the size of the largest baby previously delivered. In a primigravida the quality of the pelvis is unknown, and the uterine contractions may be less efficient than in a multigravida. Disproportion in a multigravida is usually because she has a fetus larger than any she has previously borne; in a primigravida the factor preventing vaginal delivery is likely to be inadequate uterine action. In dealing with a multigravida, therefore, it is important to obtain details of her previous labours, including for each the duration, the mode of delivery, the outcome and the birth weight of the child.

General examination. Although it is true that small women may have small babies, it is also true that small women have small pelves and a greater chance of disproportion. Any woman whose height is less than 150 cm comes into this category. Small stature is sometimes the result of poor nutrition and poor social conditions in childhood. In recent years the height of young women in Great Britain has been increasing as a result of rising standards of living, especially in the lower social classes.

Any skeletal abnormality, or evidence of previous bony or paralytic disease of the lower limbs, pelvis or spine should be noted in view of any possible effect on the shape of the pelvis.

Abdominal examination. Abdominal examination in late pregnancy should indicate whether or not the widest diameter of the fetal head has passed through the pelvic inlet. Many obstetricians now denote the relation of the head to the inlet in 'fifths' (see p. 102). When the biparietal diameter has passed through the inlet it is said that only 2/5 of the head remains above the brim, and the head is relatively immobile. In primigravidae the head normally engages between the 36th and 38th weeks. In multigravidae engagement often does not occur until labour starts.

In African races the pelvic inlet has a higher angle of inclination (p. 80) than in Caucasian and Asian races, and because of this in African women engagement of the head is uncommon before the onset of labour, even in primigravidae.

If the head is not engaged before term an attempt is made to discover it if will engage, and thus to exclude inlet disproportion. This may be done by moderate pressure on the head in a backwards and downwards direction. Another method is to raise the patient's head and shoulders half-way to the sitting position, asking her to take the weight of her trunk on her elbows while the head is palpated. Perhaps the most certain way to test whether the head will engage is to examine the patient when she is standing.

Pelvic examination. Vaginal examination in early pregnancy is chiefly performed to assess the size of the uterus and to detect any soft-tissue abnormalities. Vaginal examination should be repeated at the 36th week to examine the pelvic cavity and outlet.

The normal pelvic inlet is beyond the range of the examining fingers; only in a grossly contracted pelvis can the sacral promontory be reached. The concavity or straightness of the sacrum, and the convergence or separation of the side walls of the pelvis, may give some idea of the size of the pelvic cavity. The bony outlet can be readily palpated, and the width or the subpubic arch and the ease with which the ischial spines can be felt should be noted. The distance between the ischial tuberosities can be measured, and the antero-posterior diameter of the outlet between the lower margin of the symphysis pubis and the sacro-coccygeal joint.

The fetal head is the best pelvimeter. If it has already descended into the pelvis or can be made to do so on examination there is only the pelvic outlet left for it to pass. Pure outlet contraction is very rare, and if the biparietal diameter enters the pelvic inlet with only two 'fifths' or less of the head palpable abdominally, with the lowest point of the head at the level of the ischial spines, disproportion is extremely unlikely.

If the head will not enter the pelvis disproportion may be suspected but in many cases, with strong uterine contractions and moulding of the head, vaginal delivery will occur. Pelvic examination is of limited value in predicting the outcome as so much depends on the moulding and the efficiency of the contractions.

Diagnosis of disproportion during labour. Failure of the head to descend and of the cervix to dilate during labour may indicate unsuspected disproportion. Excessive moulding and caput formation may occur, and in some cases the caput may be felt at the level of the ischial spines even though the head has still not passed through the pelvic inlet.

In modern practice, if a partogram (p. 116) indicates that the cervix is not dilating normally the effect of an oxytocic drip is likely to be tried, unless examination shows clear evidence of disproportion. If augmentation of the uterine action does not lead to progress in cervical dilatation a diagnosis of disproportion or some other mechanical obstruction is probable.

Radiological diagnosis of disproportion. X-rays are now much less often used to investigate suspected disproportion than formerly. They have the same inability as clinical examination to predict uterine efficiency in labour, and in addition may have undesirable effects on the maternal gonads and the fetus. Present-day practice is only to x-ray the pelvis when severe disproportion is strongly suspected, and then only to use one lateral

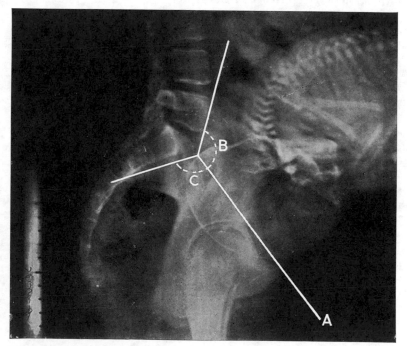

Fig. 26.10 A lateral X-ray of the pelvis, the fetus is in an occipito-posterior position. **A.** Plane of the inlet. **B.** Angle of the inclination of the pelvic brim. **C.** Angle of inclination of the sacrum.

radiograph taken in late pregnancy with the patient standing. This view allows measurement of the antero-posterior diameters of the pelvis but not of the transverse diameters. The latter can be measured by taking further views of the pelvic inlet and outlet, but these are not now thought to be justified in view of the limited information gained and the additional irradiation of the fetus. Apart from the antero-posterior diameters, the erect lateral radiograph also shows the curve of the sacrum, the angle of inclination of the pelvic brim and the degree of engagement of the fetal head.

X-rays are no longer used during labour for the diagnosis of disproportion, as they add nothing to the clinical assessment of progress.

The management of disproportion

When cephalo-pelvic disproportion is suspected as a result of antenatal examination a decision has to be taken whether or not to allow the patient to go into labour in the hope of vaginal delivery, or to deliver her before the onset of labour by elective Caesarean section.

Indications for elective Caesarean section. The indications are:
1. Disproportion so severe that vaginal delivery is unlikely.
2. Lesser degrees of disproportion when there are complicating factors such as breech presentation, previous Caesarean section, or a previous difficult vaginal delivery causing perinatal death or morbidity.
3. In older women, especially those with a long history of infertility, and women with medical complications such as diabetes.

Trial of labour. Except for the cases just mentioned, patients with disproportion should be allowed a 'trial of labour'. By this is meant that the patient's progress in labour is carefully watched for evidence of continuing progress as shown by progressive dilatation of the cervix and descent of the head. The assessment of progress is made as in normal labour by repeated abdominal and vaginal examinations, and the results are recorded on a partogram (see p. 116).

In the majority of cases of suspected disproportion good uterine contractions will bring about steady progress to vaginal delivery. In multiparous patients particularly the head may remain high until the cervix is fully dilated and then descend rapidly through the pelvis during the second stage.

Augmentation of labour in cases of suspected disproportion. Good uterine contractions are essential if mild disproportion is to be overcome. In primigravidae delay in labour caused by poor uterine action may be treated by the cautious use of an intravenous oxytocic infusion (see p. 316). Great care must be taken to avoid overstimulation leading to excessively strong contractions which may harm the fetus, or even occasionally rupture the uterus (see below). Continuous monitoring of the fetal heart rate with a scalp electrode and a ratemeter, as well as continuous recording of the uterine contractions, by the methods described on p. 411 are desirable whenever labour is being augmented, but are particularly important in cases of possible disproportion.

Deciding when a trial of labour has failed. Although no hard and fast rules can be laid down, failure to progress in a trial of labour after a period of four hours or more of good contractions suggests that the disproportion is too great to be overcome, and that Caesarean section should be performed.

The trial may also have to be terminated at any time if fetal distress develops.

Uterine rupture is a rare event in primigravidae, but less rare in multigravidae. It usually only occurs after some hours of strong contractions. The development of a Bandl's ring (p. 320), pain and tenderness over the lower uterine segment, or acute fetal distress are all indications of impending rupture and call for immediate Caesarean section.

The management of trial of labour for suspected disproportion should be under the control of an experienced obstetrician in a fully equipped unit, as considerable skill and judgment may be needed to decide how long the labour may safely continue.

Forceps delivery and disproportion. Because pure outlet contraction is uncommon a trial of labour will usually succeed once the head has passed through the pelvic inlet and the cervix has reached full dilatation. In women with android pelves disproportion is often further complicated by an occipito-posterior position of the head. Although long forward rotation of the head may occur spontaneously, arrest of the rotation with the sagittal suture in the transverse diameter of the pelvis (deep transverse arrest) or persistence of the posterior position may occur. There will then be delay in the second stage of labour. Even when the occiput has rotated anteriorly, minor degrees of disproportion may prevent the patient from delivering the fetus by her own expulsive efforts.

In such cases forceps delivery after manual rotation, or after rotation with Kielland's forceps, requires skill and judgment on the part of the obstetrician and is best conducted in an operating theatre with everything prepared to proceed to Caesarean section if difficulty arises (*'trial of forceps'*). Delivery of the head in the occipito-posterior position is sometimes preferable to difficult rotation if the vertex is below the level of the ischial spines. The obstetrician must be careful about the force he uses to effect rotation and delivery with the forceps, as there is considerable risk of causing intracranial damage by tearing the tentorium cerebelli.

Most obstetricians would not use the vacuum extractor for cases of suspected disproportion, but if it is employed the same care must be exercised as with the forceps.

In the past the risk of Caesarean section in late labour was high from sepsis and anaesthetic problems, but today section is preferred to difficult or prolonged forceps extraction.

Symphysiotomy.   Division of the ligaments holding the pubic bones together at the symphysis produces an increase in the available circumference of the pelvic ring and, by widening the subpubic arch, an increase in the available antero-posterior diameter at the outlet. The operation is hardly ever performed in Britain, but has been recommended in developing countries where some women are reluctant to agree to Caesarean section, and may not reurn to hospital for subsequent deliveries. (See p. 404.)

Craniotomy.   Destructive operations on the fetal head, which were common 50 years ago, have almost no place in modern obstetrics except when the fetal head is hydrocephalic. In the rare event of intrapartum fetal death in the presence of disproportion Caesarean section is now safer than craniotomy and extraction, procedures in which there is considerable risk of damage to maternal soft tissues.

27

Abnormal uterine action

Before considering abnormal uterine action it may be well to consider some aspects of normal uterine action during the three stages of labour.

First stage. The upper and lower uterine segments have different rôles during the first stage of labour. The upper segment plays the more active part, and shows three forms of activity—contraction, relaxation and retraction. During each contraction the upper segment compresses the uterine contents and raises the intrauterine pressure to 50 mm Hg or more at the height of the contraction, from 5 to 10 mm Hg in the interval between the contractions. The point of least resistance to the pressure is the lower segment and cervix; the lower segment therefore becomes stretched and the cervix becomes dilated. During the contraction the maternal blood flow through the placenta is temporarily arrested. Relaxation between the contractions is of the utmost importance, not only to avoid muscle fatigue, but to allow the placental blood flow to be resumed.

However, if the muscle fibres of the uterus merely shortened during the contraction and then returned to their original length when the uterus relaxed, no progress would be made. The uterus, particularly the upper segment, also *retracts*. This means that the muscle fibres remain partly shortened after the contraction. This 'rachet mechanism' allows the uterus to hold some of the advance made by the previous contraction, and to follow down any descent of its contents. By retracting the upper segment becomes progressively shorter and thicker, while the lower segment becomes more stretched and thinner. Where the two segments meet there is a circular rim running round the inside of the uterus, known as the physiological retraction ring.

In obstructed labour the lower segment becomes pathologically overstretched and thinned, and the ring between the two segments becomes very evident, and is then known as Bandl's ring (see p. 320).

The lower segment is far less active than the upper segment, although it contracts synchronously with it. Although the lower segment plays a relatively passive part in labour it has sufficient tone to transmit the pull of the upper segment to the cervix and dilate it. Thus the lower segment and cervix are drawn up over the bag of membranes and the presenting part of the fetus by the active contraction and retraction of the upper segment.

Second stage. During this stage the fetus is forced to advance down the birth canal and finally expelled by the powerful contraction and retraction of the upper segment, assisted by contraction of the abdominal muscles and the diaphragm. These forces are reflexly stimulated by pressure of the presenting part on the pelvic floor once it has passed the cervix. The patient generally experiences a desire to bear down soon after the second stage is reached, and multiparous patients may have this desire even before the cervix is fully dilated if the presenting part is able to press on the pelvic floor before the lax cervix is fully obliterated.

Third stage. The contractions of the uterus separate and expel the placenta into the lower segment and cervix, while the strong retraction of the upper segment compresses the maternal blood sinuses and prevents postpartum haemorrhage.

By measuring the changes in electrical potential at various points over the uterus and by measuring the intrauterine pressure by tocography (p. 314) the following characteristics of the action of the uterus in normal labour have been demonstrated. During a contraction the fundal part of the uterus starts to contract first, and it contracts more strongly and for a longer period than the rest of the uterus. The middle part of the uterus starts to contract a little later, and contracts less forcibly and for a shorter period than the fundal part, while the lower segment only contracts weakly. This *fundal dominance* is characteristic of normal labour.

Each contraction begins at a point near the uterine cornu on one side and then spreads as a wave through the whole myometrium. The contraction may start at the right or the left cornu constantly, or the origin may vary in successive contractions. As the contraction passes off more or less simultaneously in all parts of the uterus the duration of the contraction is longest in the upper part of the uterus where it began first.

At the onset of normal labour contractions occur at intervals of 15 to 20 minutes, and increase in frequency as labour progresses, so that by the end of the first stage they may occur every 2 or 3 minutes and each last for 60 to 90 seconds. The uterus can usually be felt to contract before the patient feels pain, and the pain ceases before the contraction has finished.

The contractions of the uterus during pregnancy are normally not painful. They differ from the contractions of labour in that they are much weaker, and the whole uterus including the lower segment contracts with about the same intensity. This pattern of contraction without fundal dominance is sometimes seen in cases of incoordinate uterine action and in 'false labour'.

Aetiological factors in cases of abnormal uterine action

Parity. The majority of cases of abnormal uterine action occur in primigravidae. It is uncommon for unfavourable uterine action in a first labour to be repeated in subsequent labours so long as the first labour ended in vaginal delivery, or at least dilated the cervix to about 7 cm or more. The resistance to cervical dilatation may be great in a first labour, and by causing relative obstruction may lead to disordered uterine action. This explanation seems more likely to be correct than one that attributes the high incidence of abnormal action in primigravidae to psychological factors such as apprehension.

Age. Abnormal action is more common in elderly than in young primigravidae, but it may occur at any age.

Maturity. Concern is felt by some obstetricians when pregnancy goes much beyond term because they believe that there is then a higher incidence of poor uterine action. Further, the possibility of reduced placental function makes prolonged labour hazardous in these cases.

Uterine overdistention caused by twin pregnancy or hydramnios is often stated to be a cause of poor uterine action. This seldom seems to be true, except possibly in the third stage of labour with twins. Postpartum haemorrhage is certainly more common in twin than single pregnancies, but with twins there is a much larger placental site.

Disproportion and malpresentation. An ill-fitting or high presenting part during labour is associated with inefficient uterine action. It has been said that trial labour is more a test of uterine action than of the fit of the head into the pelvis. An occipito-posterior position of the head with a deflexed and badly applied presenting part may be associated with ineffective and uncomfortable contractions, which have been described as 'posterior position pains'.

Psychological factors. Experience shows that it is impossible to predict the pattern labour will take in any woman in her first pregnancy. Even the most composed and emotionally well-balanced patient may have disorderly uterine action, whereas an anxious, unrelaxed and immature patient may have an easy and quick labour. The advocates of 'natural childbirth' and 'psychoprophylaxis' state that it is partly fear which causes troublesome tension, and hence pain and delay. However, statistics do not show a significant reduction in the incidence of delay in labour in those patients who have practised relaxation exercises and have attended instruction classes during pregnancy, compared to those who have done neither.

Classification of abnormal uterine action

It is difficult to define and classify the different types of abnormal uterine action, and this is reflected in the wide variety of terms used, and the varied interpretation of these terms by different authors. We have tried to avoid complexity:

A. Abnormal uterine action which may cause delay in labour.
    1. Uterine hypotonia (also described as uterine inertia)
        (a) Primary
        (b) Secondary

    2. Incoordinate uterine action

    3. Contraction ring.

B. Abnormally strong uterine action.

    1. Precipitate labour

    2. Obstructed labour.

Primary uterine hypotonia. The patient is frequently a primigravida, but the same pattern of uterine action is sometimes seen in a patient who has had several pregnancies. The pattern of uterine action and the spread of the contraction wave are normal; the only abnormality is that the contractions are weak, short and infrequent. This abnormality usually affects labour from the start, hence the term primary, and it may last throughout labour, but often the strength of the contractions improves after the membranes rupture, and also in the second and third stages. Progress is slow, but the condition of the patient is usually good for some time as the pain is slight. As long as the membranes are intact there is little danger to the mother or to the fetus, but without support her morale will eventually deteriorate.

Secondary uterine hypotonia. This is now becoming a rare condition in Britain because long labour is better managed. It usually follows prolonged labour, or excessively strong uterine action which has failed to overcome some obstruction to delivery. In the extreme case contractions cease, and labour is temporarily at a standstill. Many cases of obstructed labour in primigravidae behave like this, with alternating periods of excessive and hypotonic uterine action, before rupture of the uterus or assisted delivery takes place. In the third stage of labour the hypotonia of the uterus may cause delay in the separation and delivery of the placenta, and postpartum haemorrhage may occur from failure of effective uterine retraction.

A different type of secondary inertia may be caused by deep or prolonged general anaesthesia. Cyclopropane and halothane are especially liable to inhibit uterine action.

True secondary uterine hypotonia must be distinguished from the much more common condition in the second stage of labour in which the patient is unwilling to bear down because of fear of pain. Without the stimulus of the presenting part pressing firmly on the pelvic floor from bearing down, uterine contractions may become weak and infrequent.

Incoordinate uterine action. In this condition the contractions are irregular in time and strength. In some cases there is an increase in uterine tone, especially in the lower segment, which keeps the intrauterine pressure continuously raised above the normal interval pressure of 5 to 10 mm Hg. The raised pressure may be near the pain threshold, so that the patient either has continuous pain and discomfort, or pain is felt earlier in each contraction and stays longer. The raised intrauterine pressure will also cause gradually increasing fetal hypoxia from interference with placental blood flow.

In some cases there is reversal of normal uterine action; the upper segment contracts weakly and the lower segment shows persistent hypertonus. Under such adverse conditions cervical dilatation is distressingly slow. The disturbed uterine reflexes and the long labour are often accompanied by paralytic ileus, and abdominal distention and vomiting may occur, with electrolyte imbalance.

In modern obstetric practice delivery is assisted in cases of prolonged labour, by Caesarean section if necessary, before maternal or fetal distress occurs, but in the past some cases of incoordinate uterine action remained undelivered for several days, and there was then great danger of puerperal sepsis and a very high perinatal mortality.

Contraction ring. This is a very rare condition. There is an encircling band of muscle fibres in a constant state of spasm which is sufficient to obstruct delivery. It may occur in any stage of labour. A contraction ring in the first stage can hardly be discovered until Caesarean section is performed for delay in labour, when the ring is found. In the second stage the ring may be round the neck of the fetus and prevent delivery, even with forceps. A 'hour-glass' constriction in the third stage of labour may prevent delivery of the placenta (see p. 340).

Precipitate labour. When the uterine contractions are abnormally strong and frequent labour may be completed in a few minutes. The pattern of the contractions is essentially normal, the only abnormal feature being their strength. In some multiparous women cervical dilatation is completed almost without pain before the evident onset of labour, and then a few strong second stage contractions complete the delivery. Once a patient has had a precipitate labour all subsequent deliveries tend to be of the same type.

Obstructed labour. Here the uterine action is normal as regards the pattern of the contractions. The upper segment actively contracts and retracts while the lower segment is relatively passive but, because there is obstruction to the passage of the fetus, the uterus accepts the challenge and responds with powerful action. As the upper segment contracts almost incessantly and retracts strongly it becomes hard with thick and shortened walls as it draws the lower segment up over the fetus. The lower segment becomes dangerously thin, and will eventually rupture if help is not given. The placental circulation is obstructed by the strong retraction of the upper segment and the fetus will die.

The clinical picture and the management is described on p. 319. This condition is now very rare in Britain as intervention takes place long before this stage is reached.

Rigidity of the cervix (cervical dystocia)

For convenience this condition is described here, although few if any cases can strictly be included under the heading of abnormal uterine action.

In primary cervical rigidity the external os is unyielding through some anatomical or physiological defect. The patient is most commonly a primigravida and is not necessarily elderly. The first stage is prolonged. The cervix is well taken up and closely applied to the fetal head, but it has a firm rim which sometimes admits no more than a finger tip after many hours of labour. Occasionally a ring of cervix separates by necrosis from the pressure of the head and appears like a skull-cap on the baby's head at delivery.

Secondary cervical rigidity is caused by fibrosis due to some previous obstetric injury or some gynaecological operation such as amputation or cone biopsy. The patient is usually parous. The firm unyielding cervix may split if timely assistance is not given, and the tear may extend into the lower segment. Any patient who has had a previous cervical operation should have frequent cervical assessment during labour.

Management of prolonged labour caused by abnormal uterine action

In treating a woman in prolonged labour caused by abnormal uterine action the aim is to deliver the patient safely with her baby in good condition. If the uterine action can be made normal vaginal delivery may be possible; otherwise Caesarean section will be required. The state of the mother and fetus must be most carefully monitored in any case of prolonged labour.

Observations during labour

The art of managing a prolonged labour depends on accurate observations of the condition of the mother and fetus, and of the progress of the labour. Information must be recorded in a form that can easily be scanned, perhaps by successive attendants during a long labour.

General observations. The mother's blood pressure, pulse rate and temperature are recorded every two hours. Any alteration in the pulse rate should call for an immediate review of the case. A fluid balance chart is kept, and every urine specimen is tested for ketone bodies.

Uterine action. The action of the uterus is carefully watched. An experienced observer can feel the uterine contractions with the hand and record their frequency, regularity and duration accurately, and form an estimation of their strength. A more accurate measurement of uterine action can be made with a tocometer. An *internal tocograph* can be used after the membranes have ruptured. An incompressible plastic tube 5 mm in diameter is passed into the uterus above the fetal head into the residual pool of liquor amnii. When the uterus contracts the rise of pressure in the liquor can be recorded with a transducer onto a tracing. There is a very slight risk of introducing infection into the uterus or of injuring the placenta with this method. An *external tocograph* consists of a floating block of plastic surrounded by a guard ring which is strapped to the mother's abdomen over the uterus. When the uterus contracts its curvature alters, and the tocometer measures this change, acting as a strain gauge. It also records on a trace. Before the membranes have ruptured external tocography is the only method of recording the uterine contractions. If the patient is not moving about too much it gives almost as good a record as internal tocometry.

Cervical dilatation. If labour is proceeding normally there will be progressive dilatation of the cervix, which can be plotted against time on a partogram (see p. 116). The progress of labour is compared with that found from a study of normal primigravidae or multiparae in the same population group. Because the onset of labour can seldom be identified accurately, most obstetricians start recording at 2 cm dilatation and thereafter make an observation every 3 hours. If the cervix is opening at the same rate as that found in the normal population the patient's partogram will lie on the normal curve; if her progress is more rapid it will lie 'to the left' of the normal line; and if it is slower 'to the right'. Thus with a partogram delay in labour is often recognized at an earlier stage than by considering written notes alone, and the effect of oxytocic drugs may be tried sooner and closely watched. In cases of prolonged labour any alteration in the rate of progress can easily be observed.

Descent of the presenting part. An important indication of progress in labour is descent of the presenting part, but this chiefly occurs in the second stage of labour, and in cases of abnormal uterine action delay in labour may occur before this stage. However at each examination the station of the head should be carefully determined by abdominal and vaginal examination as described on pp. 100 – 105.

The state of the fetus. In cases of abnormal uterine action with prolonged labour fetal distress is a common complication. A continuous record of the fetal heart rate with a scalp electrode is desirable in these high risk cases.

General care of cases of prolonged labour

The observations already mentioned are appropriate for normal labour, but in prolonged labour the patient will need special support. She must never be left alone; ideally her husband is the best companion, but professional help must never be far away.

Care should be taken that the bladder does not become distended and a catheter is passed if necessary.

Apart from an occasional sip of fluid to moisten her lips, any woman in prolonged labour should not be given anything to eat or drink because of the possibility that general anaesthesia will be required, when there is a danger of inhalation of vomit. An adequate fluid intake is maintained by intravenous infusion of glucose saline if necessary.

Good analgesia is essential. An epidural anaesthetic is often helpful, and is sometimes followed by better uterine action. If systemic analgesia is used pethidine 100 to 150 mg with phenergan 25 mg may be given intramuscularly at intervals according to need. Although morphine 15 mg combined with hyoscine 0.4 mg is now seldom used because it depresses the respiratory centre of the newborn child if it is given within 4 hours of birth, there may be an occasional place for it in a long labour.

If the liquor is offensive or the patient's temperature rises a high vaginal swab is taken for bacteriological examination, and a wide-spectrum antibiotic such as ampicillin 500 mg intramuscularly 3 times daily is started, pending the bacteriological report.

If a general anaesthetic is needed the patient is given magnesium trisilicate powder 2 g in a little water to neutralize the gastric secretion. Even though the patient has not been eating, gastric juice has still been secreted and the stomach may be full because of the high pyloric tone during labour. Some anaesthetists recommend passing a gastric tube as well, and all will insist on tracheal intubation to lessen the risk of gastric contents entering the air passages.

Treatment of particular types of abnormal uterine action

Primary uterine hypotonia.   If the membranes are intact they are ruptured, and sometimes better uterine action follows. If there is no evidence of disproportion and the occiput is presenting then uterine action can be made normal by the use of intravenous oxytocin. Commonly a solution of 2 units of Syntocinon in 500 ml of 5 per cent glucose solution is used, and the rate of infusion is increased gradually, titrating the drip rate against the rate of the uterine contractions. The drip is started at 15 drops per minute, which gives an approximate dose of 3 mU/minute. If the rate reaches 60 drops per minute the concentration is increased to 8 units per 500 ml, the drip rate is reduced to 15 drops per minute and again gradually increased. The patient must be carefully watched to see that overstimulation of the uterus does not occur, and the fetal heart rate must be closely monitored, preferable with a scalp electrode and cardiographic ratemeter.

An alternative method of administration is by a mechanical pump such as the Cardiff-Pye machine, which adjusts the dose according to the tocographic record of the contractions and delivers a small bolus of oxytocic solution from time to time to the continuously running transport fluid.

When the contractions have become normal and the partogram shows that normal progress is occurring, the dose of oxytocin is not increased any further but is maintained at an effective level. It may even be possible to reduce it. In the second stage the patient is likely to be tired, and assistance with the forceps or vacuum extractor is often needed. The infusion should be kept running until the placenta has been delivered and the uterus is safely retracted.

Secondary uterine hypotonus. Careful examination is essential to make an accurate diagnosis. If the hyptonia has occurred because of some obstruction to delivery immediate Caesarean section will be required. If the patient has reached the second stage of labour delivery with the forceps is sometimes possible, perhaps after rotation of a head arrested in the occipito-posterior or occipito-transverse position, having made sure that there is no other impediment to delivery.

Incoordinate uterine action. Relief of pain with an epidural anaesthetic sometimes brings about better uterine action. It has sometimes been stated that oxytocin infusion is inappropriate treatment for these cases on the theoretical ground that the uterus is already hypertonic, at least between contractions. In practice oxytocin infusion has often proved to be both safe and effective. Certainly an oxytocic drip should be tried, with careful supervision, before resorting to Caesarean section for delay. However, in many cases Caesarean section becomes necessary because fetal distress occurs.

Contraction ring. If a ring is discovered during attempted forceps delivery or manual removal of the placenta it may relax with general anaesthesia, particularly with fluothane or cyclopropane, or after giving an inhalation of amyl nitrite (from a capsule).

Abnormally strong uterine action. This state of labour should not be allowed to develop. If the uterus is contracting strongly and regularly and progress is not being made the patient should be carefully re-examined to exlude any possible obstruction to delivery. The fetus is at high risk and if there is any obstruction this must be overcome, usually by Caesarean section, but sometimes by anaesthesia and correction of a malposition.

Cervical dystocia. When this is encountered and the cervix is less than 8 cm dilated Caesarean section is the best treatment. Only if the cervix is more widely dilated than this may the vacuum extractor be applied with gentle traction; this sometimes leads to complete dilatation and delivery. Incision of the cervix more dangerous than Caesarean section.

28

Obstructed labour

Labour is said to be obstructed when there is no progress in spite of strong uterine contractions. This may be shown by failure of the cervix to dilate or failure of the presenting part to descend the birth canal. It is a most dangerous condition if it is untreated, and can then be fatal to both mother and fetus.

Causes of obstructed labour

Obstructed labour may arise from maternal or fetal conditions, or both. The following list of the causes is long, but many of these operate in only a proportion of the cases in which they occur, and the causes marked with an asterisk are very rare.

Maternal conditions

1. Contraction or deformity of the bony pelvis.
2. Pelvic tumours
    - Uterine fibromyomata
    - Ovarian tumours
    - *Tumours of rectum, bladder or pelvic bones
    - *Pelvic kidney
3. Abnormalities of the uterus or vagina
    - *Stenosis of the cervix or vagina
    - *Congenital vaginal septum
    - *Obstruction by one horn of double uterus
    - *Contraction ring of uterus
    - *Sacculation of uterus

[handwritten margin notes: Android. Anthropoid Platypelloid Roberts Naegle]

Fetal conditions

1. Large fetus.
2. Malposition or malpresentation
    - Persistent occipito-posterior or transverse position
    - Breech presentation
    - *Mento-posterior position
    - Brow presentation

*Shoulder presentation (rare in Britain but common in countries with
   inadequate antenatal care)
*Compound presentation
*Locked twins
3. Congenital abnormalities of the fetus
   *Hydrocephalus
   *Fetal ascites or abdominal tumours
   *Hydrops fetalis
   *Double monster

Some of these causes can be detected during pregnancy so that early treatment is possible, or a plan of action can be made before labour. These conditions and their management are fully described in the appropriate
chapters; all that is given here is a description of the effects of obstructed
labour if it is left untreated.

Symptoms and signs of obstructed labour

The importance of the early detection of possible obstruction in labour is
obvious, for if labour is allowed to progress to the point of absolute
obstruction the death of the fetus is almost certain and the life of the
mother is endangered. In a primigravida complete obstruction leads within
2 or 3 days to a state of uterine exhaustion or secondary hypotonia; any
relief which this gives to the mother and fetus is only temporary. In a
multigravida obstruction becomes established much sooner and progressive thinning of the lower segment may lead to uterine rupture in less
than 24 hours.

Probably the earliest sign of impending obstruction is a deterioration in
the patient's general condition. She looks tired and anxious and behaves as
though she is beginning to lose her ability and will to cooperate. Between
the pains she seems unable to relax and her anxiety increases.

The presenting part is often above or at the level of the pelvic brim. The
membranes rupture early in labour because the presenting part is badly
applied to the lower segment. The cervix may be badly applied to the
presenting part. The liquor drains away and there is retraction of the
placental site, which causes reduction in the maternal blood flow to the
placenta, and eventual fetal death from hypoxia.

In late obstruction the patient's pulse rate and temperature rise. The
quantity of urine secreted diminishes and it is concentrated and deeply
coloured. Ketone bodies are present in the urine and acetone can also be
smelt in the patient's breath.

The possibility of obstructed labour should be suspected when labour
fails to progress. In the first stage dilatation of the cervix should be progressive, although sometimes it is not rapid even in normal cases. A partogram (p. 116) will give early warning that progress has ceased. Descent of

the presenting part should also be continuous, especially in the second stage. Any failure in the progress of labour calls for careful abdominal and vaginal examination to exclude any possible cause of obstruction, particularly in the case of previously undiagnosed disproportion or malpresentation.

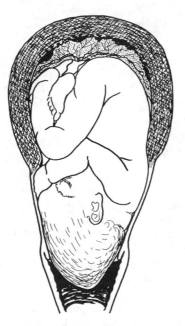

Fig. 28.1 Obstructed labour from pelvic contraction. The extreme retraction of the upper segment and the extreme stretching of the lower segment has formed a Bandl's ring. The head is greatly moulded with a large caput succedaneum.

If for some reason the diagnosis of obstruction is missed for a time the dangerous condition of over-retraction of the uterus (generalized tonic retraction) may occur. In the course of normal labour some retraction of the upper segment persists after each contraction, and the upper segment becomes slightly shorter and thicker, while the lower segment becomes stretched and thinner. If the fetus is unable to descend because of obstruction, the total length of the uterine cavity must remain constant, so that as uterine contractions continue progressive retraction causes abnormal stretching and thinning of the lower segment. The line of junction of the upper and lower segments becomes very evident and is known as the retraction ring of Bandl. It may become so high in the uterus that it can be seen or felt on abdominal examination. Eventually rupture of the lower segment occcurs.

In advanced obstructed labour the uterus is found on abdominal examination to be moulded to the shape of the fetus. It feels hard all the time and does not relax. It is tender to palpation and Bandl's ring may be evident. Fetal parts are not easily felt and the fetal heart sounds are absent. The presenting part is fixed at the level of obstruction.

On vaginal examination the vagina is found to be oedematous and feels dry. The oedematous cervix is only loosely applied to the presenting part. If the head is presenting there will be a large caput succedaneum and extreme moulding of the skull. The presenting part is tightly fixed, and even under anaesthesia cannot be pushed upward without danger of causing uterine rupture. If there is a shoulder presentation the oedematous arm of the fetus will have prolapsed, with the hand projecting from the vulva.

Treatment

Excessive retraction of the uterus should never be allowed to develop. The cause of the obstruction should have been discovered during pregnancy or in early labour, and treatment should have been applied.

When tonic retraction is present the fetus is certainly dead and the aim of treatment is to deliver the mother immediately by the safest possible method. Intrauterine manipulations are very liable to cause rupture of the abnormally thin lower segment. Internal version is particularly dangerous. In some of the cases it is possible to deliver the fetus vaginally after a destructive operation, but (except for perforation of a hydrocephalic head) these procedures are lengthy and difficult, and Caesarean section is usually less hazardous. Antibiotics, blood transfusion and modern anaesthesia have combined to reduce the risks of section in these cases.

In all cases of prolonged labour, especially if operative delivery is required, there is a high risk of puerperal sepsis, and appropriate antibiotics should be given.

Rupture of the uterus

Prolonged obstruction in a primigravida often leads to temporary cessation of uterine activity from exhaustion (secondary hypotonia), but in a multigravida it is more likely to lead to uterine rupture. In obstructed labour this usually occurs obliquely at the junction of the upper and lower segments, but occasionally the uterus splits vertically at the side near the point of entry of the uterine vessels. The peritoneum may or may not be involved. Bleeding may occur into the peritoneal cavity or may track downwards between the bladder and upper vagina. Uterine contraction may expel the fetus and placenta through the laceration into the peritoneal cavity.

The clinical picture and the treatment (which is extremely urgent) are described in the next chapter. If the patient survives the shock and haemorrhage there is a high risk of puerperal sepsis.

29

Traumatic lesions

Rupture of the uterus

Rupture of the uterus is a most serious condition. It usually occurs during labour, although it occasionally also happens during the later weeks of pregnancy.

Causes

During pregnancy the only common cause of rupture of the uterus is a weak scar after previous operations on the uterus. The higher the scar is placed on the uterus the greater is the risk. The most dangerous scar is that of 'classical' Caesarean section; this is more dangerous than a hysterotomy scar. Rupture of a lower segment Caesarean scar is uncommon during pregnancy, and rupture of a myomectomy scar or those following perforation of the uterus with a curette or cannula are rare. Rupture of the uterus during pregnancy has also followed a direct blow on the abdomen, and a perforating wound may injure the uterus.

During labour rupture may be caused by:
1. Obstructed labour. The rupture may be spontaneous or follow manipulations carried out for the relief of the obstruction.
2. Intrauterine manipulations, such as internal version or manual removal of an adherent placenta.
3. Forcible dilatation of the cervix. Rarely, a cervical tear in a normal delivery may extend up into the body of the uterus.
4. The injudicious use of oxytocic drugs.
5. A weak scar in the uterus after Caesarean section, or in rare instances after hysterotomy, myomectomy or perforation of the uterus with a curette or cannula. A lower segment Caesarean scar is safer than one in the upper segment.
6. Degeneration of uterine muscle, which is most likely to occur in women who have had numerous pregnancies.

EXCESSIVE KETOACIDOSIS.

Pathology

Ruptures of the uterus are divided into (1) complete or intraperitoneal and (2) incomplete or extraperitoneal, depending whether the peritoneal coat is torn through or not.

322

In obstructed labour rupture of the uterus generally takes place in the over-stretched and thinned lower segment, to which it may be limited, but sometimes it spreads upwards or downwards. The life of the mother is threatened by shock and intraperitoneal bleeding. There is also a high risk of peritonitis, especially when the accident occurs after long labour in which repeated examinations or intrauterine manipulations have been made. In cases of obstructed labour the fetus is nearly always dead before the rupture occurs, but in any case it will perish if complete rupture occurs.

Rupture of a scar in the uterus usually occurs during labour, but may also occur in the later weeks of pregnancy. In Britain a weak Caesarean scar is now the commonest cause of rupture of the uterus. Overdistention of the uterus, by twin pregnancy for example, will increase the risk. Healing of a uterine scar may be imperfect if gross sepsis occurs in the puerperium, or if the edges of the incision are inaccurately sutured. If the placenta is implanted over the scar the risk of rupture is increased. The scar may give way if section is repeated several times, when the latest incision is made through scar tissue left by previous operations. A lower segment scar is unlikely to rupture during pregnancy; an upper segment scar may give way in either pregnancy or labour.

A Caesarean scar in the lower segment may stretch gradually, so that the uterine wall in the region of the scar is only represented by attenuated and avascular fibrous tissue. When the weak area finally gives way there is sometimes relatively little intraperitoneal bleeding. The membranes may bulge through the rent, and will eventually give way, when the fetus or placenta may pass through it.

Symptoms and signs

Rupture through a uterine scar. In cases of rupture through a uterine scar during pregnancy the history of the previous operation will be available, and the scar in the skin will be seen, although a low transverse incision may be hidden by pubic hair. Occasionally the attenuated scar of a classical Caesarean section may be felt through a thin abdominal wall as a tender sulcus in the uterus. Rupture during pregnancy may be so gradual that the symptoms may be very slight at first, and the description 'silent rupture' has been applied to these cases. There is abdominal pain (which may be wrongly attributed to the onset of labour) but at first there is little change in the general condition of the patient. At this stage diagnosis may be difficult and it may be necessary to observe the case for a time before a conclusion is reached. If the rupture becomes complete and part of the uterine contents are extruded into the peritoneal cavity more severe pain and shock occur.

Rupture of a scar more often occurs during labour, and the scar gives way more suddenly than during pregnancy, so the symptoms are more dramatic, with severe pain and shock. Unless the contents of the uterus pass into the peritoneal cavity uterine contractions may continue. The possibility of rupture of the scar should always be considered if a patient who has had a Caesarean section suddenly complains of severe pain during labour which is not synchronous with the uterine contractions. The accident does not usually occur after a long and difficult labour, and for that reason the patient's general condition is better, and the risk of infection less, than in cases of rupture due to obstructed labour. Because pain is a good warning symptom of dehiscence of a uterine scar during labour some obstetricians hesitate to give an epidural anaesthetic to those in labour after previous section.

Spontaneous rupture during obstructed labour. The preceding labour will have been prolonged, or there will have been violent uterine action almost without intermission between the pains, so that the patient may be exhausted before the rupture occurs. There may be signs of disproportion or of a malpresentation such as a transverse lie, although these signs may have been overlooked before the accident. At the moment of rupture the patient cries out and complains of a sharp pain in the lower abdomen. Soon after the rupture she presents signs of shock, with pallor and sweating. The pulse becomes thready and rapid and the blood pressure falls. With an incomplete tear the signs of shock may not be so severe.

Slight vaginal haemorrhage is usually present. On abdominal examination there is marked tenderness. The presenting part may not be felt unless the head is impacted in the pelvis. If the fetus is completely extruded into the peritoneal cavity uterine contractions may cease, but in other cases often continue. With complete extrusion the fetus may be felt in the abdominal cavity with the retracted uterus beside it.

Rupture after intrauterine manipulations. In these cases the patient is usually anaesthetized when the manipulation, such as manual removal of the placenta is taking place, so the first evidence that anything is amiss may be a sudden deterioration in her general condition, either at the time or later when the effect of the anaesthetic wears off. In other instances the operator may discover the injury while his hand is still in the uterus. After any difficult manipulation the uterus should be examined carefully to exclude injury.

Extensive cervical lacerations. In some respects these injuries resemble the previous group, as they are usually produced with the forceps at a difficult delivery, especially if the cervix is not completely dilated, but they seldom extend far enough to open the peritoneal cavity. Brisk external haemorrhage may occur, or a large haematoma may form in the broad ligament (see p. 332). Vaginal bleeding in the third stage of labour with the uterus empty and firmly retracted should always suggest the possibility of this type of injury, which can be confirmed by visual examination. For this effective retractors and the help of an assistant will be required.

Rupture caused by oxytocic drugs. Rupture of the uterus has followed the administration of oxytocin before the delivery of the child, particularly when there was some obstruction which prevented rapid delivery. The risk is much greater in multiparae. The danger is less if the oxytocin is given as a dilute intravenous drip and the uterine contractions are carefully observed and controlled. Several cases of rupture have followed the use of buccal oxytocin.

Rupture caused by direct injury to the abdomen. In the rare cases of rupture from this cause severe shock and abdominal pain, together with the history of the accident, will suggest the possibility of visceral injury. Precise diagnosis may be impossible without laparotomy, and in case of doubt this would be well justified.

Prognosis

The maternal mortality from rupture of the uterus in cases of obstructed labour is about 7 per cent. This high mortality is because the accident usually occurs in cases of prolonged labour with much manipulation, sometimes with inefficient obstetric aid, and often with septic complications. The mortality after rupture of a Caesarean scar is much less, as the accident does not usually follow prolonged labour, and the patient is usually confined in hospital where the rupture is more quickly detected.

The fetal prognosis is bad. The perinatal mortality following obstructed labour is about 80 per cent, but less than half this in cases of scar rupture.

Dangerous intrauterine manipulations are now rarely performed, and obstructed labour is less often seen, but these difficulties are avoided by Caesarean section, so that the increased risk of subsequent scar rupture must be set against this.

Treatment

Prevention. Rupture of the uterus will be largely prevented by better obstetric care. Disproportion must be recognized early, and labour must not be allowed to continue to the stage of obstruction. An oblique lie must be corrected early but if the shoulder has become impacted, version should not be attempted: Caesarean section is the correct treatment. The cervix must not be forcibly dilated and forceps must not be applied unless it is fully dilated. Manual removal of the placenta must be carefully performed, with an external hand guarding the fundus.

A patient who has had a Caesarean section, hysterotomy or extensive myomectomy must be delivered in a hospital where all obstetric facilities are available. However, the fact that a patient has already had one Caesarean section does not mean that a subsequent pregnancy must also be

treated in this way. If the first operation was not performed for disproportion but for some non-recurrent condition, vaginal delivery should be
advised, with the proviso that if labour does not progress smoothly section
will be repeated. If the patient had an upper segment operation, or if gross
uterine infection occurred, elective section would be advisable, as it would
be in the case of a woman who had already had two or more sections.

Treatment after rupture has occurred. Before operation the
general condition of the patient must be improved as much as possible by
giving morphine, blood transfusion, and intravenous glucose solution if
necessary.

If the rupture is complete laparotomy is always necessary. Cases in
which the tear is confined to the broad ligament will not be recognized
until after delivery. If digital examination proves that the peritoneal cavity
has not been opened bleeding may be arrested by packing with gauze, but
for extensive tears laparotomy is often required.

In cases of scar rupture it is often possible to excise the edges of the rent
and resuture the uterus. The bladder is sometimes adherent to the scar and
is torn; in that case its wall must be freed and sutured in two layers and an
in-dwelling catheter inserted.

Many cases of uterine rupture during obstructed labour are best treated
by hysterectomy, as efficient suturing of bruised and ragged tissues may be
impossible. If the tear is accessible and the edges not too ragged it may be
sutured, but the risk of rupture in a subsequent pregnancy is so great that
it is usually wise to prevent this by ligating the Fallopian tubes.

Wide spectrum antibiotics are given, and paralytic ileus is treated by
giving only intravenous fluids and maintaining gastric aspiration until
bowel sounds reappear.

Acute inversion of the uterus

In this condition the body of the uterus becomes partially or completely
turned inside out after delivery of the fetus. It is an important but rare
cause of shock in the third stage of labour, which may be fatal if it is
untreated. Inversion may take place before or after the delivery of the
placenta. If it is complete the fundus of the uterus may be seen at the
vulva.

Cause

The usual cause is mismanagement of the third stage of labour by the
attendant pulling on the umbilical cord or pressing on the fundus while the
uterus is not contracting and the placenta has not separated. It is possible
for it to occur spontaneously if relaxation of the part of the wall to which
the placenta is attached permits this to be carried down by a contraction of
the rest of the uterus.

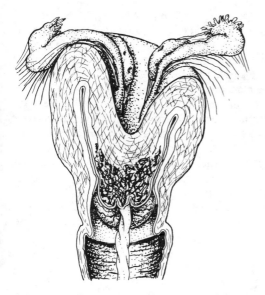

Fig. 29.1 Acute puerperal inversion of the uterus.

Symptoms and signs

The chief symptoms are those of shock, with some haemorrhage and sometimes the appearance of the uterine fundus at the vulva. As a rule shock is severe and is greater than the blood loss warrants. Pain is of variable degree. Unexplained shock during the third stage of labour should always suggest the possibility that inversion has occurred, and a vaginal examination should be made. The body of the uterus will not be felt in its usual position and the round mass of the uterus will be felt protruding through the cervix. Inversion has a high mortality if it is undiagnosed and left untreated.

In extremely rare cases the symptoms are slight and the inversion remains until the uterus involutes and is then found to be in the state of chronic inversion.

Treatment

Shock and bleeding will continue until the uterus is replaced, hence it is desirable that it should be replaced at once. The inverted fundus soon becomes oedematous, which makes replacement more difficult. As soon as the diagnosis is made the patient is anaesthetized and the uterus is replaced. If this cannot be done at once she is given an injection of morphine

15 mg. After cleansing the vulva, vagina and inverted uterus, the placenta, if it is still attached to the uterus is peeled off. The uterus is then squeezed in the hand and replaced, the part which became inverted last being replaced first, and the fundus last of all. A tocolytic agent, hexoprenaline $5\mu g$ intravenously, may allow easier replacement.

An alternative method of replacement is by fluid pressure. Sterile water is run into the vagina from a container suspended above the patient. By closing the entrance to the vagina with the hand the intravaginal pressure is raised sufficiently to replace the uterus, although very large volumes of fluid may have to be run in.

When replacement is complete further haemorrhage or recurrence of the inversion are prevented by intravenous injection of ergometrine 0.5 mg. Treatment for shock is given concurrently.

Should inversion be discovered some days after labour reposition under anaesthesia is usually possible. Hardly ever will operative division of the constricting ring or vaginal hysterectomy be needed.

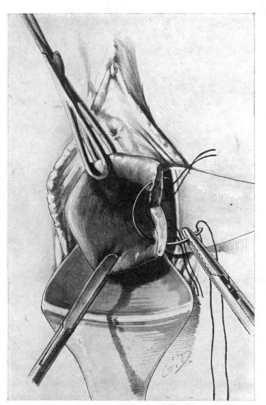

Fig. 29.2 The repair of a tear of the cervix by interrupted catgut sutures. The cervix is depicted outside for the sake of clarity.

Lacerations of the birth canal

Laceration of the cervix

Minor lacerations of the cervix occur frequently but do not cause symptoms.

Extensive lacerations may be caused by precipitate labour, application of forceps with the cervix incompletely dilated, or rapid delivery of the head with a breech presentation. A scar in the cervix from previous injury may tear. With a deep tear there is continuing haemorrhage during or after the third stage, and this goes on even when the uterus is empty and retracted. The tear must be sutured. For this the patient is anaesthetized, a wide speculum is inserted, and the anterior and posterior lips of the cervix are held with sponge forceps and drawn well down, so that interrupted catgut or Dexon sutures can be inserted through the whole thickness of its wall. While waiting for arrangements to be made, bleeding may be temporarily controlled with sponge forceps left in place.

Laceration of the perineum and vagina

These lesions are described as being of three degrees:

A first degree tear involves only the anterior part of the perineum and the related posterior wall of the vagina.

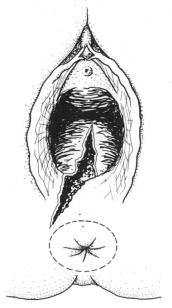

Fig. 29.3 Second degree perineal tear.

A second degree tear involves the perineum up to (but not involving) the external anal sphincter, ·with a corresponding tear in the vagina.

A third degree (complete) tear includes the anal sphincter and usually extends for 2 cm or more up the anal canal. If a third degree tear is not repaired there will be incontinence of flatus and any loose stool.

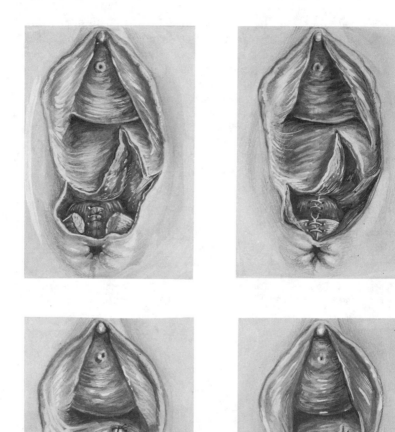

Fig. 29.4   Repair of complete perineal tear.

An extensive tear of the vagina can occur without a tear in the perineum, and the vaginal walls should always be carefully inspected after delivery. Minor lacerations can also occur on the antero-lateral vaginal wall.

Treatment of first and second degree tears. It is important to repair all perineal lacerations immediately to prevent any infection of the raw surface. Deep lacerations involving the perineal body that are not sutured or do not heal increase the possibility of subsequent utero-vaginal prolapse.

The vaginal epithelium is sutured with either a continuous suture or interrupted sutures of fine catgut or Dexon. The perineal body is repaired with slightly stronger stitches of the same material. The skin edges are brought together without tension with fine catgut or Dexon sutures. The repair should be done carefully and accurately. Unless general anaesthesia is already being used, a pudendal block (see p. 366) or local anaesthesia with 1 per cent lignocaine are employed.

Treatment of third degree (complete) tears. The operation should be done by an experienced obstetric surgeon in a properly equipped theatre with general anaesthesia and adequate assistance. The tissues heal very well if the operation is done carefully soon after delivery, but if this is not done or the tissues fail to heal the patient will have to undergo a more difficult operation later, or she will suffer from rectal incontinence.

Catgut or Dexon sutures are used throughout. The anal mucosa is first repaired with fine stitches, tying the knots inside the bowel lumen. The ends of the anal sphincter are found and carefully brought together with interrupted sutures. The vaginal epithelium is repaired from the apex of the tear, which must be identified clearly, down to the introitus. The tissues of the perineal body are approximated with interrupted sutures, and finally the skin edges are sutured without tension.

After care. Each day the perineum is washed with soap and water, and then carefully dried. Patients with extensive tears sometimes have retention of urine, for which catheterization is necessary. After repair of a complete tear if the patient cannot pass wind a flatus tube may be carefully inserted. If the bowel has not acted by the 4th day a glycerine suppository may be used, but oral liquid paraffin should not be given.

If any perineal wound becomes infected sufficient stitches are removed to permit drainage, and antibiotics are given. Bathing, preferably in a bidet, is continued until the wound is covered with granulation tissue, when secondary suture can be performed if necessary.

Fistulae

Fistulae may occur as a result of pressure by the presenting part in pro-longed labour, or by direct injury during operative procedures such as craniotomy or Caesarean section. In obstructed labour prolonged pressure between the head and the pubic bone may cause local ischaemia and subsequent necrosis of the anterior vaginal wall and base of the bladder leads to the formation of a *vesico-vaginal fistula*. Less commonly a *vesico-uterine fistula* is formed, and with very extensive necrosis the rectum may be involved. The pressure is nearly always caused by the head as other parts of the fetus are not sufficiently hard to cause necrosis.

A much more common cause of a *recto-vaginal fistula* is a complete tear of the perineum and recto-vaginal septum, in which the lower part has healed but left a defect higher up.

All these fistulae are now very uncommon in the United Kingdom, but in countries with inadequate obstetric services they are still a common cause of distressing disability. Depending on the type of fistula, the patient has urinary or faecal incontinence, and sometimes both. If the fistula is caused by operative injury the symptoms appear immediately, but if it is the result of pressure necrosis the symptoms do not appear until about the 8th day, when the sloughs separate. On examination an opening into the bladder or rectum is found.

When the wound granulates a small rectal fistula may heal, but this is unlikely with a vesico-vaginal fistula. In the case of a fistula caused by direct injury immediate repair is performed, but in those caused by ischaemic necrosis repair is not attempted for 2 to 3 months when the effects of trauma and superadded infection have subsided. Details of the surgical treatment are given in *Gynaecology by Ten Teachers* p. 87.

Haematoma of the vulva

Although this is not common it is a serious complication of pregnancy and labour. It may be due to rupture of a vulval varix, but usually it occurs without any evident preceding abnormality.

The haematoma appears fairly suddenly as a very tender purple swelling on one side of the vulva, which may become 10 cm or more in diameter. Sometimes the blood tracks upwards to form a swelling at the side of the vagina. The pain is severe, and there is often shock. If the haematoma is left it may eventually absorb, but abscess formation can occur.

If the tension in the swelling is great or if it is increasing in size it should be incised and the clot turned out. If the torn vessel can be found it is ligatured. Firm pressure is then made with a dressing and bandage. If the haematoma is noticed before delivery it may be possible to complete the delivery before dealing with it.

Broad ligament haematoma

In this uncommon accident a deep vessel is torn and a haematoma forms above the pelvic diaphragm and spreads into the base of the broad ligament, extending between the uterus and bladder or beside the rectum. It may be caused by extraperitoneal rupture of the uterus (p. 324). The bleeding most frequently occurs during or soon after labour or Caesarean section and the haematoma is discovered a few hours or days later, the presenting symptoms being pain and deterioration of the patient's general condition. The haematoma may be large enough to be palpable on abdominal examination, and it will displace the uterus upwards and to one side. The patient is often anaemic, and there may be slight fever.

A broad ligament haematoma usually undergoes gradual absorption, which will take several weeks if it is large. Infection is rare, but abscess formation may occur.

Most cases are treated conservatively. Blood transfusion may be required, and antibiotics are given. If infection occurs and an abscess forms this is opened wherever it points.

Maternal nerve injuries during labour

Foot-drop from paralysis of the dorsiflexor muscles of the leg may follow delivery.

In a few cases this is the result of pressure on the lateral popliteal nerve near the neck of the fibula by a leg support used to hold the patient in the lithotomy position. If the legs are placed outside the supports this cannot happen.

In the majority of cases it is a different type of injury involving the 4th and 5th lumbar nerve roots. This may be the result of sudden prolapse of an intervertebral disk, which may occur during labour, or of pressure on the lumbosacral cord by the presenting part near the brim of the pelvis. The lesion is usually unilateral, and it often follows difficult labour, especially forceps delivery. Apart from the foot-drop there is an area of sensory loss on the dorsum of the foot and lateral aspect of the ankle. The prognosis is good, although recovery may take several months. During that time a toe-spring is attached to lift the foot during walking, and regular physiotherapy is given.

Rarely prolonged sensory loss in the leg, without foot-drop, follows epidural anaesthesia.

30

Postpartum haemorrhage and abnormalities of the third stage

Postpartum haemorrhage is excessive bleeding from the genital tract after the birth of the child. It is conventionally defined as a loss of more than 500 ml. The haemorrhage may be immediate or *primary*, or if it occurs more than 24 hours after delivery it is described as *secondary*.

Primary postpartum haemorrhage

There are two possible sources of primary postpartum haemorrhage, the placental site and lacerations of the genital tract.

Primary haemorrhage from the placental site

Some blood must escape as the placenta separates, but usually less than 200 ml. Further loss is normally prevented by the retraction of the uterine muscle fibres which surround the vessels in the wall of the uterus and compress them until intravascular thrombosis occurs. Although a loss of more than 500 ml is arbitrarily defined as a postpartum haemorrhage, any loss which appears excessive must be treated at once. Even a small loss may be dangerous if the patient is already anaemic.

Causes. 1. *Ineffective uterine contraction and retraction.* Weak contraction of the uterus in the third stage of labour may fail to separate the placenta completely, so that it remains in the upper segment of the uterus and prevents effective retraction of the placental site. In other cases, even though the placenta has been completely separated and has been expelled, severe haemorrhage can occur if the uterus fails to maintain its retraction.

If the uterus is not completely empty retraction will be ineffective. Although it is true that a very strong contraction, for example after the intravenous injection of ergometrine, may temporarily control bleeding even if the placenta is still in the uterus, in cases in which the contractions are less strong even a retained placental cotyledon or blood clot in the uterus will interfere with retraction.

Ineffective uterine action may occur:

(a) After a long labour caused by weak or incoordinate uterine action. It will also occur in cases of long labour caused by mechanical difficulty if uterine exhaustion occurs.

334

(b) If prolonged or deep anaesthesia has been administered.

(c) If the patient is a multipara with an atonic uterus.

(d) If the uterus has been overdistended with twins or hydramnios.

(2) *Mismanagement of the third stage.* After a normal delivery, if ergometrine has not been injected at the end of the second stage, the uterus remains quiescent for a few minutes. The placenta is still completely attached, and no bleeding occurs. But if the uterus is manipulated during this interval the placenta may be partly separated, and bleeding will start and must continue until uterine contractions complete the separation and allow proper retraction to follow. Injudicious attempts to expel the placenta before complete separation has occurred are a common cause of postpartum haemorrhage, and may even cause uterine inversion (see p. 327).

3. *Abnormally adherent placenta.* Sometimes part of the placenta is abnormally adherent. In rare instances most of the chorionic villi penetrate through the decidua into the myometrium (placenta accreta). In cases of placenta praevia the placenta may have a wider area of attachment than normal, and the lower uterine segment may fail to retract strongly enough to control bleeding effectively.

4. *Hypofibrinogenaemia.* This is an occasional cause of slow but persistent and dangerous haemorrhage. It is especially associated with concealed accidental haemorrhage, but it may also occur in cases of amniotic embolism and after a dead fetus has been retained in the uterus for some weeks. In cases of accidental haemorrhage liberation of thromboplastin from placental tissue into the blood stream uses up fibrinogen. In the other cases the mechanism is less certain, but there is rapid conversion of fibrinogen to fibrin.

Clinical events. The escape of blood is usually obvious and the only question is whether it is coming from the placental site or from some laceration. In rare instances severe bleeding occurs into the cavity of an atonic uterus with only part of the blood appearing externally, but if the fundus of the uterus is abnormally high in the abdomen this will be discovered.

If haemorrhage continues the blood pressure falls and the pulse rate rises, and in severe cases pallor and air-hunger occur.

Owing to the increase in blood volume during pregnancy, and the increase in total red cell mass, a previously healthy parturient woman stands haemorrhage comparatively well, provided that the loss is not extremely rapid. However, a patient who is already exsanguinated by an antepartum haemorrhage may die if even a relatively small amount of blood is lost after delivery, and in a similar way a comparatively insignificant secondary postpartum haemorrhage may have serious effects on a patient who has lost heavily at the time of delivery.

Postpartum necrosis of the anterior lobe of the pituitary gland is a rare sequel in cases of postpartum haemorrhage in which the blood pressure has remained at a low level for some hours (see p. 342).

Prevention. The prevention of postpartum haemorrhage is very important. Anaemia must be corrected during pregnancy because an anaemic patient tolerates haemorrhage badly. Any patient with a previous history of a postpartum haemorrhage, patients with twins and grand multiparae should always be admitted to hospital for delivery.

Prolonged labour which might lead to uterine exhaustion can often be prevented by the use of an intravenous infusion of Syntocinon during labour and if such an infusion is given it should not be stopped until the third stage is safely completed. The second stage of labour should be short, and if assistance with forceps is necessary general anaesthesia is avoided whenever possible.

The corrrect management of the third stage of labour is the most important factor in avoiding postpartum haemorrhage. Intravenous ergometrine or intramuscular Syntometrine should be given immediately after delivery of the anterior shoulder of the fetus, as described on p. 124.

Treatment. Two principles govern the treatment of postpartum haemorrhage—the bleeding must be arrested and the blood volume must be restored. Bleeding from the placental site will stop when the uterus is empty and retracted. Treatment will differ according to whether the placenta is still in the uterus or has been delivered.

If the placenta is undelivered the first step must be to determine whether it has separated. The patient is placed in the dorsal position. The fundus of the uterus is rubbed gently, when it will usually contract. There are two clinical possibilities:

(a) *The placenta has separated* and been expelled from the upper into the lower uterine segment. If this is the case, when the uterus contracts it will be felt as a firm rounded mass about 10 cm in diameter, at about the level of the umbilicus, and movable from side to side. If these signs of separation are present there should be no difficulty in delivering the placenta by Brandt-Andrews method (p. 125). If the bleeding does not then stop an intravenous injection of ergometrine 0.5 mg is given. (Even if the patient has already received 0.5 mg of ergometrine at the time of delivery this dose can safely be repeated once). If the uterus does not contract well in spite of the ergometrine *bimanual compression* is immediately performed. One hand is inserted into the vagina and formed into a fist, which is placed in the anterior fornix above the cervix (Fig. 30.1). The other hand is placed on the abdomen and pressed downwards onto the posterior wall of the uterus so that it is compressed between the two hands. This is an effective but temporary method of controlling uterine bleeding, although it is uncomfortable for the patient and extremely tiring for the obstetrician. Firm pressure must be maintained until the uterus is felt to contract.

While this is in progress the placenta should be examined by an assistant to see that it is complete. If part of it is missing that will have to be removed digitally under general anaesthesia.

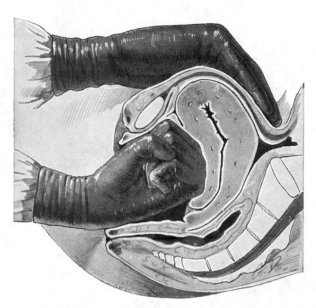

Fig. 30.1 Bimanual compression of the uterus. In the illustration the patient is in the lithotomy position and the operator is standing between the legs. Bimanual compression can be performed equally well with the patient lying on her back in the bed in the ordinary position. In these circumstances it is obviously easier for the operator to place his right hand in the vagina and his left on the patient's abdomen.

(b) *The placenta has not separated* and it remains in the upper uterine segment. If bleeding is taking place and clinical examination, which may include vaginal examination, indicates that the placenta has not separated, then *manual removal of the placenta* under general anaesthesia is immediately performed. Repeated or violent attempts to express the placenta by squeezing the uterus or pressing on it are unlikely to succeed and often produce shock. If manual removal is to be performed it is best to withhold any further injection of ergometrine until after the removal of the placenta. While the anaesthetic is being induced a catheter may be passed to empty the bladder. For manual removal the left hand is placed on the abdominal wall to locate and steady the fundus of the uterus, and then the right hand is passed into the uterus to follow the cord to the placenta. The edge of the placenta is identified, and then it is gradually separated from the uterine wall with the fingers, while the external hand serves as a guide and reduces the risk of tearing the uterus (Fig. 30.2). Only when the placenta is completely free should any attempt be made to remove it. The uterus is ex-

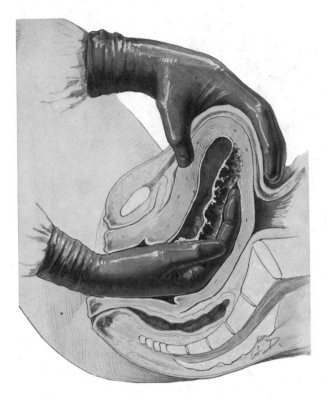

Fig. 30.2 Manual removal of the placenta.

plored carefully to ensure that no pieces of placental tissue are left behind. The beginner must realize that the site of attachment of the placenta is normally uneven and rough. The placenta is immediately examined to make sure that it is complete.

In the past manual removal of the placenta was a hazardous procedure, often performed after some delay on a shocked patient, with imperfect anaesthesia, and a grave risk of infection. Today, if the operation is performed without delay, with good anaesthetic facilities, proper resuscitation and blood transfusion services, and with antibiotic cover, the risk is slight. However, it is not an easy operation, and the beginner often diagnoses morbid adhesion of the placenta when none exists.

If bleeding still continues after removal of the placenta the same steps that have already been described under (a) above are followed, including bimanual compression if necessary. In very exceptional cases, if bleeding continues in spite of all efforts (and is not caused by a clotting defect, see below) hysterectomy may be considered as a last desperate resort.

Circulatory collapse caused by haemorrhage. In all cases of postpartum haemorrhage there is the danger of circulatory collapse, and resuscitation must be started as soon as possible, preferably *before* hypotension or tachycardia appear. Immediate blood transfusion is essential to restore the blood volume, and an infusion of plasma or saline may be started while the transfusion is being arranged. In an emergency case if the patient's blood group is not known group O rhesus negative blood may occasionally have to be used, but in every case a direct agglutination test of the donor's corpuscles and the patient's serum is essential. Dextran may interfere with the coagulation mechanism; it should only be used after a sample of blood has been collected for cross-matching, and it should not be used if fibrinogen deficiency is suspected.

The patient is kept quiet and warm, with the foot of the bed raised. Her pulse, peripheral blood pressure and central venous pressure are monitored to assess transfusion requirements.

Problems of haemorrhage in domiciliary practice. If the patient is not delivered in a unit with full facilities for blood transfusion and emergency anaesthesia the dangers are increased, and the help of an emergency obstetric unit is essential. This 'flying squad', based on a maternity hospital, consists of an obstetrician, an anaesthetist and a midwife, and carries proper equipment for resuscitation and anaesthesia. A patient who has had a postpartum haemorrhage should not be moved until she has had a blood transfusion, the placenta has been removed, and the bleeding has been controlled. There is a much higher mortality if the patients are moved to hospital with the placenta still undelivered and after inadequate transfusion.

Haemorrhage caused by clotting disorders. If bleeding persists in spite of all other treatment described, then hypofibrinogenaemia or excess fibrinolysin in the blood should be suspected. In an emergency the simple observation of failure of a sample of blood to clot in a test-tube may be sufficient to suggest the diagnosis. For discussion of investigation and treatment see p. 431.

Primary postpartum haemorrhage from lacerations

Primary postpartum haemorrhage can occur from lacerations of any part of the birth canal during labour, the commonest sites of bleeding being either the cervix or the vaginal wall. If bleeding continues after the placenta has been delivered and the uterus is firmly retracted, the vagina, cervix and lower uterine segment must be examined. This may be difficult until the patient is anaesthetized and placed in the lithotomy position. To suture a high cervical tear proper retractors and instruments are needed. If there is profuse haemorrhage from a cervical tear involving a branch of the uterine artery, this can be temporarily controlled by clamping the highest part of the tear with a sponge holder until the patient can be taken to the operating theatre.

Bleeding from tears of the lower vagina, perineum or vulva should be controlled by pressure until the tear is sutured under local anaesthesia.

Secondary postpartum haemorrhage

This occurs more than 24 hours after delivery of the child, often starting between the 5th and 10th days. It is usually caused by retention of a piece of placenta, and it is frequently complicated by intrauterine infection, with pyrexia. Secondary postpartum haemorrhage may also be caused by separation of an infected slough which has formed in a cervical or vaginal tear, or in a lower segment Caesarean wound. A rare cause is infection and sloughing of a submucous fibromyoma.

Treatment.   Under general anaesthesia the uterine cavity is explored with the finger to discover and remove any placental tissue. The cervix often remains open when there is something retained in the uterus. The appropriate antibiotic is chosen according to the result of cultures from a uterine swab.

Delayed delivery of the placenta and membranes

The normal process of separation and expulsion of the placenta has already been described (p. 76). Separation is usually complete within 10 minutes of the delivery of the baby. Retention of the placenta within the uterus for more than 30 minutes is now regarded as abnormal.

Causes

The causes of delayed delivery of the placenta are:

1. **Ineffective uterine action.**   If the uterine action is not sufficient to separate the placenta there will be no bleeding; the placenta is simply retained. If the placenta is partly separated and retraction is impaired there will be postpartum haemorrhage.

2. **Contraction ring (hour-glass constriction of the uterus).**   In this condition a localized constriction just above the lower uterine segment prevents expulsion of the placenta. Bleeding is seldom heavy. It may occur after prolonged labour with intrauterine manipulation. A more generalized spasm, involving the lower as well as the upper segment may occur after administration of ergometrine or Syntometrine. If ergometrine is given, as in the active management of the third stage of labour, it is always advisable

to deliver the placenta directly it has separated to avoid any risk of its retention.

3. **Morbid adhesion of the placenta.** The placenta normally separates in the plane of the spongy layer of the decidua. Rarely this layer is poorly defined and the chorionic villi are adherent to the myometrium (*placenta accreta*) in part or the whole of the placental site. If the villi have penetrated even more deeply into the muscle the condition is called *placenta increta*. There is no proper line of cleavage and separation does not occur when the uterus contracts. Deficient formation of the decidua may occur over a Caesarean or other scar in the uterus.

Treatment

The cause of delayed delivery of the placenta can only be ascertained by examination under anaesthesia. If the delay is accompanied by postpartum haemorrhage the treatment is urgent and is that already described above.

In the absence of bleeding intervention can be delayed for 30 minutes, but soon after that the placenta should be removed manually under general anaesthesia. If ergometrine was given at the time of delivery it is best to wait for at least this time so that any effect of the drug will be less.

If a contraction ring is present this will be felt as a tight band. Inhalation of amyl nitrite (supplied in small glass capsules) or anaesthesia with fluothane or cyclopropane should relax the ring sufficiently for the placenta to be removed.

If during manual removal partial placenta accreta is encountered the placenta can usually be removed. Placenta increta is very rare, and then no plane of cleavage at all will be discovered. The placenta can be left in place to separate by necrosis, but in most cases the operator will have torn the placenta and started bleeding, so that hysterectomy may be the safest course.

Antibiotics should be given and blood transfusion if there is bleeding.

Retention of the membranes

Part of the membranes may be found to be missing when the placenta is examined after its delivery, but this is not a matter for concern. Even large pieces of chorion will separate and be discharged spontaneously.

Shock in obstetrics

Obstetric shock does not differ significantly from surgical shock, and results from depression of many functions, in which reduction of effective circulation volume and blood pressure are of basic importance. The consequent inadequate perfusion of all the tissues leads to oxygen depletion and the accumulation of metabolites.

Most cases of shock in obstetrics are associated with severe haemorrhage, especially when there is also trauma or prolonged anaesthesia. It usually results from a combination of factors, for example prolonged labour may be associated with electrolyte imbalance, general anaesthesia and trauma during operative delivery. Concealed accidental haemorrhage can cause severe shock, and in the third stage of labour postpartum haemorrhage may occur. Maternal exhaustion, especially if combined with infection, will increase the effect of other factors.

Less frequent causes of shock include rupture of the uterus (p. 332), acute inversion of the uterus (p. 326), amniotic embolism (p. 431), pulmonary embolism (p. 436), and adrenal haemorrhage (p. 236). Bacteraemic shock is an additional form of shock (p. 139).

Prolonged postpartum shock and hypotension may cause ischaemic necrosis of the anterior lobe of the pituitary gland (see below).

Treatment. Unless prompt resuscitation is undertaken death may occur rapidly. It is essential to restore the blood volume as quickly as possible by intravenous infusion. If blood is not immediately available transfusion with saline or reconstituted plasma is started while it is being obtained.

Constant monitoring of the pulse rate, arterial blood pressure and central venous pressure is required to regulate the circulatory balance. Oxygen is sometimes required, and a small dose of morphine if there is severe pain. Attempts to raise the blood pressure by administration of vasoconstrictor drugs are usually wrong. If the limbs are pale and cold vasoconstriction is already present, and further vasoconstriction may only decrease the venous return still further. In many of these cases there is a risk of infection, and broad-spectrum antibiotics may be given intravenously.

Postpartum pituitary necrosis

Severe postpartum collapse due to haemorrhage may be followed by ischaemic necrosis of the anterior lobe of the pituitary gland. Thrombosis occurs in the vessels which supply the anterior lobe, and necrosis of the whole lobe occurs, except for a thin rim of tissue which may survive at the surface of the lobe. Death may occur soon after delivery, but if the patient survives she will show the clinical picture of Simmonds's disease (sometimes also known as Sheehan's syndrome). All the endocrine functions of the anterior lobe of the pituitary gland are disturbed. There will be failure of lactation due to lack of prolactin. Because of lack of thyrotropic hormone the patient becomes lethargic, abnormally sensitive to cold, and usually gains weight. Her basal metabolic rate falls, and her glucose tolerance is increased. Because of lack of corticotrophic hormone she will also have asthenia, a low blood pressure, and will respond poorly to infection. Lack of gonadotrophic hormones will lead to genital atrophy, with superinvolution of the uterus, amenorrhoea, and atrophy of the breasts.

Less severe cases may only have part of this complex clinical picture, and in very rare instances a further pregnancy has followed, with regeneration of the pituitary gland.

Prompt treatment of collapse due to postpartum haemorrhage should prevent this disastrous complication. Once the necrosis has occurred substitution therapy may maintain the patient in fair health. For the hypothyroidism thyroxine will be required. For the failure of suprarenal function suprarenal cortical hormones are given. There is no useful purpose in giving gonadotrophic hormones, but testosterone has been found to supplement the action of cortical hormones.

31

Premature labour and premature rupture of the membranes

Premature labour

This is arbitrarily defined as labour occurring before the 37th week of pregnancy. About 10 per cent of hospital deliveries occur prematurely.

Causes

In many cases no cause can be found.

Spontaneous premature rupture of the membranes may occur before term from a variety of causes (see p. 346) including incompetence of the cervix, and in the majority of these cases delivery soon follows.

Premature labour may occur in cases of multiple pregnancy, hydramnios and accidental antepartum haemorrhage. Labour usually, but not invariably, follows fetal death within 3 weeks.

Labour may follow direct trauma to the uterus, and occasionally appears to be the result of acute emotional disturbance or severe fright. With maternal infection which causes high fever premature labour may occur.

Artificial induction of premature labour may be necessary for a number of conditions which threaten intrauterine fetal death, for example pre-eclampsia, hypertension and proteinuria, maternal diabetes, antepartum haemorrhage and haemolytic disease; and is occasionally required for maternal indications, for example rising hypertension.

Prevention

Early admission of cases of pre-eclampsia and hypertension to hospital for rest may reduce the need for early induction of labour. Although it has been claimed that rest in bed will reduce the risk of premature labour in twin pregnancies there is little statistical evidence to support this. In cases of hydramnios repeated paracentesis may prevent premature labour.

A history of previous mid-trimester abortion of a normal fetus may be an indication that the cervix is incompetent. Investigation of this possibility is more conclusive in the non-pregnant state than during pregnancy (p. 140) but in any patient with a history of repeated premature labour or abortion the insertion of an encircling suture in the cervix during early pregnancy may be considered.

Treatment

The patient is admitted to a hospital where there are facilities for specialized care for a premature infant. A vaginal examination is made to determine whether liquor is escaping and whether the cervix is dilated. An external tocograph is useful for recording uterine activity.

Drugs are available which will inhibit uterine contractions. Most obstetricians would not use these if the pregnancy had reached the 35th week. If the membranes have ruptured there is also some risk of intrauterine fetal infection and this may sway the decision against attempting to delay delivery, unless the fetus is so small that it has a high risk of neonatal death. On the other hand, a short delay of 24 to 48 hours before delivery may permit the administration to the mother of dexamethasone with the hope of encouraging the surfactant activity of the fetal lung (p. 466).

Drugs which may be used to inhibit uterine action. Opinions differ about the effectiveness of these drugs. Some controlled trials have thrown doubt upon their value, but many clinicians believe that they are useful.

β-sympathomimetic drugs. These include isoxsuprine, orciprenaline, salbutomol and ritodrine. As an example, ritodrine is added to 5 per cent glucose in water to give a solution containing $100 \mu g/ml$. Intravenous infusion is started at $50 \mu g/minute$ and increased by $50 \mu g/minute$ every 20 minutes until the contractions of the uterus are inhibited or $400 \mu g/minute$ has been reached. Infusion is continued for 2 hours after contractions have ceased, usually for a total of $6-12$ hours. Thereafter ritodrine 15 mg 6-hourly is given by mouth for 4 weeks, or until the 36th week of gestation has been reached. If cardiovascular side-effects such as hypotension and tachycardia occur they may be treated with propanolol 1 mg intravenously.

Alcohol. A dilute solution of ethanol given intravenously for some hours will inhibit uterine action, but the side-effects include nausea, vomiting, restlessness and disorientation.

Inhibitors of prostaglandin synthesis are under trial.

Management of labour. If the pregnancy has passed the 35th week, or if at an earlier stage it is evident that attempts to inhibit uterine action have failed, then prompt delivery is the aim. Before the 33rd week Caesarean section may be considered as it will avoid the risks of birth trauma; after that time vaginal delivery is usually advised.

During labour pain relief should be by epidural block rather than by drugs such as pethidine which may cause respiratory depression in the newborn infant. An episiotomy is performed to minimize compression of the fetal head during delivery, and in a primigravida gentle forceps extraction with Wrigley's forceps may be advantageous. Everything must be ready for the resuscitation and care of the premature infant.

Premature rupture of the membranes

This refers to spontaneous rupture of the membranes before the onset of labour. Labour is likely to follow soon afterwards, and while this is of little significance if the pregnancy is near term, at an earlier stage a small fetus will be delivered, with increased perinatal mortality. If labour does not occur for some days after the membranes rupture bacteria may invade the uterine cavity and cause intrauterine infection of the fetus. There is also a risk of prolapse of the cord.

Causes

There is no evidence that the membranes are weak or abnormal.

Premature rupture of the membranes may occur in cases of multiple pregnancy and hydramnios. With malpresentations such as a transverse lie the presenting part does not fit into the pelvic brim and premature rupture of the membranes is a theoretical possibility; in fact this seldom occurs unless labour has started.

Incompetence of the internal os of the cervix may be caused by forcible surgical dilatation of the cervix for termination of pregnancy or the treatment of dysmenorrhoea, or by obstetrical injury. The cervix dilates painlessly, the membranes bulge through it, and their eventual rupture is followed by mid-trimester abortion or premature labour.

Very rarely there is an intermittent escape of clear fluid throughout pregnancy (*hydrorrhoea gravidarum*). The cause is often obscure. Exudation of fluid from the exposed but intact membranes sometimes occurs in cases of cervical incompetence. Fluid loss is said to occur in cases of circumvallate placenta (p. 152).

Diagnosis

The patient notices the escape of fluid, and sometimes speculum examination will show that this is coming through the cervix.

Sometimes the difficulty is to make sure that the escaping fluid is not urine. If it is liquor, microscopical examination may show fetal squames, lanugo hairs or vernix. If the urine is tested and contains no protein, discovery of protein in the escaping fluid suggests that it is liquor. Cervical mucus has a different consistency.

Management

The patient is admitted to hospital. A vaginal examination is made with sterile precautions to obtain a sample of the fluid, to assess cervical dilatation, to discover the presentation and to exclude prolapse of the cord. An ultrasonic scan may be required to confirm the period of gestation.

If the pregnancy has passed 36 weeks it is best to expedite labour with an intravenous oxytocin drip. Before 35 weeks it may be more prudent to delay labour until the fetus is more mature. The patient is kept at rest in bed and given a broad-spectrum antibiotic such as ampicillin. Some liquor may be obtained by amniocentesis (rather than by testing that which is escaping) for determination of the lecithin-sphingomyelin ratio (p. 369) as an index of the maturity of the fetal lungs.

If there is any uterine activity this may be inhibited by giving one of the drugs mentioned above. If the fetal lung is immature the mother is given dexamethasone 12 mg orally, then 6 mg daily in divided doses.

32

Presentation and prolapse of the umbilical cord

Descent of the umbilical cord below the presenting part occurs about once in 300 births, and constitutes a grave risk to the fetus because of obstruction to the circulation in the umbilical vessels.

Two types of descent are described. The cord is said to be *presenting* when it lies below the presenting part in an intact bag of membranes (Fig. 32.1), and *prolapsing* when the membranes have ruptured. Sometimes the cord lies beside the head but cannot be easily felt on vaginal examination (occult prolapse). This may cause fetal distress, the cause of which is not evident at the time.

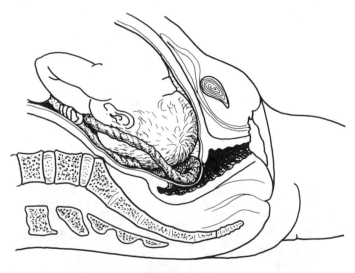

Fig. 32.1 Presentation of umbilical cord.

Causes

Descent of the cord is more likely to occur when the presenting part does not fit well into the lower uterine segment. In normal cases the well-flexed head engages before the onset of labour or soon after this, and tends to prevent prolapse of the cord. Prolapse is particularly likely to occur with malpresentations such as a flexed breech or shoulder presentation, and occasionally with a brow, face or even an occipito-posterior position of the vertex. It is more likely to occur when the head is free above the pelvic brim, sometimes because of pelvic contraction. Prolapse of the cord may occur with a premature or small fetus, and in twin pregnancy.

Excess of liquor amnii, by permitting greater mobility of the fetus tends to encourage malpresentation, and when the membranes rupture a sudden gush of liquor may carry a loop of cord down into the vagina. In some cases of descent the cord is unduly long, or is attached to a low-lying placenta.

Diagnosis

Presentation of the cord is seldom discovered. This may be because it is less common than prolapse of the cord, and also because patients are not invariably examined vaginally at the onset of labour. A presenting cord can be felt through the intact bag of membranes, and the pulsation of its vessels should be recognized. (Pulsation may also be felt in cases of vasa praevia, in which there is a velamentous insertion of the cord. See p. 156.) Slowing of the fetal heart may be noted when the head is pushed into the brim in cases of presentation of the cord, but slowing may also occur in cases of placenta praevia or vasa praevia, or simply as a result of compression of the head.

In prolapse of the cord the diagnosis is easy as a loop of cord is felt in the vagina, or may even present at the vulva. It should be a rule that every patient is examined vaginally as soon as possible after rupture of the membranes, whether she is having contractions or not, in order to exclude or diagnose prolapse of the cord. The loop of cord should be felt to see if pulsations are present, but even if the cord is compressed so that pulsations are absent the fetus may yet be alive, and fetal heart sounds may be audible on auscultation of the abdomen.

Whenever presentation or prolapse of the cord is diagnosed, the degree of dilatation of the cervix should be noted, and the cause sought. The possibility of twins, malpresentation or contracted pelvis should be considered.

Prognosis

Presentation or prolapse of the cord does not itself increase the risk to the mother, except for the possible increased risk of complications such as malpresentations or contracted pelvis, but descent of the cord often calls for speedy delivery by forceps, breech extraction or Caesarean section, and these procedures increase the maternal risk to some extent.

The prognosis for the fetus is grave; stillbirth or neonatal death occurs in about 20 per cent of cases. It is said that the fetal prognosis is worst when the head presents as it is more likely to compress the cord than the breech or shoulder. The outlook for the fetus has been improved by the more frequent use of Caesarean section in cases in which the cervix is not fully dilated.

Treatment

If the fetus is alive the treatment is immediate delivery.

If the cervix is not fully dilated this will be by Caesarean section. While preparations for the operation are being made immediate steps are taken to relieve pressure on the cord. Even if pulsation cannot be felt in the cord the fetal heart may still be heard on auscultation or detected with ultrasound. Two or more fingers are inserted into the vagina and the presenting part is pushed as far out of the pelvic cavity as possible and held there. Attempts to replace the cord are usually unsuccessful and also produce spasm in the cord vessels; they should not be made.

If the cervix is fully dilated and there is a cephalic presentation with no complicating factor such as malpresentation or contracted pelvis immediate delivery with the forceps is performed. If there is a breech presentation the presenting part is very unlikely to be deep in the pelvis, and Caesarean section may be preferable to breech extraction, but the latter may be chosen for a flexed breech that is not unduly large. For other malpresentations which would require correction before vaginal delivery is possible, Caesarean section is wisest.

If it is certain that the fetus is dead, unless there is some other problem such as a contracted pelvis, labour is left to continue to eventual vaginal delivery. Analgesic drugs, including morphine, can be freely given.

33

Fetal distress during labour

During each uterine contraction the maternal blood flow through the placenta is impeded, the venous outflow before the arterial supply. The fetus is usually unaffected by this, but if uterine contractions are prolonged or if there has been previous impairment of placental function then fetal hypoxia occurs. As a result the carbon dioxide concentration in the fetal blood rises and respiratory acidosis occurs with a fall in pH. In severe hypoxia the fetal tissues meet their energy requirements by anaerobic glycolysis, burning up glycogen but producing lactic acid in the process, and this causes further depression of the pH by metabolic acidosis. Although the fetus will withstand and recover from degrees of hypoxia and acidosis which would be fatal in an adult, if the pH falls below about 6.9 death is inevitable.

Coincidentally with the changes in hydrogen ion concentration the fetus shows clinical signs of distress. This is an ill-defined term, and distress may not invariably be due to hypoxia, although this is the commonest cause. The first effect of hypoxia is a rise in fetal heart rate from sympathetic action. Fetal tachycardia in cases of hypoxia is of varying degree, but a rate persisting at well above 160 beats per minute has considerable significance. Fetal tachycardia may also occur if the mother has high fever or is dehydrated, but in all other cases this sign must be regarded as evidence of fetal distress.

If the hypoxia persists and is of more severe degree the fetal heart rate will slow after each uterine contraction, and there will also be persistent bradycardia. Any case with slowing below 120 beats per minute should be carefully assessed, and urgently if the rate falls below 100, or if there is cardiac irregularity.

Initial slowing of the fetal heart rate is probably a vagal effect, and vagal activity may also lead to contraction of the bowel and the passage of meconium into the liquor. However, it should be noted that premature fetuses, even if fatally hypoxic, seldom pass meconium.

Unfortunately the correlation between many of these clinical signs of fetal distress and real hypoxia is not very strong. Even the most serious combination of these signs, bradycardia with the passage of meconium, is found to be associated with a significantly hypoxic fetus in only 25 per cent of instances, so that if action were taken on these signs alone it might be unnecessary in three-quarters of the cases.

Continuous monitoring of the fetal heart rate. Ordinary auscultation of the fetal heart rate suffers from several limitations. It has to be performed intermittently, and alterations may occur in the intervals between observations. If the heart is being auscultated for 60 seconds every 15 minutes that leaves 14 out of 15 minutes when changes may not be observed. Further, the main stress that affects the fetal heart rate is a uterine contraction, yet it is at this time that many doctors and midwives fail to hear the heart. Unless auscultation takes place very soon after the contraction any change due to the stress will be missed. In consequence efforts have been made during the last 20 years to record the fetal heart rate continuously, even during contractions. This can be achieved by several methods:

1. In phonocardiography a carbon microphone is held on the mother's abdomen by a wide elastic belt where it picks up the fetal heart sounds. This works well enough when the patient is still, but as labour progresses and the patient moves a good deal the microphone picks up too much background noise, and this method is now seldom used during labour.

2. With pulsed ultrasound the fetal heart rate can be recorded by using the Doppler effect when a pulse source and receiving head is placed on the

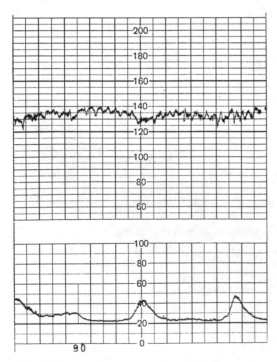

Fig. 33.1 Fetal heart rate. Normal trace.

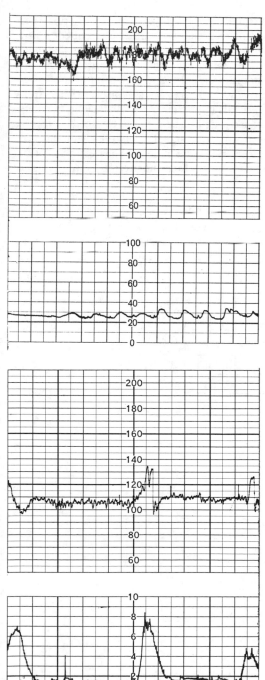

Fig. 33.2
Fetal tachycardia.

Fig. 33.3
Fetal bradycardia.

mother's abdomen. An ultrasonic pulse is passed into the fetus; those waves that hit moving fluid are returned at a different frequency from those reflected back from static objects, and the pulsations of the fetal heart can be recognized. The combined head is less affected by movements and external sounds than the phonocardiograph.

3. The best method currently available is to record the electrical activity of the fetal heart. When the cervix is more than 2 cm dilated and the membranes have ruptured a scalp electrode can be fixed to the fetal scalp; this largely eliminates difficulties arising from signals from the electrical activity of the maternal heart. With a ratemeter a continuous estimate of the fetal heart rate is recorded on a trace on which the uterine contractions are also recorded with a tocometer.

Conventionally a range of 120 to 160 beats per minute is taken as the normal heart rate during labour, but with better recording methods it is found that in most cases the rate is within a range of 130 to 150 beats per minute. Both base-line tachycardia (Fig. 33.2) and base-line bradycardia

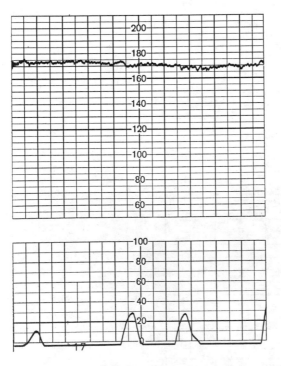

Fig. 33.4   Fetal heart rate. Loss of beat-to-beat variation.

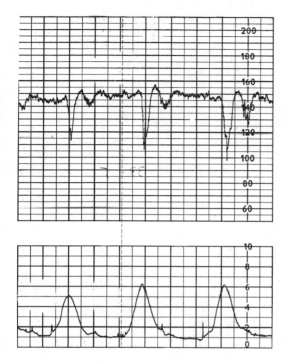

Fig. 33.5 Fetal heart rate. Early decelerations.

(Fig. 33.3) have a significant association with chronic fetal hypoxia. Probably in most instances the heart first beats faster and then slows down if
the stress continues.

Continuous records of the fetal heart rate normally show continuous
minor variations, with a range of about 10 beats per minute. This beat-to-
beat variation is the response of the heart to a variety of factors, including
vagal and sympathetic stimuli, catechol amines and oxygen tension. Loss
of beat-to-beat variation (Fig. 33.4) implies that the cardiac reflexes are impaired, either from the effect of hypoxia or of drugs such as diazepam
(Valium). Loss of beat-to-beat variation is often of serious significance.

Stress to the fetus during labour occurs during a uterine contraction, and
the response of the fetal heart rate to contractions is shown on the
ratemeter trace. With each contraction the rate often slows, but it returns
to normal soon after removal of the stress. These early decelerations or
'dips' in the heart rate start within 30 seconds of the onset of the contraction and return rapidly to the base-line rate. They are not of serious

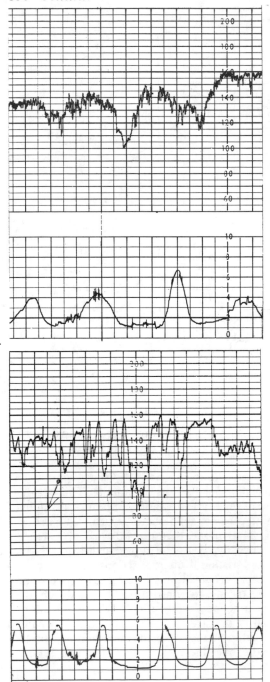

Fig. 33.6
Fetal heart rate.
Late decelerations.

Fig. 33.7
Fetal heart rate.
Variable decelerations.

significance as a rule, and indicate that while the fetus is undergoing some stress the cardiac control mechanisms are responding normally (Fig. 33.5).

Figure 33.6 illustrates a more serious condition. Here the fetal heart takes some time to respond to the stress of the uterine contraction, with the onset of the late deceleration more than 30 seconds after the beginning of the uterine contraction, and a slow return to the base-line rate. Such late decelerations are commonly caused by hypoxia. They must be considered seriously and their exact significance checked by taking a sample of fetal blood at once from the fetal scalp to determine its pH (see below).

In practice variations in the fetal heart rate may be complex and difficult to interpret. Figure 33.7 shows variable decelerations with no consistent relationship to uterine contractions. These are sometimes caused by compression of the umbilical cord between the uterus and the fetal body, or because it is looped round some part of the fetus. Provided that they do not persist for more than a few minutes they may have little significance, but

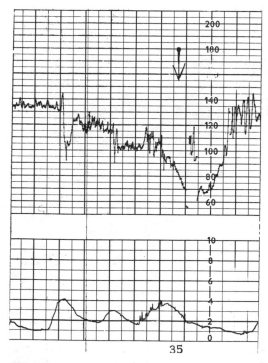

Fig. 33.8 Trace of fetal heart rate showing the effect of overstimulation of the uterus with oxytocin. The drip was turned off at the point marked with the arrow.

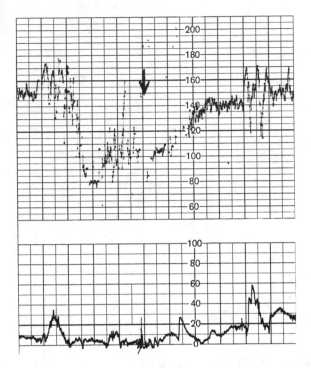

Fig. 33.9 Trace of fetal heart rate showing the effect of maternal supine hypotension. At the point marked with the arrow the mother was turned onto her side. As her blood pressure returned to normal the fetal bradycardia ceased.

persistence for more than 15 minutes would call for an urgent fetal blood sample.

Overstimulation of the uterine muscle with oxytocin will cause prolonged uterine contractions and severe changes in the fetal heart rate. (Fig. 33.8.) However, if the mother lies on her back, compression of the inferior vena cava by the uterus may impede the venous return, depress the cardic output and reduce placental blood flow. The effect of asking the mother to lie on her side should always be observed (Fig. 33.9.) If the changes in the fetal heart rate still persist myometrial overactivity may well be the cause.

A rare cause of a slow fetal heart rate is congenital heart block. It carries a bad prognosis as it may be associated with other congenital cardiac abnormalities. The condition may be recognized by noting that the rate has always been slow, even in pregnancy, and by observing that the slow rate does not vary during labour.

An increase in the fetal heart rate can occur with intrauterine infection or with maternal pyrexia from any cause.

Precise continuous recording of the fetal heart rate in relation to uterine contractions is a great advance in monitoring the fetus during labour, but it should not be assumed that such traces are absolute indications for intervention. Any suggestion that the fetus is hypoxic should be checked by determining the pH of the fetal blood before Caesarean section is undertaken. The most serious pattern of heart-rate changes, namely fetal bradycardia with loss of beat-to-beat variation and late decelerations, is associated with significant fetal hypoxia in about 65 per cent of cases. Even among these there will therefore be about 35 per cent of cases in which fetal blood sampling will show that immediate intervention is not necessary.

Fetal blood sampling. During labour after the membranes have ruptured spontaneously or have been ruptured artificially a sample of fetal blood can be obtained for evaluation of its acid-base status. It is possible to measure the partial pressure of oxygen, but this fluctuates very quickly, and the pH gives a better indication of the metabolic state of the fetus. The blood is obtained by passing an endoscope through the cervix and then us-

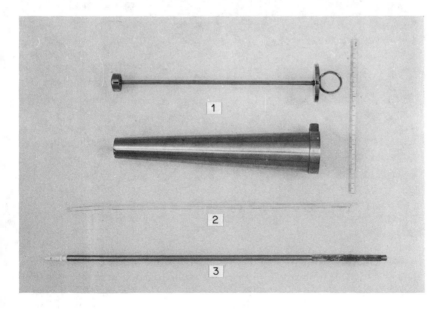

Fig. 33.10 Instruments for fetal blood sampling. 1. Amnioscope and obturator. 2. Glass tube for aspiration of blood. 3. Long-handled bladeholder (see Fig. 33.11) for incision of scalp.

ing a very small blade held in a suitable handle to make a small incision in the fetal scalp. A drop of blood is drawn into a long fine tube. With 0.2 ml of blood the pH can be determined immediately with a micro-Astrup machine.

Fetal blood sampling during labour is of value in excluding hypoxia in cases with clinical suspicion of fetal distress, so that unnecessary Caesarean section may be avoided. If the pH is above 7.25 there is no hypoxia *at the time of the observation*, although the test has no predictive value. In doubtful cases a progressive fall in pH below 7.20 in successive samples during the first stage of labour is highly significant, but in the second stage a pH of 7.15 may be accepted as the lower limit of normal. Sampling is seldom performed during the second stage, because by this time it is usually simpler to deliver the fetus suspected of being hypoxic with forceps.

The state of the fetus is best monitored during labour by a combination of continuous recording of the fetal heart rate with blood sampling when

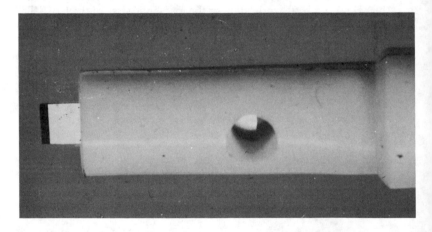

Fig. 33.11   Enlarged photograph of blade. The small square white blade is 2 mm long and the wide shoulder prevents deeper penetration of the scalp.

necessary to confirm any suspicion of hypoxia. Obviously such monitoring is only possible in well-equipped and well-staffed units. In such units about a third of the patients are usually judged to need continuous monitoring. At present continuous fetal heart rate monitoring is widely used in Britain, but fetal blood sampling is less often performed. These methods do not cause an increased work load for the staff, because they may reduce the Caesarean rate for unreal fetal distress. In some respects they make surveillance of the patients easier, but they must never be allowed to interfere with the close personal relationship between patients in labour and the staff. If women who are judged to have high risk pregnancies are transferred to units with good facilities for monitoring better management of fetal hypoxia will result, with a reduction in both perinatal mortality and morbidity.

34

The relief of pain in labour

It was an obstetrician, James Young Simpson, who first used chloroform for the relief of pain during labour. Even for operative delivery anaesthesia was not available until 1847. Dr Snow administered chloroform to Queen Victoria during the births of her two youngest children, and 'chloroform á la Reine' became popular for analgesia during normal labour.

The amount of pain experienced during labour appears to vary enormously from patient to patient. A few women find that labour is almost painless, but the majority have pain that they describe as severe. Some will manage with minimal doses of analgesic drugs while others demand much more.

During the first stage of labour pain is felt with each uterine contraction. The pressure in the uterus between contractions is of the order of 10 mm Hg. During a first stage contraction the pressure is about 50 mm Hg. Most patients do not feel pain until the pressure reaches 25 mm Hg; the beginning of the contraction can be felt with the hand or recorded with a tocograph before the patient feels pain. The pain is believed to be caused by ischaemia of the myometrium, which occurs when the blood flow is arrested or impeded by the contraction.

The nerve pathway for the pain of uterine contractions is the hypogastric plexus and then the pre-aortic plexus, entering the cord as high as the 11th and 12th dorsal segments via the posterior nerve roots.

Pain is also caused by dilatation of the cervix, and this is severe at the end of the first stage. Probably sensory impulses from the cervix enter the cord via the sacral roots; pain towards the end of the first stage is often referred to the sacral region.

The upper vagina distends easily, and this does not seem to cause much pain, but during the second stage, when the head is stretching the vulval orifice, severe pain is felt which is different from that of uterine contraction. Pain impulses from the vulva and perineum are carried by the pudendal nerves, and to a small extend in the ilio-inguinal nerves.

During the antenatal period patients should be told about the stages of labour in simple terms, avoiding technical words and the jargon of the labour ward. It is particularly important to explain that the first stage of labour is long compared to the second, and that during the first stage the neck of the womb is being opened up, and that there will be no sensation of progress or descent of the baby. In a normal second stage the patient will be encouraged by feeling the descent of the baby and the realization that the end of labour is not far away. The severity of pain may not be altered by explanation, but fear of the unknown and fear that the labour is not progressing normally can greatly add to distress.

There are those who believe that if the patient is tense this will impede the progress of labour, and that if she is relaxed labour will be both quicker and less painful. While it is agreed that a tense pelvic floor might delay delivery, there is nothing to show that dilatation of the cervix will be affected by the general state of the patient. However, it is probable that the patient who relaxes completely and rests between pains is conserving her energy, and will be able to make stronger voluntary efforts in the second stage.

Various courses of antenatal exercises have been recommended; if they give the patient confidence they are useful and helpful, although there is little or no scientific evidence that they have any other effect on the course of labour. It is wrong to tell women that if only they follow some pattern of exercises or relaxation that they will have little pain and that labour will be quick and normal; when this sometimes proves to be untrue disappointment may turn into anxiety and recrimination.

Patients should be told about the various means of relieving pain, and that these will be available on demand. Secure in the knowledge that help is available many women will not ask for any analgesic until the first stage is well advanced. Drugs should never be given in a routine fashion, but always with respect for the patient's wishes and need. During antenatal instruction classes the patients should visit the labour ward and if possible meet the staff who will look after them there, and be given a demonstration of such equipment as the gas and oxygen machine.

During labour women should never be allowed to feel that they have been left alone and deserted. A sensible and affectionate husband can give much support and comfort, provided that he has also been given a little instruction and told what to expect. The knowledge that a trusted doctor or midwife is present or immediately available will make labour more tolerable.

The ideal analgesic

An ideal analgesic for labour will not harm or endanger the mother or the fetus. In particular it:
1. Should not interfere with uterine action
2. Should not lead to more operative intervention
3. Should not depress the respiratory centre of the newborn infant
4. Should be easy to administer and be foolproof
5. Should be predictable and constant in its effects.

Analgesia in the first stage of labour

Three methods are in common use during the first stage:

(1) Drugs which are given by intramuscular injection. This method is simple and convenient. Oral administration of drugs during labour is unsatisfactory because absorption is so unreliable.

(2) An anaesthetic agent which is inhaled. This method is not suitable for use over long periods, and is therefore only used in the latter part of the second stage; it is more appropriate for the second stage.

(3) An epidural or caudal block. This gives compelete relief of pain, but requires skill in injection, and has a few hazards.

Analgesic drugs.   Over the years many drugs have been used, but *pethidine* is now in almost universal use. It is a synthetic drug which is less effective than morphine in relieving pain, but has less depressant effect on the respiratory centre of the newborn infant. However, it is untrue to say that it has no depressant effect, and it should not be given if delivery is expected within 2 hours. The usual dose is 100 – 150 mg intramuscularly, and 50 – 100 mg can be repeated after 2 hours. In an average labour the total dose should not exceed 400 mg. It is sometimes combined with promezathine (Phenergan) 25 – 50 mg, or with promazine hydrochloride (Sparine) to increase the sedative effect. Pethidine sometimes has an emetic effect; this can be counteracted with metoclopramide (Maxolon) 10 mg intramuscularly.

Morphine sulphate 15 mg, sometimes combined with hyoscine 0.4 mg, is seldom used today for normal labour because of its effect on the infant's respiratory centre, but in cases in which the fetus is dead or grossly abnormal (e.g. anencephalic) such drugs will give good pain relief.

Respiratory depression in the newborn from pethidine or morphine can be counteracted by injecting naloxone (Narcan neonatal) into the umbilical vein. The preparation contains 0.02 mg/ml, and the dose is 0.005 mg/kg.

Inhalation analgesia.   See below.

Epidural block.   This is usually started in the first stage, and it is then effective throughout labour. It is preferable to spinal anaesthesia during pregnancy, because the latter causes vasomotor paralysis of the lower part of the body, and if this is combined with interference with the venous return by the large uterus sudden and severe hypotension may occur. The anaesthetic is injected into the epidural space through a Tuohy needle which is usually inserted between the 1st and 2nd lumbar spines. Lignocaine (Xylocaine) 1 per cent is used. A polythene catheter is threaded through the needle and left in the epidural space so that further injections of the anaesthetic can be given as required. The injection calls for some skill and experience of the method, and whoever gives it must maintain continuous supervision and be prepared to deal with immediate complications such as hypotension, or temporary respiratory paralysis from accidental intrathecal injection. Long-term neurological sequelae such as weakness or paraesthesia of the legs or bladder disturbances are very rare.

In some hospitals today epidural anaesthesia is provided for more than half of the patients in normal labour, but a 24 hour service makes heavy demands on anaesthetic staff (or on the obstetricians if they choose to master the technique and give the injection themselves). With epidural analgesia the incidence of forceps delivery will be increased because voluntary expulsive efforts are often ineffective, but apart from this there are no adverse fetal effects. Uterine tone is good, and the risk of postpartum haemorrhage is reduced.

Epidural anaesthesia is excellent for cases of prolonged labour from incoordinate uterine action, for vaginal operative procedures such as rotation and forceps delivery of a head in the occipito-posterior position, for breech delivery, for severe cases of pre-eclampsia and for Caesarean section.

Caudal analgesia is an alternative method of introducing an extradural block. A malleable needle is inserted through the sacral hiatus into the sacral canal, and a catheter may be left in the extradural space to continue the injection. The lumbar route is now generally preferred.

Analgesia for the normal second stage of labour

Two methods are in common use:
(1) Intermittent inhalation of anaesthetic mixtures.
(2) Regional block.

Intermittent inhalation methods. *Nitrous oxide mixtures.* If an anaesthetist is available nitrous oxide and oxygen can be given as required with the pains. Because most women cannot have the services of an anaesthetist for normal labour, in 1934 Minnett introduced the first machine for self-administration of a mixture of nitrous oxide and air. The patient applied the mask to her face with each pain, and as long as she kept her finger on the valve hole each inspiration drew in the mixture. For effective analgesia at least 50 per cent concentration of nitrous oxide is needed and then 50 per cent of air contains insufficient oxygen to prevent hypoxia. Later machines were designed to deliver mixtures of gas and oxygen.

All these machines have been superseded by the Entonox machine. This has gas cylinders containing a mixture of nitrous oxide and oxygen in equal proportions. The cylinders must not be kept below room temperature, because at lower temperatures the gases separate out. Successful self-administration depends on the patient fitting the mask accurately to her nose and mouth, and closing the valve properly with her finger. She should take a deep breath as soon as the pain starts. Careful preliminary instruction is essential.

Trichlorethylene (Trilene). Freedman devised the first machine for self-administration of mixtures of trichlorethylene and air. Later modifications

(Emotril and Tecota machines) deliver a very constant mixture of 0.5 per cent trilene by volume in air. These machines are small and portable. They produce satisfactory analgesia in most patients without affecting the strength of the uterine contractions or adversely affecting the infant.

Regional block.   This method has many advantages. It does not affect the baby's respiratory centre, nor the uterine action. Except for epidural analgesia, the services of an anaesthetist are not required. In comparison with general anaesthesia it is much safer during labour because the risk of the unprepared patient inhaling vomit is avoided. Furthermore many women like to be fully conscious during delivery. Methods in general use include:

Epidural analgesia.   This has been described.

Pudendal block.   This simple method can be used for normal delivery, including repair of an episiotomy or perineal tear, for forceps delivery or vacuum extraction, for breech and twin delivery. The pudendal nerve is derived from the 2nd, 3rd and 4th sacral nerves. These roots unite above the level of the ischial spine. The nerve passes out of the greater sciatic foramen posteriorly to the ischial spine and re-enters the pelvis through the lesser sciatic foramen. It then enters the pudendal canal where the vessels lie lateral to the nerve. The nerve divides into:

1. The inferior haemorrhoidal nerve, giving branches to the anal sphincter and the skin around the anus.

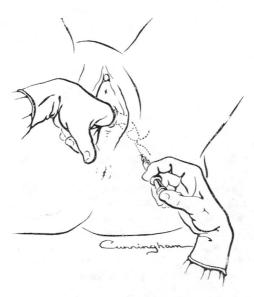

Fig. 34.1   Pudendal block. The index finger of the left hand helps to direct the needle to the correct position.

2. The perineal branch, supplying the perineal muscles and the skin of the perineum and labia majora.

3. The dorsal nerve of the clitoris, supplying the clitoris and labia minora. Fibres from the posterior femoral cutaneous nerve and from the ilio-inguinal nerve also reach the perineum.

Lignocaine hydrochloride 1 per cent is used throughout (without adrenaline). The total amount injected should not exceed 50 ml. A skin weal is raised halfway between the anus and the ischial tuberosity. The index finger of the left hand is inserted in the vagina and the right ischial spine is located. A 20 cm 20 gauge needle is passed through the weal and directed towards the ischial spine with the guidance of the vaginal finger. The needle is directed just posteriorly to the inferior tip of the spine. The plunger of the syringe is withdrawn to make sure that the needle is not in a vein and about 5 ml of lignocaine solution are injected. The needle is inserted a further centimetre and, after testing for intravasation by withdrawing the plunger again, another 5 ml of lignocaine are injected. The process is repeated on the left side.

Some prefer to insert the needle through the vaginal wall rather than the perineal skin.

Pudendal block is usually combined with local infiltration of the vulva, a weal being raised at the fourchette and lignocaine injected here and on each side, extending well forward in both labia majora. If the local infiltration is carried out before the pudendal block it will reduce the discomfort of the manipulations required for the block.

The anaesthetic takes effect in about 5 minutes.

Perineal infiltration. If an episiotomy is required in advanced labour with the presenting part well down, direct infiltration of the line of incision with lignocaine 1 per cent is employed.

Anaesthesia for operative delivery

For operative deliveries numerous anaesthetic techniques are available. Whenever possible, for vaginal delivery an epidural or pudendal block is used, but sometimes general anaesthesia is unavoidable. For lower segment Caesarean section some abdominal relaxation is required and general anaesthesia (including the use of a relaxant, see p. 399) is generally employed, although it is possible to perform the operation under lumbar extradural block or regional infiltration of the abdominal wall. Whatever method is used, morphine and allied drugs which may depress the respiratory centre of the newborn infant should not be given for premedication.

The danger of general anaesthesia in obstetrics. The Reports on Confidential Enquiries into Maternal Deaths in England and Wales show that a number of fatalities occur every year from complications of general anaesthesia. Most of these are caused by inhalation of vomit when solid particles obstruct the bronchioles, or by acid secretion causing intense bronchial spasm (Mendelson's syndrome). It is extremely dangerous to give a general anaesthetic if the head of the obstetric bed cannot be lowered immediately if vomiting occurs, and without proper suction apparatus ready.

Although the responsibility for the technical details of general anaesthesia during labour does not fall to the obstetrician, it must never be forgotten that any patient in labour may unexpectedly need an anaesthetic. Solid food should never be given to women in labour, but during labour there is gastric stasis and the stomach may contain food which has been taken many hours before. The passage of a gastric tube is sometimes prudent before an emergency anaesthetic, and in all cases magnesium trisilicate powder 2 g in a little water may be given before induction of anaesthesia. A most useful preventative measure against inhalation of vomitus during induction of anaesthesia is cricoid pressure. As the patient is falling asleep and the relaxant that is commonly used is taking effect, an assistant pushes the cricoid cartilage back against the cervical vertebrae so as to compress the oesophagus and prevent regurgitation into the pharynx until the cuffed endotracheal tube is passed and inflated.

Should vomiting occur the head of the patient must be lowered at once and turned on one side so that vomit can flow out of the mouth. The pharynx is immediately cleared with suction apparatus. If inhalation has occurred the patient must be carefully observed afterwards lest there should be collapse of the lungs. If Mendelson's syndrome develops 500 mg of hydrocortisone is given intravenously and oxygen used as required. Further injections of hydrocortisone 250 mg 6-hourly may be required, and prophylactic antibiotics are given.

An administrative problem is that emergency obstetric anaesthesia is often required at inconvenient hours, or when senior anaesthetists are already engaged with other work. In large obstetric units provision of anaesthetic cover at all times for the labour ward is a necessity, not only for the comfort but for the safety of the patients.

35

Obstetric operations

Amniocentesis

Amniocentesis means the insertion of a needle into the amniotic sac through the abdominal wall in order to withdraw some of the fluid. It is performed after the 14th week.

Indications for diagnostic purposes

1. **Haemolytic disease.** Rhesus immunization causes destruction of fetal red cells and an excess of bilirubin enters the liquor amnii. Spectrophotometric analysis of the liquor is effected by scanning with light of wave-length between 700 and 300 mμ. Bilirubin causes absorption at 450 mμ and the degree of change of optical density is a measure of the bilirubin content. Tests carried out repeatedly between 20 and 36 weeks serve as a guide to the treatment necessary.

2. **Maturity of the fetal lungs.** Lecithin is secreted from the fetal lungs into the amniotic fluid during the second half of pregnancy. Lecithin is a constituent of surfactant, which is necessary for normal lung expansion after birth (p. 466), and the lecithin concentration in the liquor is an index of the maturity of the lungs. Because the total volume of the liquor varies greatly and the dilution of lecithin will therefore vary, the concentration of lecithin in the liquor is usually expressed in relation to the concentration of sphingomyelin, which is fairly constant. If the lecithin-sphingomyelin ratio (L/S ratio) is greater than 2 the production of surfactant is likely to be adequate.

3. **Duration of pregnancy and fetal maturity.** Creatinine is excreted into the liquor in fetal urine. As the kidneys mature the creatinine level rises, and a level of 16 mmol/l (2 g/100 ml) indicates a probable maturity of 36 weeks or more.

The liquor may be centrifuged to obtain a smear of fetal epithelial cells, which are stained with Nile Blue sulphate. After 36 weeks mature cells containing orange-yellow fat are seen against the background of blue-stained cells. If there are more than 10 per cent of orange cells the maturity is likely to be more than 36 weeks, and 38 weeks or more if there are more than 50 per cent.

4. **Fetal hypoxia.** Discovery of green-stained liquor suggests that there has been an episode of fetal hypoxia, during which the fetus passed some meconium into the liquor.

5. **Detection of fetal abnormalities.** (a) *Chromosomal studies.* Fetal amniotic cells can be grown in tissue culture for chromosomal analysis. The culture and study of the cells takes 2 or 3 weeks. There is no point in chromosomal studies unless the purpose has been fully explained to the parents, and they have decided that termination of the pregnancy is desirable if the abnormality under investigation is found.

The most important group of fetuses needing investigation are those at risk of having Down's syndrome. The risk reaches 1 in 50 with mothers aged 40 or more, and investigation is also required when there has already been an affected child (see p. 502).

Prediction of fetal sex would permit selective abortion of female fetuses with X-linked disorders such as Duchenne muscular dystrophy, and male fetuses when the mothers are carriers of such conditions as haemophilia.

(b) *Chemical studies.* In cases of open neural tube defects an excess of α-fetoprotein may be discovered in the liquor. Levels above 20 μg/ml indicate the presence of a defect, but the results need careful interpretation. It is possible to screen all pregnant women for the serum level of α-fetoprotein, and then those with a level above the 95th centile can be offered amniocentesis and ultrasonic scanning.

Antenatal enzyme assay of amniotic fluid or cultured fetal cells will detect some rare inborn metabolic disorders.

Indications for therapeutic purposes

Amniocentesis may be performed to relieve severe or acute hydramnios (p. 175). It is part of the procedure for intrauterine fetal transfusion for haemolytic disease (p. 453) and for the intra-amniotic injection of hypertonic saline or of prostaglandins for termination of pregnancy.

Procedure

A preliminary ultrasonic scan is recommended to locate the site of the placenta and the position of the fetus. The patient empties her bladder and lies supine. Using a strict surgical technique, the skin is infiltrated with a local anaesthetic over the site of puncture, which should be between the fetal limbs. A spinal needle with a stylet is inserted into the amniotic cavity, which is usually entered at a depth of about 4 cm. The stylet is withdrawn and clear liquor should flow up the needle; 20 ml of fluid are withdrawn with a syringe. If blood is encountered it may be necessary to relocate another clean needle. Liquor for spectrophotometry is placed in an amber container to avoid exposure of the bilirubin to light; genetic samples are placed in a polystyrene container.

The procedure is not free from risk. In early pregnancy abortion may occur. Later, accidental antepartum haemorrhage or damage to fetal vessels on the surface of the placenta may cause fetal death. The needle may pierce some part of the fetus. There is a small risk of inducing rhesus isoimmunization, and for that reason 50 μg of anti-D gammaglobulin should be injected if the mother is rhesus negative. The risk of fetal death from amniocentesis is greatest in early pregnancy, and may then be as high as 2 per cent. Parents must be warned of this.

External version

Turning the fetus with both hands on the mother's abdominal wall is known as external version. Nearly always the head is brought to present (cephalic version), but occasionally this is not possible in cases of transverse lie, and then breech presentation is chosen as second best (podalic version).

Indications

External version is most commonly performed to turn a breech presentation or a transverse lie to a cephalic presentation in the antenatal clinic, usually between the 34th and 36th weeks of pregnancy, although it is sometimes possible later.

It is also performed before the delivery of a second twin, if that is found to be lying transversely before the membranes of the second sac have ruptured. For this particular case many obstetricians would choose podalic rather than cephalic version (see p. 183).

Contraindications

External version should not be attempted if there has been any antepartum haemorrhage for fear of causing further placental separation. Some would regard hypertension as a contraindication because it is occasionally associated with antepartum haemorrhage.

External version is not possible with twin pregnancy; the other fetus will not allow space for turning.

Version is pointless if the patient is to be delivered by Caesarean section, but it may be performed in cases of doubtful disproportion so that a trial of labour may then be conducted. If there is a Caesarean scar in the uterus only very gentle attempts at version are permissible.

Technique

The technique is described on p. 283. Only gentle version is safe; force must never be used. Version may fail because the fetus has become too big, or because there is a deficiency of liquor. The patient may have difficulty in relaxing her abdominal muscles, so that the fetus cannot be grasped. Persistent attempts at version will only cause bruising, with tenderness and even less relaxation. Failure often occurs if the breech is deeply engaged in the pelvic brim and the legs are extended.

Version under anaesthesia. Anaesthesia is only indicated if it will eliminate the factor causing failure. It can overcome contraction of the abdominal muscles, but most anaesthetics (including relaxants) have no effect on the tone of the uterus. An exception is fluothane (Halothane), but this occasionally causes toxic jaundice. By removing the patient's pain reflexes anaesthesia adds considerably to the dangers of version, and particular care must be used to avoid excessive force. Anaesthesia is less often used now than formerly.

Immediately after successful cephalic version the head is high above the pelvic brim, but this must not be taken to imply that the pelvis is contracted. One advantage of using anaesthesia is that clinical assessment of the pelvis can be made at the time by vaginal examination.

Risks

When version is performed by an experienced obstetrician in selected cases without anaesthesia there is very little risk. However, version can cause partial placental separation and accidental antepartum haemorrhage, rupture of the membranes and premature labour if it is injudiciously employed, particularly with anaesthesia.

Induction of labour

Indications

The indications for induction of labour include *some* cases of:
1. Pre-eclampsia and essential hypertension
2. Postmaturity
3. Antepartum haemorrhage
4. Hydramnios
5. Unstable lie
6. Diabetes mellitus
7. Haemolytic disease
8. Fetal abnormality
9. Fetal death.

Details of the indications for induction for these conditions are set out in previous chapters, and still other indications will occasionally arise. It is important that induction should only be carried out for sound obstetric or medical reasons, and always in what is judged to be the best interest of the mother and fetus. A few patients will have exceptional domestic or social problems which are very important to them and for which they request induction, and the doctor must consider such requests carefully, but in no circumstances should induction be undertaken just for the convenience of the hospital or its staff.

Methods

Today nearly all inductions are performed by (1) administration of oxytocin or prostaglandins or (2) artificial rupture of the membranes (amniotomy), and the two methods are often combined.

If the fetus is dead amniotomy is undesirable because of the possible entry of bacteria to colonize the dead tissue, and prostaglandins or the intra-amniotic injection of hypertonic urea are used.

Induction with oxytocic drugs. Drugs used for the induction of labour may be given alone; or they may be given before, at the same time or after amniotomy. The dose must be carefully adjusted according to the uterine response; otherwise unduly strong uterine action may endanger the life of the fetus or even rupture the uterus.

Grossly excessive doses of oxytocin also have an antidiuretic effect and may cause serious water retention.

Intravenous oxytocin infusion. Oxytocin is best administered by intravenous drip. This has the advantage that the drug acts continuously and that the dose can be accurately regulated according to the response of the uterus. It is essential that the patient is kept under constant observation. The uterine contractions should be recorded with a tocograph and the fetal heart rate wth a ratemeter, as described in Chapter 33, p. 351. The drip fluid contains 2 units of natural oxytocin (Pitocin) or, more commonly, 2 units of synthetic oxytocin (Syntocinon) in 500 ml of 5 per cent glucose solution and is started at 15 drops per minute (about 3 mU/min). The rate of infusion is gradually increased until satisfactory contractions occur at 3 to 4 minute intervals. If the uterus proves to be relatively insensitive it is better to double the concentration of oxytocin rather than to increase the rate of drip above 60 drops per minute. When the contractions are regular the oxytocin solution can sometimes be turned off, but the drip is continued slowly with glucose solution until the end of the third stage, so that oxytocin infusion can be resumed at any time.

Prostaglandins. Prostaglandins E_2 and $F_{2\alpha}$ may be given by intravenous infusion for the induction of labour, but they do not appear to have any advantage over oxytocin when used at or near term, and the side-effects, particularly nausea and vomiting make them unacceptable to patients. Prostaglandin pessaries (PGE_2, 3 mg) inserted into the vaginal fornix are most effective in inducing labour if the cervix is ripe, and they may also be used to ripen the cervix before amniotomy. They have no side-effects.

Artificial rupture of the membranes. This is a reliable method of inducing labour even when it is used alone, but it is now common practice to combine it with the use of oxytocin or prostaglandins. Complications and failures are few if the pregnancy is near or past term, if the head is engaged in the pelvis, and if the cervix is soft.

Anaesthesia is seldom necessary. After emptying her bladder, the patient is placed in the lithotomy position, and the vulva is swabbed with antiseptic lotion and cream. After draping the area with sterile towels the operator, wearing a mask and sterile gloves and gown, makes a vaginal examination to confirm that the presentation of the fetus is normal. A finger is passed into the cervical canal and then swept round inside the uterus to separate the membranes from the lower segment as widely as possible. This in itself is an important factor in the induction, perhaps because it causes liberation of prostaglandins locally. Under the guidance of the fingers a pair of Kocher's artery forceps are passed through the cervix to seize and tear the bag of membranes. If the head is high an assistant should push it down from above; this not only makes the amniotomy easier by making the bag of membranes tense, but diminishes the risk of prolapse of the cord. Once the membranes have been ruptured the presenting part will descend as uterine contractions begin.

After amniotomy alone labour will usually begin within 8 hours, but if labour is not in progress within 3 hours it is now the practice to begin an oxytocic drip, as already described.

Risks of induction

With the combination of amniotomy and oxytocin infusion failure of induction is now very rare. If labour does not start for some hours there is a slight risk of infection, and ampicillin 250 mg would then be given 6-hourly by injection. Loss of the forewaters does not delay labour, but rather appears to increase the rate of cervical dilatation. In rare cases in which labour has not started 12 hours after amniotomy and oxytocin infusion Caesarean section would be seriously considered.

The fetal risk is chiefly that of the condition for which the induction was performed. If there is any fear of placental insufficiency the fact that any meconium staining of the liquor can be seen after amniotomy is an advantage of the method.

Intra-amniotic injection of hypertonic urea

After fetal death induction by intra-amniotic injection of hypertonic solutions was formerly preferred to amniotomy, but induction with prostaglandins may now be chosen. Because of the danger of inadvertent injection of concentrated saline into a vein, a solution of urea is safer. A spinal needle is inserted into the amniotic cavity and about 200 ml of liquor is withdrawn and replaced with an equal volume of 40 per cent urea solution. It is essential to ensure that this is not injected into the tissues or the peritoneal cavity. Anaesthesia is not used, and if the patient complains of abdominal pain the injection is immediately stopped.

Episiotomy

This refers to an incision in the perineum to enlarge the introitus. Although it is a minor operation it increases the safety of many obstetric procedures, and can reduce the duration of the second stage of labour.

Indications. The indications for episiotomy are:

1. *Whenever the perineum threatens to tear.* Episiotomy is often indicated in primigravidae when the head is about to crown, and in multiparae when the perineum is scarred after suture at a previous delivery. An escape of blood from the introitus is often an indication that the vaginal wall is tearing, even if the perineal skin is still intact. Occasionally the perineum begins to split in the centre; an incision is even more urgently needed in this circumstance.

The perineum is more likely to tear with delivery of the head in the persistent occipito-posterior position than in the occipito-anterior position because in the former the larger occipito-frontal diameter distends the vulva (see Fig. 9.13, p. 87).

With an android pelvis the subpubic angle is reduced, and the head may be displaced backwards, causing increased tension in the perineum.

If there has been a previous operation for a complete perineal tear or a colporrhaphy episiotomy is required.

2. *When there is delay in delivery* with the head pressing on the perineum.

3. *Forceps delivery.* Episiotomy is commonly required for forceps delivery, but by no means always if the light Wrigley forceps are used. It is sometimes necessary before the introduction of the hand into the vagina to discover the cause of delay or to rotate manually a head which is in the occipito-posterior position.

4. *Breech delivery.* Episiotomy is performed when the breech is distending the perineum. The reasons are (a) to reduce the risk of intracranial haemorrhage, (b) to avoid the need for the breech with extended legs to undergo lateral flexion over the perineum and (c) to anticipate and make easier the bringing down of extended arms.

5. *Fetal distress.* Episiotomy can be life-saving when fetal distress occurs at the perineal stage of delivery.

6. *Prolapse of the cord.* If the cord prolapses with rupture of the membranes late in the second stage of labour, and especially if the patient is a multipara, the head may be showing when the complication is discovered. By encouraging the patient to push and incising the perineum the fetus can often be delivered before forceps are available.

7. *Premature labour.* Episiotomy should be routinely performed in cases of premature labour to reduce the risk of intracranial injury.

Technique.   The operation varies from an incision about 1 cm long to one extending the whole length of the perineum but swinging to one side to avoid the anal sphincter (Fig. 35.1). The incision should keep to the midline as far as possible because the tissues heal better here than when the incision is placed laterally, and there is less bleeding.

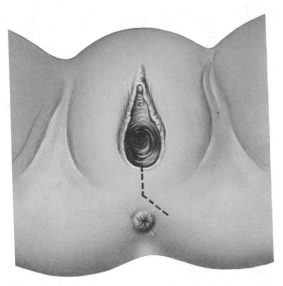

Fig. 35.1   Episiotomy. An incision is shown which starts as a median episiotomy and has then been extended laterally.

The operation may be done under general anaesthesia, epidural or pudendal block which has been previously instituted; otherwise local anaesthesia by infiltration with 10 ml of lignocaine (Xylocaine) 1 per cent is used. The incision is best made during a contraction when the presenting part is distending the perineum. Straight scissors with blunt points are used. The external sphincter ani must not be cut; if the episiotomy needs to be very extensive it should curve out laterally to avoid the sphincter. Occasionally there is free bleeding from a small vessel; this must always be arrested by pressure or the application of an artery forceps.

Suturing should be done with care. The tissues are highly vascular and heal obligingly well. Every effort must be made to avoid unsutured spaces in which lochia may collect and infection begin. Care must be taken to bring the upper limit of the vaginal incision into view and suture it. It is the usual practice to use fine catgut or Dexon throughout, with a continuous suture for the vagina first, then interrupted sutures for the perineal body, and a subcuticular suture for the skin of the perineum. 'Tension' stitches of nylon or thread increase discomfort, probably do not improve healing, and require to be removed after 5 days.

Daily bathing is advised; otherwise the wound is kept as dry as possible and left alone. Sometimes local discomfort is the most irksome feature of vaginal delivery and then mild analgesics are required, and the use of an infra-red lamp may help.

Delivery with the forceps

The original obstetric forceps were invented by one of the two elder Chamberlen brothers who came of a Huguenot family that settled in England in about the year 1600. The invention was kept secret in the family for over 100 years and passed from the third Chamberlen brother, Peter, down to his grandson Hugh who died in 1728. For nearly another hundred years, until 1818, the original forceps lay hidden beneath the floorboards of a box-room in Woodham Mortimer Hall, Essex, which had been the family home for 80 years. Knowledge of the use of the forceps leaked out with varying degrees of completeness and accuracy during the early part of the 18th century.

The Chamberlen forceps consisted of two blades, curved to fit the fetal head, with short handles, the two halves being strapped together where they crossed because they had no lock. In 1723 Chapman improved the forceps by lengthening the shank between the blade and the handle. In 1744 William Smellie devised the double-slotted English lock which allowed easy application and gave additional strength. The pelvic curve was added by Levret of Paris in 1747.

A new type of forceps was introduced by Christian Kielland in 1915; their purpose is not only traction but also rotation of the head. Finally, light short curved forceps were introduced by Wrigley in 1935 for the particular purpose of outlet application.

The forceps is used to apply traction to the head of the fetus in a pelvis of adequate size, never to attempt to overcome disproportion. With Kielland's forceps the head may also be rotated into a more favourable position before traction is applied. The forceps are designed to fit the head; if applied to the breech they are liable to slip with resulting injury to fetal or maternal soft parts.

The presentations suitable for the forceps operation are vertex, face with the chin anterior, and the after-coming head of the breech. The vertex may have the occiput anterior or posterior, but with the latter certain additional factors, referred to later, must be taken into account.

Indications for the use of the forceps

Before using the forceps there should always be a clear indication that good will come from their use and that the instrument is not merely being used to expedite delivery in a normal labour. The aim is always to give *assistance*, usually because of one or more of the following: (1) Delay in the second stage of labour, (2) impending or established maternal distress or (3) impending or established fetal distress. It is absolutely essential that a careful abdominal and vaginal examination is made before deciding that forceps delivery is necessary and safe.

Delay in the second stage of labour. In primigravidae the second stage of labour should not last for much over 1 hour, and in multiparae is often much shorter, usually being less than 30 minutes. A second stage is considered to be delayed if these limits are exceeded, but this is only a general guide and if progress is not being made assistance should be given sooner.

Conditions likely to cause delay in the second stage of labour:
(1) Inadequate uterine contractions and poor voluntary effort
(2) Rigid pelvic floor and perineum
(3) Large fetus
(4) Persistent occipito-posterior position or deep transverse arrest of the head.
(5) Other malpresentations such as face presentation or brow presentation. Forceps are also used for delivery of the aftercoming head of a breech presentation, even in the absence of any delay.
(6) Contraction of the pelvic outlet.

A common cause of delay in the second stage of labour is the resistance of the pelvic floor, but it should be treated by episiotomy rather than by the application of forceps.

Maternal distress. If the patient becomes distressed during the second stage assistance is given. Distress may arise from causes which are not purely obstetric, and in cases of heart disease or severe pulmonary disease the forceps or vacuum extractor should always be applied unless the second stage is passing quickly, and in severe pre-eclampsia or eclampsia the stress of expulsive efforts should be avoided. For such cases the forceps or vacuum extractor should, whenever possible, be applied under epidural or pudendal block analgesia.

The signs of maternal distress may be broadly divided into mental and physical, although the former are bound to be present to some degree when the latter have appeared. Mental distress occurs in patients who have had a long tedious first stage and are in no condition to cooperate in aiding expulsion during the second stage. In some cases the patient is moaning and apathetic, in others restless and uncooperative. This usually means that analgesics have been too sparingly used.

The signs of physical distress are a rising pulse rate and a slightly raised temperature. If labour has been long the patient will look tired and say so, but if distress has arisen as a result of obstructed labour the contractions are strong, there are no signs of progress and the patient shows restless anxiety.

Fetal distress. The following conditions may cause fetal distress during the second stage of labour:
(1) Prolapse of the cord, or a tight loop or knot in it.
(2) Placental insufficiency from pre-eclampsia or essential hypertension, antepartum haemorrhage or postmaturity.
(3) Prolonged or difficult labour.
(4) Uterine infection.

Prolapse or presentation of the cord is mentioned first because the threat to the fetus is serious and immediate. The subject is dealt with in Chapter 32, p. 348. If the cervix is fully dilated and the fetus is alive expeditious forceps delivery is required.

Anything that interferes with fetal oxygenation will cause fetal distress. With gross placental lesions such as separation or infarction there may be severe fetal distress, but diminished utero-placental blood flow may occur to a lesser degree in cases of postmaturity and maternal hypertension. Apart from prolapse of the cord, less acute cord compression may arise from tightening of a knot or a loop around the fetal neck.

Each uterine contraction temporarily impedes the maternal blood flow to the placenta, and in long labour, or in cases in which much retraction of the upper segment of the uterus occurs, fetal hypoxia may eventually arise.

The signs of fetal distress are changes in the fetal heart rate or rhythm and the appearance of meconium in the liquor. These signs and the methods of monitoring the fetal heart rate are discussed in Chapter 33, p. 351. Examination of a sample of fetal blood will also allow a diagnosis of hypoxia to be made, but in the second stage of labour it is more practical to effect delivery without further delay.

The sudden appearance of meconium in the liquor amnii is also a sign of fetal distress. It is due to intestinal peristalsis in the impending asphyxia. The appearance of meconium-stained liquor can be misleading, for if it is seen when the membranes rupture it indicates that distress has taken place at some time, but has not necessarily persisted; counting the fetal heart rate will usually decide this point. Stale meconium stains the liquor a pale green colour; fresh meconium is much darker. Meconium is often passed by a fetus during breech delivery because of compression of the fetal abdomen in the pelvis.

When there are signs of fetal distress in the second stage of labour delivery should be effected at once. While preparations for delivery are being made oxygen is given to the mother in the hope of improving the supply to the fetus. In forceps delivery for fetal distress, episiotomy reduces the risk of adding intracranial stress to the fetal asphyxia. Full preparations must be made for resuscitation of the baby.

Conditions which must be fulfilled before application of forceps

To apply forceps safely and successfully certain conditions must be fulfilled:

(1) *The presentation must be suitable*. The forceps can only be used to extract the head of the fetus when it presents as a vertex or as a face with the chin anterior (leaving aside the use of forceps for the aftercoming head of a breech). A brow or a mento-posterior face presentation must be corrected before forceps can be used for extraction. The forceps must be applied accurately to the sides of the fetal head; otherwise dangerous compression of the head will occur causing intracranial stress and haemorrhage, and very likely the attempt to deliver will fail.

(2) *The head must be engaged*. If the head is not engaged in the second stage this may be because of cephalopelvic disproportion or because the head is extended. The 'high forceps' operation, with the head above the brim, is never attempted now as it is very dangerous and Caesarean section is safer.

(3) Even with the head engaged the *pelvic outlet must be of adequate size*. If the subpubic angle is narrowed there must be room in the posterior sagittal diameter (p. 82).

(4) *The cervix must be fully dilated*. If it is not there will be difficulty in applying the forceps without including and tearing the cervix. More traction will be required to overcome the resistance of the cervix. The attempt to deliver may fail because the factor which prevented cervical dilatation may be uncorrected. (In the hands of an experienced operator, with the head in the occipito-posterior position, once the malrotation has been corrected a residual anterior lip of cervix can be pushed up over the forceps before traction is applied to effect delivery).

(5) If the forewaters are still present the *membranes should be ruptured* before application of the forceps.

(6) *The bladder should be empty*. A catheter is passed to empty the bladder before forceps delivery, not only to avoid any risk of injuring it but also to remove its inhibiting influence on retraction of the uterus after delivery, and thus to reduce the risk of postpartum haemorrhage.

(7) *The uterus should be contracting*. Only very rarely is uterine exhaustion so pronounced as to result in complete inactivity. If there is an indication to effect delivery before the contractions have returned spontaneously, oxytocin may be given by continuous intravenous infusion and then delivery completed with forceps. Intravenous ergometrine should be given as soon as the fetal shoulders are born.

Types of obstetric forceps

Forceps in use today include (1) short curved forceps, (2) long curved forceps, (3) Kielland's forceps and (4) parallel shank forceps. Each of these instruments consists of two halves meeting at the lock. Each half has a

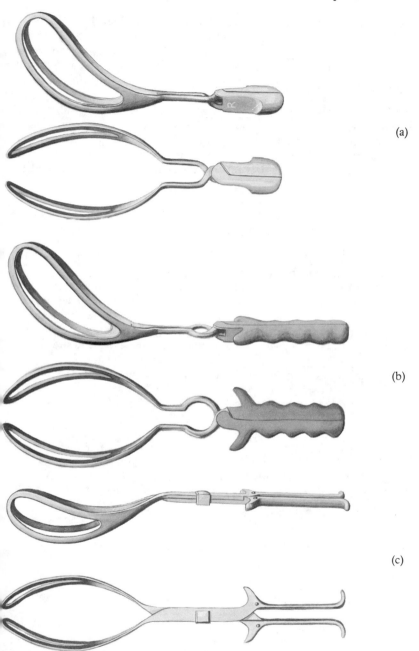

(a)

(b)

(c)

Fig. 35.2 (a) Short curved (Wrigley's) forceps. (b) Long curved forceps. (c) Kielland's forceps.

blade which is joined to the handle by a shank. The blades have two curves; the cephalic curve in which the blade is curved to fit the fetal head, and a curve on the edge, the pelvic curve, to correspond with the curved axis of the pelvis. The length of the handles and shanks varies with the different forceps, and the type of handle differs too. Kielland's forceps have special characteristics.

Short curved forceps. This instrument, designed by Wrigley in 1935, is for use in the low or outlet forceps operation. The shank is short (2.5 cm) and the whole instrument is light.

Long curved forceps. The total length is 35 cm, with shanks of 6.5 cm, and the instrument is relatively heavily built. It can be used for delivery of a head from the pelvic cavity.

A modification of this instrument that was formerly used was the axis traction forceps. In this angled rods led from the junctions of the blades and shanks to a second handle. This axis traction mechanism enabled the operator to pull backwards as well as downwards when the head was at the level of the pelvic brim. Such a 'high forceps' operation is not now performed, so axis traction rods are not required.

Kielland's forceps. The advantage of this instrument it that is allows accurate cephalic application, no matter what the position or level of the head in the pelvis. If the occiput is posterior or lateral the application is made and then the head can be rotated with the forceps to bring the occiput anterior. The forceps have a lock which allows one blade to slide on the other in the long axis, and thus permits the blades to lie at different levels when applied to a head which is lying transversely and is tilted. The other special characteristic is the pelvic curve. This is initially in a backward direction and then it quickly begins its forward sweep, but the tips of the blades never quite reach the plane of the shanks and handles (Fig. 35.2(c)). It is this feature which makes rotation with the forceps possible.

Parallel shank forceps. The Shute forceps is similar to Kielland's forceps, but the shanks are joined by an adjustable screw which permits the distance between the blades to be varied according to the size of the head with little divergence of the tips of the blades. The risk of slipping is thus eliminated and compression forces are reduced to a minimum.

Preliminary steps before the application of forceps

The obstetrician prepares himself and his instruments as for any other operation.

Some form of anaesthesia will be required. This may take the form of pudendal block, caudal or epidural analgesia, or general anaesthesia. Pudendal or epidural block should be used whenever possible in preference to general anaesthesia. A general anaesthetic should only be given by someone experienced in dealing with the complications which may arise. Unless it is reasonably certain that the patient's stomach is empty a stomach tube must be passed before the anaesthetic is begun. It is essential that a suction apparatus is available, and that the head of the obstetric bed can be lowered without delay in case of unexpected gastric regurgitation. Prolonged general anaesthesia may increase the risk of postpartum haemorrhage and depress the respiratory centre of the newborn infant.

The lithotomy position is best, provided that expert anaesthesia is available and that the head of the bed can be lowered quickly. In exceptional emergency cases when these facilities are not available and pudendal block is not sufficient anaesthesia the patient may be given a general anaesthetic and delivered in the left lateral position, but manipulation and forceps extraction is then more difficult.

After swabbing the vulva and perineum with an antiseptic solution, sterile towels are put in position and the bladder is emptied with a catheter. A careful preliminary vaginal examination is made. It must first be established that the cervix is fully dilated. The level and position of the head is then determined. If the sutures and fontanelles are obscured by caput formation it may be necessary to insert the whole hand to feel for an ear; the pinna will be directed toward the occiput. Episiotomy may be needed for this. Finally the size of the pelvic outlet is assessed. This is not always easy, but the points to note are the prominence of the ischial spines, the width of the subpubic arch, and the length of the sagittal diameter from the lower border of the symphysis pubis to the sacro-coccygeal joint.

If all these points are satisfactory and the occiput is near to the midline in front the forceps can now be applied, but if it is lying obliquely or transversely manual rotation will be needed first, unless Kielland's forceps are being used, when the head may be rotated with the forceps. If the occiput is posterior, unless the head is so low that the perineum is already being stretched, it is almost always best to rotate the occiput to the front before the head is delivered. The disadvantage of not doing so is the increased risk of intracranial stress and of extensive perineal laceration that goes with delivery of the head in the occipito-posterior position.

If the head has not descended to the pelvic floor then a more serious cause for delay is possible. A flattening of the sacrum might be felt, or the head might be found to be seriously deflexed or extended. If there was any serious doubt about the size of the pelvis with the head arrested at this level Caesarean section would be the safest course, but if there was a malposition without pelvic contraction then forceps delivery would be carried out after correction of the position of the head.

Application of the ordinary patterns of obstetric forceps

The left blade of the forceps is applied first. The fingers of the right hand are passed into the vagina. The left blade of the forceps is held between fingers and thumb of the left hand by its handle, and passed between the

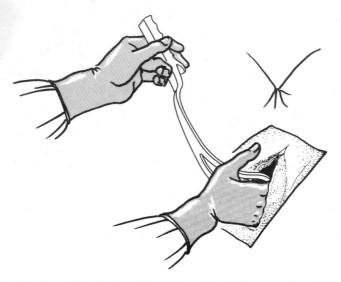

Fig. 35.3   Application of forceps. Insertion of the left blade.

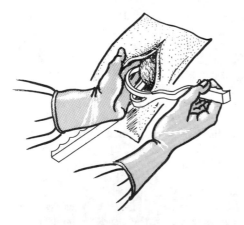

Fig. 35.4   Application of forceps. Insertion of the right blade.

fetal head and the palmar surfaces of the fingers of the right hand (Fig. 35.3). The handle is held well over the mother's abdomen, and inclined to the mother's right side, so that it is almost parallel with her right inguinal ligament. As the blade passes up into the birth canal the handle is carried backwards and towards the midline, thus following the direction of both the pelvic and cephalic curves of the instrument. After ascertaining

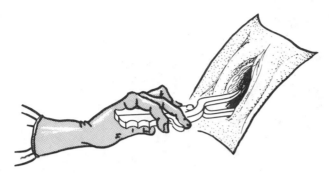

Fig. 35.5 Forceps articulated before traction.

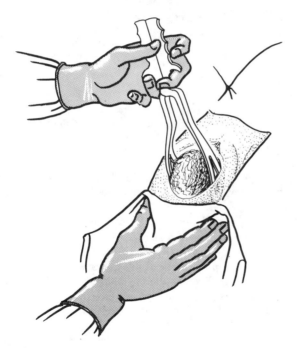

Fig. 35.6 Delivery with the forceps.

that the blade lies next to the head and in the correct position the fingers of the right hand are withdrawn.

The fingers of the left hand are now introduced along the right side of the pelvis, and the right blade of the forceps is held as before and passed in a similar manner. Its external visible portion will thus lie above and across

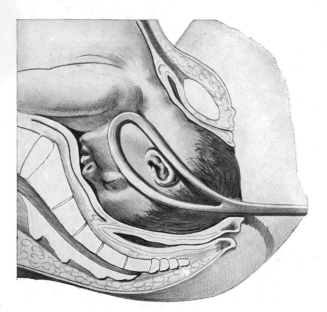

Fig. 35.7   Position of the blades of the forceps during extraction of a vertex presentation. The blades of the forceps lie in the submento-vertical diameter and grasp the biparietal diameter.

the handle of the left blade. The shanks are now pressed backward against the perineum and the handles should lock and come to lie in a horizontal position.

Occasionally difficulty may be experienced in locking the forceps. This may be caused by relatively trivial faults such as not passing the blades to the same depth, or allowing one to rotate after its introduction. A more serious possibility is that the position of the head has not been diagnosed correctly, and that the instrument has been applied to a head in the oblique or transverse diameter of the pelvis. If the forceps will not lock, or if the handles will not close together, the blades must be removed and the position of the fetal head re-examined.

The standard curved forceps must always be applied correctly to the fetal head, with the parietal eminences lying within the fenestrations of the blades and the sagittal suture lying midway between the blades. These forceps must also be correctly placed in the pelvis. It does not matter if the head is slightly oblique in the pelvis, with the occiput pointing less than 45° away from the midline. With such a slight degree of obliquity the head and forceps will turn into the midline as traction is applied, but if the head is more oblique than this its position *must* be corrected before the ordinary type of forceps are applied to it. The ordinary forceps should never be used to rotate the head more than 45°.

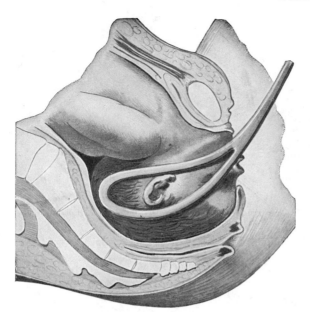

Fig. 35.8   Position of the blades of the forceps during extraction of head in mento-anterior position. The blades of the forceps lie in the occipito-mental diameter and grasp the head in the bizygomatic diameter.

Application of forceps to a face presentation.   If the head is delayed in the pelvic cavity and there is a mento-anterior position the forceps may be used to assist delivery (Fig. 35.8). If there is a mento-posterior position delivery with the forceps is only possible after the chin has been rotated forwards. This is possible manually or by the expert use of Kielland's forceps, but it may be safer to treat this uncommon condition by Caesarean section.

Application of forceps to the aftercoming head.   The forceps is applied to the aftercoming head in breech delivery as a routine procedure (see p. 287).

Extraction with the forceps

The operator sits facing the perineum. Traction is applied to the handles of the forceps in a backward and downward direction in the axis of the birth canal. Traction is intermittent, and each pull should only last for a few seconds. As the head descends the handles are gradually raised to about 45° above the horizontal, when an episiotomy is performed through the stretched perineum (unless this has already been done). The head is then gently guided through the vulva until crowning takes place with the handles of the forceps in vertical position. The forceps blades are then removed before delivery of the face by manual extension of the head.

Excessive force should never be used. Slow intermittent traction permits progressive safe moulding of the head and reduces the risk of intracranial injury.

The use of Kielland's forceps

Kielland's forceps should only be used by those who have been trained in their use. In inexperienced hands this is a dangerous instrument, and may be the cause of severe vaginal lacerations if it is used incorrectly.

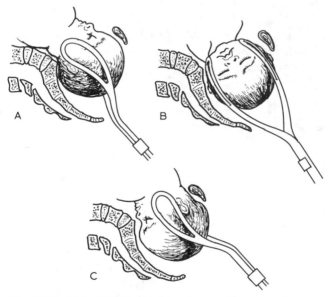

Fig. 35.9   Use of Kielland's forceps.   **A.** Application to head in occipito-posterior position before rotation.   **B.** Application to head in occipito-lateral position before rotation.   **C.** Position of forceps after rotation.

Before applying the forceps the exact position of the head in the pelvis must be determined. To avoid error the operator is advised to hold the articulated instrument before the vulva in the position to be taken up when it is applied to the head. The blade which is to be inserted first is selected, and the other blade is put aside. If the head lies antero-posteriorly or only slightly obliquely the application of the forceps is not difficult. The forceps are always applied *correctly to the head*, so that if the occiput lies posteriorly and it is intended to rotate it with the forceps, the forceps must be applied with the pelvic curve in the reverse direction so that *after* rotation the curve will be correctly orientated to the birth canal.

Unlike ordinary forceps this instrument can be applied to a head lying transversely in the pelvis and there are special methods of application for this. In both methods the anterior blade is applied first. In the *wandering method* the anterior blade is guided into the lateral side of the pelvis beside the head, with the cephalic surface of the blade properly facing the head. It is then slid gently round the pelvis, keeping as close as possible to the head and passing over the forehead until it comes to rest fitting the anterior parietal eminence. The posterior blade is then introduced behind the head, to fit the posterior parietal eminence.

The *direct method* of application is only used when the head is low down and the fit is not too tight. The tip of the anterior blade, with the handle as far back as possible, is applied to the side of the head anteriorly and then slipped over the anterior parietal eminence behind the symphysis pubis, with the cephalic surface of the blade kept as close as possible to the head while it is in transit. The posterior blade is then inserted behind the head over the posterior parietal eminence.

For *rotation of the head* force is never used, and it should be done with three fingers of one hand only. Rotation is first tried at the level of arrest, but if this is not immediately easy the head should be elevated slightly and rotation tried again. Sometimes rotation will be easier after traction has brought the head down to a roomier level of the pelvis. *Traction* is made in the line of the handles and is exerted with only two fingers hooked over the proximal shoulders of the handles. Rotation and traction are never done together, although spontaneous rotation sometimes occurs during traction and should not be impeded. The handles should never be compressed together, as this will have a crushing action on the head.

The dangers of forceps delivery

Some of the dangers of forceps delivery are due to the circumstances calling for the operation rather than to the operation itself. For example, delivery with forceps is commonly called for at the end of a long tedious first stage of labour because of either maternal or fetal distress or both.

The risk of general anaesthesia in an unprepared patient is great if the anaesthetist is inexperienced and proper equipment is lacking.

Some of the dangers of forceps delivery may be summarized thus:

Mother:	Infant:
Dangers of general anaesthesia	Intracranial haemorrhage
Lacerations of cervix, vagina or perineum	Facial palsy
Postpartum haemorrhage from uterine atony or lacerations	Cephalhaematoma
Puerperal genital infection	

Spastic diplegia is sometimes attributed to instrumental delivery. It is improbable that intracranial haemorrhage will have this effect; if the haemorrhage is not fatal complete recovery is likely. On the other hand, prolonged cerebral hypoxia may well leave permanent damage; forceps may have been used in such a case but could hardly have caused the hypoxia.

Bad results from forceps delivery usually result from bad forceps delivery. The dangers will be minimal when proper regard is given to the indications for the operation, and when the exact position of the head is determined by a preliminary vaginal examination, and any necessary correction of the position of the fetus is made before traction. Good anaesthesia and basic obstetric skill are no longer exceptional refinements, but are the essentials on which safe forceps delivery must depend.

Failure to deliver with forceps

Fortunately failed forceps delivery is now rare in Britain, for the dangers to both mother and baby are serious, and are directly proportional to the lack of skill and the force employed during the unsuccessful attempts at delivery. The serious criticism is not so much against attempting to apply forceps or attempting traction, but against *persisting* in such endeavours in the face of obvious difficulties.

The causes of failure to deliver with the forceps are mostly commonplace; either the cervix is not fully dilated or the head is in a malposition, usually with the occiput posterior. Attempts to apply forceps with the head not yet engaged fortunately are not often made nowadays, for the dangers are even greater.

Severe laceration of the cervix may be caused by attempts to apply forceps with the cervix incompletely dilated, either because the blades are applied outside the cervix or because the head is forcibly dragged through it. Sometimes an extensive tear of the upper vagina is caused by attempts to rotate the head with the long curved forceps. If the obstruction is at the brim the uterus itself may be perforated by a blade of the forceps. A complete tear of the perineum into the anal canal comes from a combination of roughness and misapplied force. The effect on the patient of these obstetric insults, even if she has avoided a badly given or prolonged general anaesthetic, is to cause shock from trauma or haemorrhage, or both. Sepsis is likely to follow.

The fetus may suffer intracranial haemorrhage and it may be dead on admission or die soon after ultimate delivery; or there may be permanent cerebral damage, sometimes partly from hypoxia. If only the preliminary vaginal examination was always carried out carefully the serious damage done in many cases of failed forceps delivery would be avoided.

Such a case must be carefully reassessed. Not infrequently a more experienced operator is able to effect an easy delivery with forceps after correcting a malposition. In other cases Caesarean section has to be performed.

Vacuum extractor (ventouse)

The idea of extracting the fetal head by means of a vacuum cup applied to the scalp has been considered since Younge in 1706 tried a glass suction cup, but the first practical instrument was designed by Simpson in 1849, although little use was made of it. The modern vacuum extractor was introduced by Malmström in 1954. Opinions differ about the value of this method of assisting delivery. In some clinics, particularly on the European continent, the vacuum extractor is preferred to the forceps, but it is less often chosen in Britain and America.

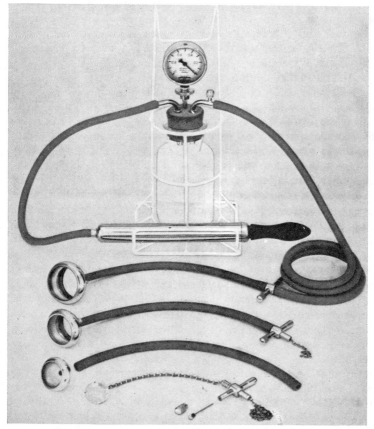

Fig. 35.10 The vacuum extractor. (Allen & Hanbury's Ltd.) In this pattern the cup is attached to a rubber tube which can be connected to the vacuum pump. Within the cup and the tubing is a chain device to allow traction to be applied.

Malmström's extractor (Fig. 35.10) consists of a metal suction cup attached by a chain, which runs through a rubber tube, to a metal handle. The rubber tube is connected by further tubing to a glass container with a pressure gauge and a hand pump. The suction cups are made in three sizes, 40, 50 and 60 mm in diameter, and the largest possible cup is used, according to the dilatation of the cervix.

Method of use

Local infiltration of the perineum with lignocaine 1 per cent is usually the only anaesthetic needed, and this is a great virtue of the method.

The cup is introduced sideways into the vagina by pressing it backwards against the perineum. It is then guided into place on the scalp, taking care that neither the cervix or any part of the vaginal wall comes between the cup and the scalp. While the obstetrician holds the cup in the correct position an assistant uses the pump to create a vacuum, gradually inceasing the negative pressure by 0.1 kg/cm² at 2 minute intervals, until 0.8 kg/cm² is attained. Failure to maintain the vacuum indicates that either the cup is incorrectly applied or that the apparatus is faulty. The negative pressure causes an artificial caput succedaneum or 'chignon' to be formed within the cup and when the vacuum reaches 0.8 kg/cm² the cup is completely filled with scalp, ensuring maximum adhesion, and traction can be started.

Traction on the handle is made as nearly vertically as possible, because an oblique direction of traction will tend to pull it off. Traction is made intermittently with the uterine contractions, the direction of pull changing as the head descends through the birth canal. Unless there is obvious descent during 3 or 4 contractions the use of the ventouse should be reconsidered.

After delivery the vacuum is reduced as slowly as it was created as this tends to diminish the risk of damage to the scalp. Immediately after removal of the cup the baby has an unsightly 'chignon' where the cup was applied, but this rapidly diminishes and within a few hours only a faint ring can be seen.

Indications

These are similar to those for the use of obstetric forceps. If the occiput is not anterior the extractor may still be used. It is applied as near to the vertex as possible, and with traction forward rotation of the occiput often occurs. However, many obstetricians would prefer to use Kielland's forceps or to perform manual rotation in such a case.

The ventouse may also be used to accelerate dilatation of the cervix in cases of prolongation of the first stage of labour. The cervix must be sufficiently dilated to allow application of the cup, and the utmost care must be taken to see that there is no disproportion or other impediment to delivery. When the application is prolonged the vacuum must be reduced to 0.2 kg/cm^2 for 1 minute in every 5 minutes to permit circulation through the scalp. Suitable cases for the use of the extractor during the first stage of labour are few. If the cause of delay is weak uterine action the contractions should improve with an oxytocic infusion; if the cause of delay is obstruction Caesarean section is the proper treatment.

Contra-indication

The vacuum extractor cannot be applied to the breech or face.

In urgent cases of fetal distress the operation takes too long, and forceps delivery is preferred.

There is some doubt as to its safety when used on premature babies. Some obstetricians believe that there is an increased risk of intracranial haemorrhage, and that forceps are safer because they protect the head from compression by the soft tissues of the birth canal.

Necrosis of the scalp, cephalhaematoma, subaponeurotic haematoma and intracranial haemorrhage have all been reported after vacuum extraction, but in a number of these cases the cup had been injudiciously applied for long periods and strong traction had been applied to overcome some degree of disproportion.

Internal version

Version is described as external when it is achieved by manipulation applied to the abdomen. In internal version a hand is passed through the cervix, which must be fully dilated or nearly so, into the uterus to turn the child. It is always podalic version, and one or both legs are brought down as part of the operation. The patient must always be deeply anaesthetized. It is a difficult and hazardous procedure for both mother and child.

Before Caesarean section and forceps delivery were introduced internal version was the only way out of many obstetric difficulties. Today almost the only indication is for the correction of a transverse lie of a second twin when external version has failed.

Internal version is extremely dangerous when labour has been in progress for some time and the lower segment is stretched and thin because of the risk of uterine rupture.

Figures 35.11 and 35.12 show the method of performing internal version.

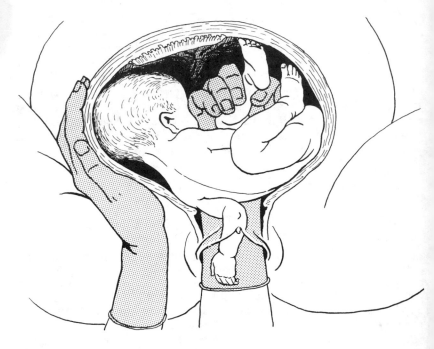

Fig. 35.11   Internal podalic version. Stage 1. Shoulder presentation. In a shoulder presentation it matters little which hand the operator uses internally. In this case he has introduced the right hand to grasp the leg of the fetus and bring it down. His left hand, working outside the sterile sheet, is coaxing the head out of the iliac fossa.

Caesarean section

Caesarean section is the operation by which the fetus is delivered through an incision in the uterus after the 28th week of pregnancy. (A similar procedure before that time is referred to as hysterotomy).

History

The origin of the operation is uncertain, but it is of great antiquity. There are references to it in Rabbinical writings of about 140 B.C., but it is known to have been practised on the dead pregnant woman long before this. Traditional Roman history (written seven centuries later) states that the second king of Rome, Numa Pompilius (762–715 B.C.), forbade burying a woman who died during labour until the fetus had been cut out. This law later became the *Lex Caesarea*, and the term Caesarean section is said to have arisen from this.

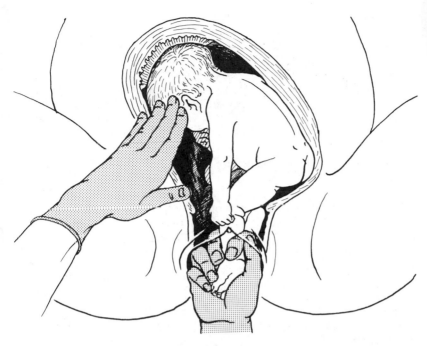

Fig. 35.12 Internal podalic version. Stage 2. Shoulder presentation. The leg is being brought down causing the back to rotate forwards. The head has almost reached the fundus.

Works on Caesarean section were published in the sixteenth century, but faced with the difficulties of controlling bleeding and sepsis, and in the absence of anaesthesia, the mortality remained high, and even in the beginning of the nineteenth century Osiander wrote: 'Of the women who undergo Caesarean section more than two-thirds die . . . . Before, then, undertaking this procedure one should allow the patient to draw up her will and grant her time to prepare herself for death.'

As it was believed that sutures could not be buried in the tissues without causing sepsis, there was the problem of the open wound pouring infected lochia into the peritoneal cavity, with inevitable peritonitis. Porro of Padua temporarily solved it by following section by subtotal hysterectomy, and marsupializing the cervical stump in the abdominal wound. The Porro operation was abandoned when Kehrer in 1881 devised a satisfactory method of suturing the uterine wound with silk. Although the mortality fell in elective cases there was still a very high mortality after incision of the upper segment in patients who were in labour.

In 1906 Frank of Cologne devised an operation which not only employed transverse abdominal and lower segment incision, but excluded the lower segment from the general peritoneal cavity by suturing the upper edge of the parietal peritoneum to the upper edge of the utero-vesical peritoneum. In the next few years the lower segment operation gained popularity, and was soon found to be safe during labour, even without any attempt to close off the field from the general peritoneal cavity.

Indications

A list of indications for Caesarean section can easily be devised, but in many cases there is more than one indication. As the danger of the operation has diminished there is a tendency for it to be performed more often for fetal indications such as distress during labour, placenta praevia, severe pre-eclampsia, diabetes mellitus, haemolytic disease and prolapse of the cord.

A few indications are 'absolute' in the sense that delivery by any other method would be extremely dangerous, for example gross disproportion or placenta praevia, but in most cases the indications are 'relative' when it is thought that the balance of maternal and fetal dangers will be reduced by section rather than vaginal delivery. The indications include:

Faults in the birth canal. (1) *Cephalopelvic disproportion.* Gross obstruction to delivery from pelvic contraction will obviously justify Caesarean section; it is in the more common borderline cases that judgment is required. Trial of labour is discussed on p. 360. A trial often has to be terminated because of fetal distress, or because of abnormal uterine action. It is not always certain what is causing delay in labour, but when a patient has been in labour for some hours, with cautious augmentation of labour (p. 411), and cervical dilatation is not progressing, no matter for what reason, Caesarean section should not be delayed.

If a trial of labour in a previous pregnancy is judged to have failed because of disproportion, delivery should be by elective section shortly before term.

In obstructed labour with a dead fetus, now fortunately very rare in Britain, a difficult decision may have to be made. Craniotomy is best if the head is accessible, but with a high head lower segment section may be safer.

(2) *Pelvic tumour.* Impaction of an ovarian cyst (p. 248) or a fibromyoma (p. 245) in the pelvis are indications for section.

(3) *Cervical or vaginal stenosis* are rare complications of surgical procedures for which section may be required. It is emphasized that if the cervix fails to dilate the usual cause is poor uterine action or disproportion rather than any fault in the cervix.

Section is advised after operative repair of a fistula, or successful treatment of stress incontinence, but after most repair operations vaginal delivery after episiotomy is preferable to section.

(4) With a *double uterus* obstruction during labour may occur because the unimpregnated horn lies below the presenting part, because the narrower part of the uterus fails to dilate, or because of a vaginal septum.

Fetal malpresentations. Caesarean section is the best treatment for a *brow presentation* with the head at the level of the pelvic brim, and it may be justified for an impacted *mento-posterior face presentation*. It is performed for a *shoulder presentation* if the fetus is alive in preference to internal version, and for some cases of *locked twins*.

In the case of a *breech presentation* section is justified if the mother is an elderly primigravida or has previously been infertile, or if there is disproportion or an android pelvis. It is usually wise to operate during labour if the breech does not descend onto the pelvic floor after some hours of regular contractions.

In exceedingly rare cases of *conjoined twins* section may be required.

Abnormal uterine action. The place of Caesarean section in cases of abnormal uterine action is discussed in Chapter 27, p. 309. In many cases of abnormal uterine action there may also be some mechanical difficulty, and precise diagnosis of the cause of delay may be uncertain, but if a patient has been in labour for more than 12 hours, the membranes are ruptured, and there is no progress with an oxytocic infusion, section should be considered.

A contraction ring is a very rare indication for section during the first stage of labour, but is not usually diagnosed until it is discovered at the operation.

Antepartum haemorrhage. Caesarean section is the best treatment for both mother and fetus in all cases of *placenta praevia* except those of Type I.

Section is seldom performed in severe cases of *accidental haemorrhage* because the fetus is usually dead. In unusual cases in which the fetus is alive but bleeding is continuing Caesarean section is justified. Placental separation, even if it is slight, is a major threat to fetal survival, and during labour section may become necessary for fetal distress.

Other maternal indications. For cases of cardiac or respiratory disease, and indeed most intercurrent medical disorders, assisted vaginal delivery is preferable to Caesarean section unless there is some obstetric impediment to easy delivery. Section should never be performed merely to permit sterilization; this is better done 6 weeks later by laparoscopy.

Fulminating pre-eclampsia may have to be treated by section if the chances of speedy vaginal delivery are small. The patient may not go into labour after induction, or the severity of the hypertension may demand delivery before the 34th week in a primigravida, when induction is uncertain. In other cases of pre-eclampsia, essential hypertension or renal disease section is performed in the fetal interest, as will be mentioned in the next section.

Fetal indications. In cases of *diabetes mellitus* the fetus is usually delivered before term, and often by section (p. 226).

If *placental insufficiency* is suspected because of inadequate fetal growth, maternal hypertension or proteinuria, or previous fetal death the tests described on p. 252 are carried out. Many cases are treated by induction of labour before term, but if labour does not follow, if the fetus is very small, or if fetal distress occurs during the first stage of labour section is the best method of delivery.

Fetal distress may occur during labour in cases of postmaturity or hypertension, in cases of long labour or abnormal uterine action, or without explanation. Whatever the cause, if there is clinical evidence of fetal distress during the first stage of labour, confirmed by monitoring of the fetal heart rate and by scalp blood sampling, Caesarean section is urgently performed.

Prolapse of the cord when the cervix is not sufficiently dilated to allow immediate vaginal delivery is treated by emergency section.

A *bad obstetric history*, when the patient has had several stillbirths or neonatal deaths, may be a sufficient indication for Caesarean section, and the selection of the best time for this may call for much judgment.

Caesarean section should not be routinely performed in the case of an *elderly primigravida*, but if there is an additional factor such as minor disproportion, a breech presentation, hypertension or even postmaturity, this may justify section.

Repeated Caesarean section

If a patient has had a section there is a risk of rupture of the scar in any subsequent labour. If the indication for the section persists, for example a contracted pelvis, the operation should obviously be repeated. If, however, the indication was a non-recurrent one, for example placenta praevia, then the risk of a second elective operation outweighs the risk of rupture of a lower segment scar at vaginal delivery. When a patient has had more than one previous section the indication for repetition of the operation may be stronger.

The upper segment scar is less secure than the lower segment scar, and after an operation of the former type (now rarely performed) it is wise to repeat the section.

Technique of Caesarean section

In the past the classical procedure was a vertical incision in the upper uterine segment. This incision was attended by free bleeding, could not be covered with a free layer of loose peritoneum, and gave an insecure scar which might give way during a subsequent pregnancy or labour. It is seldom performed today.

The standard procedure is now the transperitoneal lower segment operation with a transverse incision in the uterus.

With any operation the best results are obtained when there is ample time to prepare the patient, but the need for Caesarean section may only become evident during the course of labour. If section is elective it should be performed a few days before the expected date of labour, but if there is doubt about the maturity it may be wiser to wait until labour begins.

Anaesthesia for Caesarean section. Section often has to be performed at inconvenient times, but the services of a skilled anaesthetist should be insisted on. Deaths from avoidable complications of anaesthesia still make a tragic contribution to maternal mortality statistics. In emergency cases the patient may be ill-prepared. It may be necessary to pass a gastric tube and empty the stomach before anaesthesia, and magnesium trisilicate 2 g, shaken up in a little water, may be given orally or left in the stomach after passing the gastric tube, to reduce acidity.

Morphine and allied drugs which may depress the respiratory centre of the newborn infant should not be used for premedication. For the welfare of the fetus the patient should not be under the influence of the anaesthetic longer than is absolutely necessary before the operation begins, and all preparations for the operation must be completed before inducing anaesthesia. The induction is often performed on the operating table.

The anaesthetist must be able to insert a cuffed intratracheal tube. A very common technique is to induce sleep with a small dose of intravenous thiopentone, to obtain relaxation with an injection of scoline and, after insertion of a cuffed intratracheal tube, to maintain anaesthesia with nitrous oxide and oxygen.

An alternative method is to use a lumbar extradural block. Spinal anaesthesia is unsuitable as the paralysis of the vasomotor control of the lower part of the body, combined with the reduction in venous return from the pressure of the uterus on the inferior vena cava when the patient is supine, may cause dangerous hypotension.

Regional infiltration of the abdominal wall can be employed, but this method is time-consuming and not suitable for apprehensive patients.

Other pre-operative precautions. The bladder is emptied with a catheter before the operation is started. An intravenous glucose-saline drip is set up. A litre of cross-matched blood should be available (although not necessarily used). In cases of placenta praevia, when blood loss may be heavy, this is essential.

Lower segment Caesarean section

The peritoneal cavity is opened by a low transverse or vertical sub-umbilical incision. Some operators like to pack off the operative field with moist gauze, making sure that the end of the roll is left out of the wound with an artery forceps attached. A wide Doyen's retractor is inserted into the lower end of the wound. The peritoneum of the utero-vesical pouch is divided transversely for about 10 cm and the bladder is gently pushed

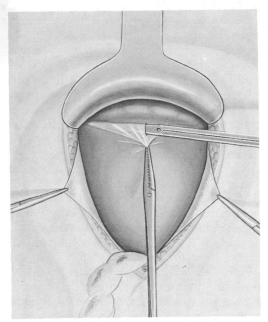

Fig. 35.13   Lower segment Caesarean section. The loose peritoneum over the lower segment is being lifted up before it is incised.

down off the lower segment. A transverse incision about 2 cm long is made in the midline of the lower segment and deepened until the membranes bulge (Fig. 35.14), but the amniotic sac should be kept intact at this stage if possible. Two index fingers are slipped into the incision and by separating them it is split transversely to an extent of about 10 cm. The membranes are ruptured and the head is delivered by slipping a hand beside it and applying first one blade of Wrigley's forceps and then the other. The head is delivered gently with the forceps. If the patient is in strong labour and the head is deep in the pelvis, or wedged in the brim in rare instances, an assistant may be needed to push the head up from below with fingers passed into the vagina. As the head is delivered the anaesthetist injects ergometrine 0.5 mg intravenously. The shoulders are carefully delivered, easing them out of the wound to avoid dangerous lateral splitting of the uterine wound. The fetus is held head downwards at about the same level as the placenta while the mouth and pharynx are cleared of fluid with a soft catheter attached to a suction apparatus. The cord is clamped and divided and the infant is handed over to the care of an assistant.

The placenta soon separates and is delivered through the wound. The uterine cavity is explored to confirm that the placenta is complete. Unless

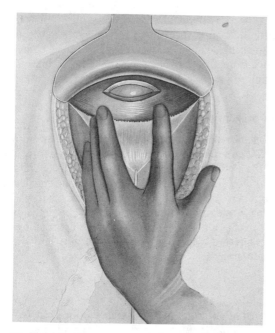

Fig. 35.14 Lower segment Caesarean section. The lower segment is being exposed and a short incision made through it down to the membranes.

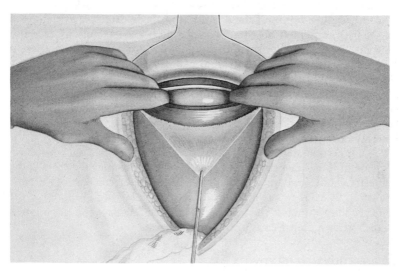

Fig. 35.15 Lower segment Caesarean section. The incision in the lower segment is being enlarged by finger traction.

the cervix is known to be dilated a finger is passed down through it to ensure drainage. The uterine incision is sutured with two layers of catgut or Dexon. It is important to secure complete haemostasis and to remove any blood, liquor and vernix from the peritoneal cavity. The abdominal wound is closed in the ordinary way.

Upper segment Caesarean section

Although the operation is often still described as 'classical' it has been completely replaced by the lower segment operation, except possibly for a case of transverse lie of the fetus with the arm prolapsed, or if a fibromyoma prevents access to the lower segment. A paramedian incision is made. The uterus is incised vertically in the midline of the anterior wall of the upper segment and the membranes are ruptured. The fetus is grasped by the feet and delivered in a manner similar to breech extraction. The incision in the uterus is closed with two layers of catgut, and the abdomen is closed in the ordinary way.

Sterilization

Sterilization may be performed at the time of Caesarean section, but section is never done just to give an opportunity of sterilizing the patient. It is sometimes advised if a patient has had two or more sections on the grounds of the increased risk of section over normal delivery, and it may be recommended for various medical reasons.

The irreversible nature of the operation must be carefully explained to both the patient and her husband, who should both sign consent. It is also important, because of the risk of litigation, always to point out that there is a very small percentage of failures, no matter what method is used.

Because it is not possible to guarantee that any baby will survive and thrive, unless there are very strong medical reasons to advise against further pregnancy it may be wise to postpone sterilization until the baby is 4 to 6 months old and has been weaned, when it can be performed by diathermy coagulation of the tubes by a laparascopic method.

The most certain method of sterilization at the time of Caesarean section is excision of the interstitial part of each tube, but this may be attended by free bleeding and the Pomeroy method is often preferred. Part of the tube is drawn up into a loop and a plain catgut ligature is tied tightly round the base of the loop, which is then excised. Within a few days the catgut gives way and the two sealed ends of the tube separate.

Caesarean hysterectomy

Hysterectomy at the time of Caesarean section is rarely indicated, although it carries little additional risk except on account of the condition which led to it. The technique differs little from that of an ordinary hysterectomy.

The tissues are more vascular, but the tissue planes separate easily. It is occasionally indicated in cases of:

(1) Rupture of the uterus if there is gross damage to the uterine blood supply or evidence of severe infection.

(2) Fibromyomata. When a patient has to be delivered by section because of multiple or large fibromyomata, hysterectomy may be considered (see p. 246).

(3) Carcinoma of the cervix. Cases that have reached late pregnancy may be treated by Caesarean section followed by Wertheim's operation (see p. 249).

(4) Concealed accidental antepartum haemorrhage. If persistent bleeding occurs from the uterus and from any incision or needle puncture it is likely to be caused by hypofibrinogenaemia (p. 431), and treatment of this rather than hysterectomy is usually indicated.

Postoperative care after Caesarean section

A patient who has had a Caesarean section is looked after in the same way as any patient who has had a major abdominal operation. Possible complications will be mentioned in the next section.

Dangers of Caesarean section to the mother

It is estimated that the maternal mortality after Caesarean section is seven times greater than after vaginal delivery. The risk to the mother is affected by the indication for the operation, her health before and during labour, whether there have been previous attempts at delivery and the length of labour, and the skill of the surgeon and anaesthetist. The risks in lower segment Caesarean section performed as a planned procedure are low, about 0.2 per cent, but if emergency cases are considered the risk is higher, possibly 0.8 per cent (see p. 523).

Immediate risks. We have already emphasized the risks of anaesthesia in an unprepared patient with an inexperienced anaesthetist.

Blood transfusion must always be readily available for patients undergoing section, particularly cases of placenta praevia. When emergency section is performed anaemia and shock must first be treated by blood transfusion.

Serious infection is uncommon in planned operations, but still may occur if section is performed after labour has been in progress for some time or any other attempt at delivery has been made. Severe postoperative ileus is now rare.

Pulmonary embolism may occur after Caesarean section, and this and anaesthetic complications now account for most of the fatalities. It is more likely in obese and anaemic patients. Early ambulation and anticoagulant treatment will play an important part in reducing the danger.

Remote risks. Rupture of a Caesarean scar is relatively rare after lower segment section, and then usually occurs during labour. An upper segment scar is more likely to rupture, and may do so during pregnancy as well as during labour (see p. 322). Any patient who has had a Caesarean operation should be under the care of a hospital obstetric unit for every subsequent delivery.

Intestinal obstruction from adhesions is now exceedingly rare since the upper segment operation has been given up.

Dangers of Caesarean section to the fetus

Caesarean section has an inherent small hazard for the fetus, although the conditions for which the operation is performed may explain much of the increased perinatal mortality. Anaesthetics cross the placental barrier and may depress the respiration of the newborn. Respiratory problems may occur with premature babies or those of diabetic mothers.

Occasionally when section is planned to be done near term the duration of gestation is erroneously estimated. The routine use of ultrasonic scan, if this becomes available, should eliminate this risk.

It is possible to cause intracranial damage by delivering the head without proper care when it has to be brought up from the pelvis, or even by delivering it through too small a uterine incision.

Symphisiotomy

In this procedure the symphysis pubis and the pubic ligaments are divided with a tenotomy knife passed through a small suprapubic incision under local anaesthesia. The transverse diameter of the pelvic brim may be enlarged by as much as 2.5 cm by this, and any enlargement is available at any subsequent labour.

In some primitive communities failure to deliver a child vaginally is regarded as a moral failure on the part of the patient, and not only so, but a patient may not return to hospital for subsequent delivery after Caesarean section, and disastrous scar rupture may occur far from help.

Symphysiotomy has seldom been employed in Britain, but has had its advocates in developing countries.

Destructive operations

Craniotomy

This may be performed for (1) hydrocephalus or (2) obstructed labour with a dead fetus.

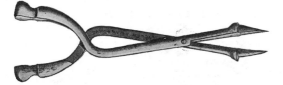

Fig. 35.16 Oldham's perforator.

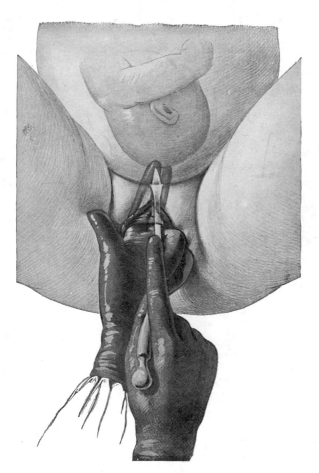

Fig. 35.17 Perforation of the fetal skull. Stage 1. Showing the perforator guided to the child's head by the index and middle fingers of the left hand of the operator. The head in the figure is not fixed and would be held at the brim by an assistant.

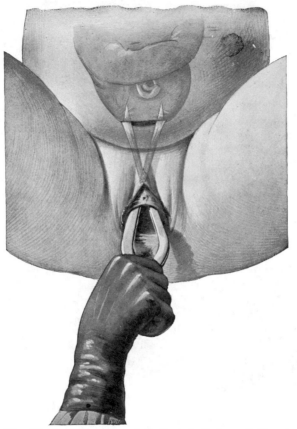

Fig. 35.18   Perforation of the fetal skull. Stage 2. Showing the perforator pushed in as far as the shoulders of the blades, the handles approximated and the blades separated.

Hydrocephaly.   In these cases it is often sufficient to pass a wide-bore needle into the head and draw off the cerebrospinal fluid. This may be done through the abdominal wall. It can also be done through the cervix when that is about 5 cm dilated. After withdrawal of the fluid the head may collapse sufficiently for spontaneous delivery to occur.

If the fetus presents by the breech the aftercoming head can be collapsed after the trunk has been delivered by passing a metal cannula up through the spinal canal (via a spina bifida if one is present).

If spontaneous delivery does not follow tapping, traction is applied to the scalp with Morris toothed forceps.

Craniotomy in cases of disproportion or malpresentation. When the fetus is dead but conditions are unsuitable for vaginal delivery with forceps, for instance in cases of disproportion or of impacted mento-posterior face presentation, craniotomy may be considered, but unless the head is already in the pelvic cavity it is now generally held that lower segment Caesarean section is a safer alternative. Craniotomy consists of two steps:

(1) *Perforation of the head.* Oldham's perforator (Fig. 35.16) consists of two halves, joined by a bolt. Each half has a shouldered cutting blade, a shank and a handle. The method of using it is shown in Figs. 35.17, 35.18. A bone (not a suture or fontanelle) is perforated by a twisting movement. The blades are then separated by closing the handles. After separating the handles the instrument is rotated through 90° and the handles are closed again. The brain tissue is aspirated with a suction curette.

Perforation of a face presentation is performed through the orbit. For the aftercoming head of a breech the trunk is drawn forwards or backwards to fix the head.

(2) *Extraction of the head.* If the head is already in the pelvic cavity traction on the scalp with toothed forceps, or the application of ordinary obstetric forceps, should be sufficient to effect delivery after perforation. In the past the very dangerous operation of cranioclasm of a high head was performed, using heavy instruments to crush the head or to remove the bones of the skull piecemeal.

Decapitation

Decapitation of a dead fetus may be necessary in cases of impacted shoulder presentation, in some cases of locked twins and of double monsters.

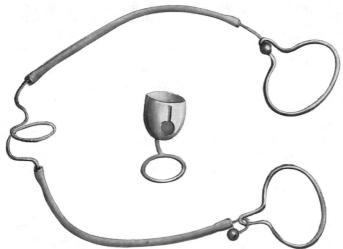

Fig. 35.19 Blond-Heidler wire saw and thimble. This consists of a wire saw covered by rubber except for a few inches at its centre. A loop-type steel wire traction handle slips on to each end for sawing. The other part of it is a thimble slotted on the side to carry one end of the saw and bearing a loop on its summit.

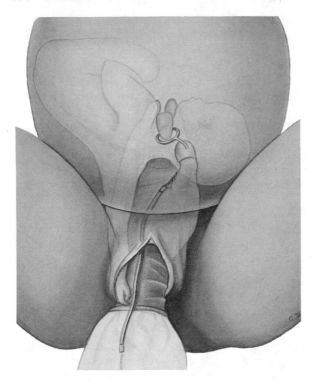

Fig. 35.20   Introducing the Blond-Heidler saw. The thimble is worn on the thumb of the hand introducing the saw and is readily transferred to the middle finger of the same hand which is curved over the fetal neck and slipped into the loop on the thimble. The thimble carrying the saw is thus transferred from the operator's digit in front of the neck to his digit behind it.

The Blond-Heigler saw has been devised for decapitation of the fetus with an impacted shoulder presentation. It consists of a wire saw with a protective covering except for a few centimetres at its centre. A thimble can be attached to one end and this is carried over the fetal neck with the thumb. (Figs. 35.19 – 35.21.) The loop on the thimble is caught by a finger of the same hand (on the other side of the neck). The wire saw having been carried over the neck, the handles are applied, and the neck is divided. The trunk is delivered by traction on the prolapsed arm. The head is guided into the pelvic brim by fundal pressure and a finger in the mouth and delivered with forceps.

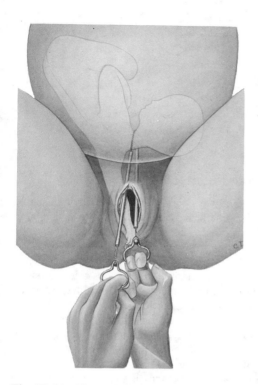

Fig. 35.21 Blond-Heidler saw in position. When in place the saw is used to divide the neck.

Cleidotomy

With a very large dead fetus, or a postmature anencephalic fetus, difficulty with the delivery of the shoulders may occur. If the manoeuvres described on p. 122 fail the clavicles can be divided with a strong pair of straight scissors with blunt points.

36

Oxytocic drugs

Posterior pituitary extract and Syntocinon

Extracts of posterior pituitary gland were found to have an oxytocic action by Dale in 1906 and were used in obstetrics by Blair Bell three years later. Such extracts contain (1) antidiuretic hormone (vasopressin) and (2) oxytocin (Pitocin).

Antidiuretic hormone (ADH) controls water reabsorption in the renal tubules. It also stimulates intestinal peristalsis. In large doses in animals it causes hypertension, but in therapeutic doses in man it has little effect on the blood pressure, although capillary constriction occurs.

Oxytocin is an octapeptide. It causes contraction of the myometrium and also of the myoepithelial cells of the breast. Preparations of oxytocin also have some antidiuretic and hypertensive effect, and with prolonged and excessive doses water intoxication may occur.

The response of the myometrium to oxytocin is relatively slight until late pregnancy, when in response to physiological doses strong but rhythmical contractions occur (unlike the prolonged spasm produced by ergometrine). However, abnormally large doses of oxytocin will cause sustained contraction, which can arrest the placental blood flow, and cause fetal hypoxia or even death. There have been a number of cases of uterine rupture after administration of oxytocin. This is not so much a condemnation of the drug as of the mode of administration. If the treatment is properly supervised so as to produce contractions which are no stronger than those of normal labour the risk of rupture is no more than in spontaneous labour. Clearly there is some risk of rupture if the patient has a Caesarean scar, when even more careful supervision is required.

An increase in neonatal hyperbilirubinaemia has been reported after the use of oxytocin to induce or augment labour. The reason for this is uncertain, but it is possible that oxytocin causes osmotic swelling of erythrocytes, reducing their plasticity so that they are easily destroyed.

Oxytocin is destroyed in the gastro-intestinal tract and is therefore usually administered by intravenous infusion. The dose is measured in units, based on a standard preparation. A synthetic preparation, Syntocinon, is now used, containing 10 units per ml. Some absorption does occur through the buccal mucosa, and oxytocin so absorbed is not destroyed. Buccal Pitocin tablets are available, but are now rarely used because absorption is erratic and reversal of action is not possible.

Clinical uses of oxytocin. Syntocinon or oxytocin is used:

1. *To induce labour.* Oxytocin is most effective as term is approached or passed, but it has some effect even in cases of missed abortion or vesicular mole (for which high concentrations can be used). It is more effective to give the oxytocin after the membranes have been ruptured, but some obstetricians prefer to give it for a few hours before rupturing the membranes, especially if the head is high or the cervix is unfavourable. (see below.)

2. *To augment slow labour.* A Syntocinon infusion may be used to accelerate labour if there is delay from inadequate uterine action (see below) but care must be taken to exclude mechanical obstruction as a cause of the delay.

3. *In the third stage of labour.* Syntocinon may be used for the prevention or treatment of postpartum haemorrhage (see p. 334). A preparation that is often used for intramuscular injection in the third stage of labour is Syntometrine, 1 ml of which contains 5 units of Syntocinon and 0.5 mg of ergometrine.

4. *During therapeutic abortion.* Oxytocin is sometimes used to enhance uterine contractions during therapeutic abortion induced with prostaglandins.

5. *During lactation.* Buccal Pitocin has been used to increase milk ejection but with doubtful success.

Method of administration for induction or during labour. Any patient receiving intravenous or buccal oxytocin must be under continuous supervision. The fetal heart rate must be counted at intervals of not more than 15 minutes, and a record must be kept of the frequency and strength of the uterine contractions, ideally by tocography with a continuous fetal heart ratemeter. Infusion pumps regulate the flow of the solution of oxytocin more accurately than a gravity drip. A common method is to mix 2 units of Syntocinon in 500 ml of 5 per cent glucose solution, and to start running this at 15 drops per minute. This gives an approximate dose of 3 mU/min. The dose is gradually increased at 15 minute intervals according to the strength and frequency of the uterine contractions. This can be done by manual control of the infusion, or by using an automatic system such as the Cardiff-Pye infusion pump, by which a starting dose of 1 mU/min is stepped up and regulated according to the tocographic record of the uterine contractions. Once contractions are regularly occurring the rate of infusion can often be decreased, but it should be kept running until the third stage of labour is completed. If at any time there is evidence of fetal distress or hypertonic uterine contractions the infusion is immediately stopped.

Ergometrine

In the middle ages epidemics of ergotism (St. Anthony's fire), with gangrene of limbs and toxic effects on the central nervous system used to occur after eating rye which had been infected by a fungus, *Claviceps purpurea*. It was found that an infusion of infected rye would expedite labour. Various vasoconstrictors such as ergotamine and ergotoxin were extracted from crude ergot, but it was not until 1932 that Chassar Moir and Dudley separated ergometrine, the substance which is responsible for the strong action of ergot on the uterus. Ergometrine has an almost specific action on the myometrium, with only a slight general vasoconstrictor action, although this may cause a rapid rise in blood pressure in patients who are already hypertensive.

Ergometrine maleate may be injected intravenously, intramuscularly, or given by mouth. After intravenous injection of 0.5 mg a strong uterine contraction occurs within 40 seconds, and persists for 30 minutes. After intramuscular injection the time before the uterus contracts is about 6 minutes, and even if hyalase is added to the injection the time will be 4 minutes. Therefore if ergometrine is to be used for postpartum haemorrhage, or in the active method of management of the third stage of labour, it should be given intravenously. As an alternative a mixture of Syntocinon 5 units and ergometrine 0.5 mg (Syntometrine) may be given intramuscularly. The Syntocinon will act in about 2 minutes, and its action will be followed and maintained by that of the ergometrine.

Ergometrine is also used in the treatment of abortion and at Caesarean section.

If the uterus remains flaccid after one dose of 0.5 mg of ergometrine a second similar dose may be given, but not more as occasional cases of severe peripheral vasoconstriction have been reported. If oxytocic action is still inadequate a Syntocinon infusion can be used in such a case.

The risk of causing a further rise of blood pressure in a patient who is already hypertensive during labour has already been mentioned. Syntocinon alone is given in such a case, and ergometrine is only used if haemorrhage occurs. It has also been suggested that ergometrine should be withheld in cases of cardiac disease, but there is little evidence of any risk.

Ergometrine should never be given to expedite the delivery of a living child as the uterine spasm which it produces will stop the placental blood flow, and there is also a risk of uterine rupture.

Ergometrine is sometimes used in the puerperium if the loss is unduly heavy, but it is futile to give it with the hope of increasing the rate of uterine involution; it causes contraction, not involution.

Prostaglandins

The name prostaglandin was given by von Euler in 1936 to a factor found in seminal fluid which stimulated smooth muscle and lowered the blood

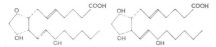

Fig. 36.1 Prostaglandins $F_{2\alpha}$ and E_2.

pressure. It was found that this was not a single substance, and an extensive group of chemically related long-chain hydroxy fatty acids have now been described. Prostaglandins have been found in many tissues and body fluids, and their physiological significance is still uncertain, but two (E_2 and $F_{2\alpha}$) have potent oxytocic effects on the pregnant uterus. Because $PGF_{2\alpha}$ has been found in decidua, in amniotic fluid during labour, and in maternal venous blood during labour it has been suggested that it may play a physiological role during labour.

It has been shown that there is a rapid increase in plasma levels of PGF after amniotomy or vaginal examination, perhaps from release of PGF from the adjacent decidua. Prostaglandins are also thought to play a part in the process of ovulation, in luteolysis, and in the regulation of the fetal circulation by controlling the tone of the umbilical vessels and of the ductus arteriosus after birth (see p. 456).

Clinical uses. Synthetic forms of PGE_2 and $PGF_{2\alpha}$ are available for clinical use. Depending on the purpose for which they are to be used they can be administered intravenously, extra- or intra-amniotically, intravenously or orally. The clinical uses include:

1. *Induction of labour.* PGE_2 or $PGF_{2\alpha}$ may be given intravenously in increasing doses with a similar success rate as for intravenous Syntocinon, but the side effects of vomiting and diarrhoea may be troublesome, and therefore Syntocinon is preferred if this route is used. Prostaglandins in tylose paste may be administered extra-amniotically by injection through the cervix. The simplest method, which is both effective and usually free from side effects, is to place pessaries containing 3 mg of PGE_2 high up in the vagina.

2. *Therapeutic termination of pregnancy.* To induce mid-trimester abortion prostaglandins may be given intra- or extra-amniotically. Over 90 per cent of patients will abort within 48 hours.

In cases of missed abortion or of fetal death the uterus can be evacuated by extra-amniotic injection of prostaglandins.

37

Puerperal pyrexia

Until recently puerperal pyrexia was defined as a rise of temperature to or above 38°C (100.4°F) within 14 days of labour or miscarriage irrespective of the cause, and the doctor was required to notify all such cases to the local medical officer of health. Notification is no longer required.

The causes of puerperal pyrexia are:
1. Birth canal infection (puerperal sepsis)
2. Urinary tract infection
3. Breast infection
4. Thrombophlebitis
5. Respiratory tract infection
6. Other causes of pyrexia.

With the decreased incidence of birth canal infections, urinary infections are now the commonest cause of puerperal pyrexia. In about 15 per cent of cases of puerperal pyrexia no cause is established for the rise in temperature on clinical or bacteriological examination, and the temperature returns to normal without a precise diagnosis being made.

1. Birth canal infection (puerperal sepsis)

Childbed fever was the scourge of the first obstetric hospitals where the mortality from it became so great that a patient was held to be fortunate if she survived her stay in hospital. It was not realized until the middle of the nineteenth century that the cause of epidemic puerperal infection was lack of cleanliness on the part of the attendants, who carried the infection from one patient to another. At this time Semmelweis in Vienna observed that puerperal fever was more common among patients delivered by medical students who had attended postmortem examinations than among cases delivered by midwives. He believed that the fever was caused by products of decomposition and showed that washing the hands in chlorinated lime water reduced the incidence of infection. It is tragic that his contemporaries did not accept his work.

When Pasteur proved that surgical infection was caused by micro-organisms, antiseptics (and later asepsis) were introduced into obstetric practice and quickly diminished the risks of infection, but it still remained the most important cause of maternal mortality.

In 1935 the sulphonamide group of drugs was discovered and produced dramatic results in the treatment of the most lethal type of infection, that due to the haemolytic streptococcus. Pencillin and the other antibiotic drugs have still further reduced the dangers of infection, the great majority of causes occurring today being of the mild localized type. Puerperal sepsis, once the most important cause of maternal mortality, now accounts for only 7 per cent of all deaths (0.008 per thousand maternities), and many of these follow abortion rather than delivery at term.

Although the incidence and severity of birth canal infection has fallen so dramatically in recent years there is danger in complacency. There is evidence to suggest that the virulence of organisms such as the haemolytic streptococcus varies from time to time, and that we are now in a period of relative avirulence. New strains of organisms resistant to the commonly used drugs appear from time to time and cause outbreaks of serious infection. It is only by strict attention to asepsis and the maintenance of a high standard of obstetric practice that they can be controlled.

Aetiology. When the placenta separates from the uterine wall a raw area is left which may be regarded as an extensive but superficial wound.Further down the birth canal other wounds may be left as a result of delivery; thus the cervix is occasionally torn, the fourchette is commonly torn in first confinements, and sometimes the perineum also. These wounds may become infected, and the symptoms and physical signs resulting therefrom constitute the disease which is termed puerperal sepsis.

Bacteriology. In practice it is found that only a few organisms cause puerperal birth canal infections; they are:

Endogenous   Coliform organisms.
             Streptococcus faecalis.
             Anaerobic streptococcus.
             Clostridium welchi.
Exogenous   Haemolytic streptococcus (group A).
             Staphylococcus aureus.

The endogenous organisms are present in the patient's body before the onset of labour. They are only liable to cause infection in debilitated patients, or following injury to the birth canal such as may occur as the result of a difficult forceps delivery or manual removal of the placenta. Such infections are almost always localized to the pelvis. In very exceptional cases a localized infection due to the anaerobic streptococcus may spread into the pelvic veins and cause lung abscesses from septic emboli, or cause thrombosis of the femoral vein (white leg). A clostridial infection may cause collapse, jaundice and haemoglobinuria. These rare infections may be rapidly fatal. They occur in the presence of much bruising and tissue damage or the retention of a macerated fetus.

The exogenous organisms come from other infected patients or from attendants who have an infection or are carriers. The organisms may be conveyed to the birth canal of the woman in labour by the hands of attendants, by droplet infection from coughing, sneezing or even, in the case of the haemolytic streptococcus of group A, from infected dust.

Patients and attendants suffering from colds and sore throats are liable to harbour haemolytic streptococci or staphylococci in their noses and throats, but a small proportion of healthy individuals are also found to be carrying these organisms. In either event the organisms can also be cultured from the hands. Haemolytic streptococci can be divided into several groups according to the Lancefield classification. Group A is the only one responsible for serious infections, and it caused the severe epidemics with many fatalities in the past. Mild localized infections occur with Group B organisms. Both types are sensitive to sulphonamides, penicillin and most other antibiotics.

With virtual elimination of the haemolytic streptococcus as the cause of serious infection owing to a probable diminution in its virulence, combined with its sensitivity to penicillin, the main danger is now from the staphylococcus because of the increasing incidence of resistant strains.

After the introduction of the antibiotics it was anticipated that serious infection would become a thing of the past—it would only be necessary to administer an antibiotic to cure every type of infection. Unfortunately this has not proved to be true because of the ability of organisms to produce strains resistant to the antibiotics, and the widespread use of antibiotics leads to the emergence of these. Laboratory tests show that organisms originally sensitive have now become resistant. An antibiotic kills bacteria by interfering with their metabolism in a specific way. Resistant strains arise spontaneously by mutation. Resistance depends on the acquisition by bacteria of an alternative chemical process by which its metabolism can be maintained, or by the production of an enzyme to destroy the antibiotic, for example penicillinase produced by resistant staphylococci.

As already stated, normal healthy persons may be carriers of staphylococci so that a considerable number of strains are present among the medical and nursing staff and patients in any hospital. Before the widespread use of penicillin only a very small proportion of these strains was naturally penicillin-resistant, so that the great majority of infections were caused by sensitive strains. The introduction of penicillin treatment resulted in the sensitive strains being practically eliminated whilst the resistant strains were encouraged to flourish. The result is that the incidence of carriers of resistant strains of staphylococci among hospital staff has now risen greatly, and these resistant strains are harboured in dust and bedding. Staphylococci may colonize the umbilical stump of the newborn child, and organisms from this site may spread to other infants in the nursery. Infection with penicillin-resistant strains of staphylococci is not only of importance in puerperal sepsis, but also in breast infections, and these organisms are also a source of danger to the newborn.

Pathology.   After the organisms have entered the tissues subsequent events depend on (1) the virulence and powers of invasion of the organisms, (2) the resistance of the patient, (3) the amount of tissue trauma and (4) the speed with which effective chemotherapy or antibiotic treatment is begun.

Depending on the spread of infection three degrees of severity are recognized:

a. In the mildest cases the infection remains localized to the birth canal, in perineal, vaginal or cervical lacerations or at the placental site.

b. Direct spread of infection may take place from the vagina or cervix into the pelvic cellular tissue to cause pelvic cellulitis; infection may spread from the uterine cavity to involve the Fallopian tubes and pelvic peritoneum, giving rise to acute salpingitis and pelvic peritonitis.

c. When the organisms are particularly virulent, as in the case of the haemolytic streptococcus group A, the infection may involve the general peritoneal cavity to cause a general peritonitis, or spread into the blood stream to produce septicaemia. The synovial membranes lining the cavities in remote parts of the body are liable to be infected, for example the pleura, the pericardium or joints. When there is an overwhelming infection of this sort the patient rapidly becomes acutely ill from the effect of toxins formed by the organisms, but the local inflammatory response at the site of entry of the organisms in the birth canal may be minimal, and a perineal laceration, for example, may look quite clean.

Symptoms and signs. The earliest and most important sign of puerperal sepsis is fever. There may be a slight and transitory rise of temperature associated with the activity of labour but thereafter the puerperium should be apyrexial. The fever of puerperal sepsis may appear within 12 hours of delivery, more often within 24 hours, and only exceptionally later. The rise of temperature may be abrupt, occasionally accompanied by a rigor, or it may be step-like, taking several days to reach its maximum. Coincidentally with the fever the pulse rate is raised and the patient feels hot, with headache and backache.

Spread to the pelvic peritoneum is shown by lower abdominal pain and tenderness on examination of the uterus and adnexa. Pelvic cellulitis causes persistent pyrexia and a mass to one or both sides of the vagina and uterus which may take several weeks to resolve.

In cases of general peritonitis the patients are severely ill with a rapid thready pulse, abdominal pain and distention, vomiting and diarrhoea. There is generalized tenderness and few, if any, bowel sounds. The fever is usually persistently high, but in the very worst cases and terminally it may be slight.

In septicaemia, however, rigors are common with continuous high fever. The patients are very ill and there may be no localizing signs. A high vaginal swab and blood culture are of paramount importance in diagnosing these cases.

Diagnostic examination. Pyrexia following labour or miscarriage and persisting for more than 24 hours must always be assumed to be due to an infection of the birth canal until this has been excluded by bacteriological examination. In every case a general clinical examination should be made, including the throat, chest, breasts, abdomen, renal angles and legs. Involution of the uterus may be delayed and it is often tender on abdominal examination. The perineum should be examined to see if any lacerations or an episiotomy are infected. If so they will not be healing normally, and there will be swelling with surrounding redness and a purulent exudate. A vaginal swab should then be taken and a midstream specimen of urine collected for examination and culture. In taking the vaginal swab no antiseptic cream or lotion should be applied to the vulva. Although a more accurate assessment of the bacteriology can be made from a swab taken from the cervix it may be difficult to pass a speculum to visualize the cervix. The bacteriologist should not only report on the organisms found, but perform sensitivity tests against the various antibiotics, so that effective therapy can be chosen as soon as possible. The finding of pathogenic streptococci in the vaginal swab should always be regarded as significant. Other organisms, such as staphylococci, coliforms and non-haemolytic streptococci are commonly found in the vagina in the absence of clinical infection. The lochia may be purulent and foul-smelling, when coliforms and anaerobic streptococci are commonly found, but it is important to realize that virulent haemolytic streptococcus group A infections may spread to the general peritoneal cavity or cause septicaemia with relatively few local abnormal physical signs, and lochia which is not offensive. If the severity of the illness or the type of fever leads to suspicion of septicaemia blood is taken for culture, preferably when the temperature is at its height or during a rigor. Several blood cultures are sometimes needed to establish a diagnosis.

In salpingitis the Fallopian tubes and ovaries are swollen and inflamed with adherent omentum and bowel, but the tenderness of these structures in the recto-vaginal pouch makes them difficult to distinguish on bimanual examination. In most cases of pelvic cellulitis a vaginal examination will show induration of the parametrium extending out to the lateral pelvic wall. If it is unilateral it may push the uterus to the other side of the pelvis. With extensive cellulitis the whole pelvis feels solid, and the induration may even be palpable in the lower abdomen.

Prevention.   It is the duty of the medical attendant to take every possible precaution to prevent infection from an outside source during labour. Patients are advised to abstain from coitus in the last week or two of pregnancy. For vaginal examinations during pregnancy sterile gloves should be used. During labour vaginal examinations should only be done when necessary, and trauma at delivery should be reduced to a minimum. The risks of exogenous infection are diminished by the usual aseptic technique with instruments and towels, and the use of a mask, sterile gloves and gown.

A constant watch must be kept on the medical and nursing staff to exclude from the department any persons with obvious sources of infection such as sore throats, paronychiae, boils or whitlows. In the event of the occurrence of more than a sporadic case of puerperal infection it is essential that swabs are taken from all those working in the department so that the source of infection can be traced and removed. Infected patients must be isolated.

Dust is an important source of cross-infection. It can be kept down to a minimum by using vacuum cleaners instead of brushes, oiling floors and frequent washing of walls. Blankets collect dust and the woollen variety are difficult to sterilize; they should be replaced by the terylene type. Bed-pans must be sterilized after use, and soiled vulval pads should be burned in an incinerator with the minimum of delay.

The prevention of endogenous infection is a far more difficult problem. It is impossible to sterilize completely either the vagina or vulva. In normal circumstances the vagina does not contain organisms of high virulence, but the vulva and perianal region are covered with intestinal organisms such as *E.coli* and *Strep.faecalis*. These organisms are potentially pathogenic, and it is impossible to pass anything, even a sterilized instrument, into the vagina without conveying organisms from the introitus into it. To minimize this risk the vulva and perianal region are swabbed with an efficient antiseptic such as chlorhexidine before making a vaginal examination. When any vaginal operation is necessary during labour the same technique should be employed as in an operating theatre; after swabbing the vulva with antiseptic the surrounding skin, especially the perianal region, is covered with sterile towels.

Although the indiscriminate use of antibiotics for prophylaxis is to be condemned because it encourages the production of resistant organisms, such treatment may be considered after premature rupture of the membranes or amniotomy if labour has not started within 24 hours. Antibiotics may also be given in a case of long labour, especially if this is terminated by Caesarean section. The antibiotic chosen should be safe for mother and fetus; ampicillin or a cephalosporin such as cephalexin (Keflex) are often used.

Treatment. The patient must be isolated. If the pyrexia occurs in domiciliary practice the patient should be transferred to hospital where all facilities for nursing and diagnosis and treatment are available. She must be made comfortable by good nursing, with analgesics if she has pain and sedatives to ensure rest. The fluid intake must be adequate. Haemoglobin estimations should be done every 2 or 3 days because anaemia is often associated with severe sepsis, and transfusions of fresh blood may be required. Antibiotic treatment will be chosen according to the infecting organism and its sensitivities. If the patient is not very ill the bacteriological report can be awaited, but in many cases treatment is started immediately with co-trimoxazole (Septrin) or with a broad-spectrum antibiotic such as ampicillin or cephalexin (Keflex) and subsequently modified if necessary.

If there is an infected perineal wound the stitches are removed. Operative treatment has little place and is usually confined to exploration of the uterine cavity to remove infected pieces of placenta. It is sometimes necessary to drain a pelvic abscess by an incision in either the posterior vaginal fornix or rectum. Pelvic cellulitis may sometimes result in an abscess which points above the outer end of the inguinal ligament and needs drainage there.

2. Urinary tract infection

Infection of the urinary tract is the commonest cause of puerperal pyrexia, and is generally caused by *E.coli*. The infection is almost always introduced by catheterization, which is frequently necessary during labour and sometimes in the puerperium. Apart from catheterization, the bruising of the tissues during delivery may be sufficient to give rise to recurrence of a pre-existing chronic and symptomless infection.

Diagnosis.   This is made by examination of a mid-stream specimen of urine or on a specimen obtained by suprapubic bladder puncture. Part of the specimen is sent to the laboratory for bacterial culture and sensitivity tests, but immediate examination of a drop under the microscope will often settle the diagnosis; a large number of pus cells in the field makes the diagnosis of a urinary infection certain. Symptoms such as dysuria and frequency are often equivocal, since they may occur after delivery when there is no infection, and may be absent in the presence of infection.

Treatment.   In order to prevent urinary infection catheterization should not be performed unnecessarily, and then only with strict aseptic technique. When there is a history of recent urinary infection a prophylactic course of sulphadimidine or ampicillin may be given during labour and the first 4 days of the puerperium.

In the established case the fluid intake must be at least 3 litres in the 24 hours. Sulphadimidine 1 g is given 4-hourly up to a total of 25 g. If the sensitivity tests show that the organism is resistant to the sulphonamide group of drugs an appropriate antibiotic is used; this is often ampicillin.

3. Breast conditions

Acute mastitis or a breast abscess may cause puerperal pyrexia (see p. 423).

4. Thrombophlebitis

The commonest time for pyrexia from this cause to appear is at about the 10th day after delivery. The fever is slight except in cases of extensive ilio-femoral thrombosis, and those cases caused by pelvic infection.

The aetiology and pathology of thrombophlebitis during pregnancy and the puerperium are described in Chapter 39 (p. 433). Apart from the usual type of case of deep venous thrombosis which starts in the veins of the calf and which is caused by stasis rather than bacterial infection, it is possible that in some cases of puerperal sepsis the initial thrombosis is in the deep veins of the pelvis. Anaerobic streptococci may occasionally invade pelvic veins, proliferate in blood clot, and then give rise to septic emboli which pass to the lungs or other sites with episodes of high fever.

5. Respiratory tract infection

When an anaesthetic has been given during labour, post-anaesthetic chest complications such as basal collapse or bronchopneumonia may occur.

6. Other causes of pyrexia

Tonsillitis, influenza, or any of the acute specific fevers may occur in the puerperium, as well as surgical conditions such as appendicitis. A general clinical examination should always be made.

38

Disorders of the breast in the puerperium

Engorgement of the breasts

At about the end of the third day after delivery the breasts become engorged with blood and secretion of milk begins. If the baby does not empty them sufficiently they rapidly become overdistended. The breasts are enlarged and covered with distended veins; the skin over them may be slightly congested. They are very tender, and feel hard and knotty. Nodules of enlarged breast tissue may be palpable in the axilla. The pain may prevent the patient from sleeping.

Treatment

Prophylactic treatment of the breasts during pregnancy will help to promote successful breast feeding by preventing engorged breasts, with the risk of subsequent infection (see p. 59).

In the early stages of engorgement the baby may be able to take enough milk to relieve the congestion, but once the condition is fully established the congestion and pressure on the ducts prevent the flow of milk and the infant from emptying the breasts. A little milk should be manually expressed before putting the baby to the breast as this will help to promote an easy flow of milk. Sometimes the mother cannot tolerate this, and then an electric breast pump which produces rhythmical negative pressure in a soft rubber breast cup may give relief. Hot fomentations are also helpful in relieving the pain of the acute stage, and a sedative should be given at night. Adequate support of the breasts is essential.

Cracked nipples

The nipple may become sore and painful from two conditions. One consists of loss of the epithelium covering a considerable area of the nipple, with formation of a raw area which is very tender. The other is a small deep fissure situated at either the tip or the base of the nipple, which is also very painful. The two conditions may exist simultaneously, and are referred to as cracked nipples.

After delivery a flat nipple, or one that is not kept aseptic and dry, tends to become sore. If there is not sufficient milk in the breast a hungry baby will suck too vigorously and its gums cause abrasions of the epithelium. It has been stated that another cause is leaving the baby too long at the breast, but with demand feeding (p. 476) this does not seem to occur. The nipples may also become sore if, when the baby is suckled, the mother does not depress the breast away from the baby's nostrils with her fingers, because if the baby cannot breathe through its nose it has to drop the nipple repeatedly and then take it up again. Thrush is another occasional cause of soreness of the nipple.

Cracked nipples cause tenderness and pain during suckling. There is also a risk of a mammary abscess forming, as the ducts are not emptied because of pain and engorgement is unrelieved, and perhaps also because the raw area allows access for infecting organisms. The baby may draw blood from a fissure into its stomach with the milk, and if the blood is regurgitated it may give rise to a false diagnosis of gastric haemorrhage.

Treatment

During the first three days the child should be put to the breast for only a few minutes, and must never be allowed to sleep with the nipple in its mouth. At the end of each feed the nipple must be cleaned and dried.

A cracked nipple will heal spontaneously if the trauma that produced it ceases. The first essential of treatment is therefore rest, and the baby must not be put to the breast on that side until the crack has healed. Meantime the breast is emptied by manual expression or by electric breast pump. When breast feeding is recommenced the baby should only be put to the breast for a few minutes at first, otherwise the nipple will crack again. If the lesion is recognized at an early stage it may heal within 48 hours, but once the crack has become extensive or indurated healing will be far more difficult, and in many cases breast feeding cannot be re-established.

Various local applications have been recommended. Any such application must not stick so that it drags away any newly formed epithelium when it is removed, and it must not be harmful to the baby so that it has to be cleaned off before a feed. Flavine in liquid paraffin is a suitable and harmless antiseptic, which will not adhere.

Acute puerperal mastitis

The infecting organism is almost always *Staphylococcus aureus*, frequently of the resistant phage type 80. All that has been said about the prevalence and problems of infection with this organism in puerperal sepsis applies equally to breast infections. In addition the baby is a frequent source of infection to its mother's breasts. It has long been known that breast infections were liable to occur in association with skin infections of the baby, and that such infections spread rapidly in a nursery unless isolation and careful aseptic techniques were practised. The umbilical cord is a common site for infection, and must be inspected daily.

Bacteriological investigations carried out in epidemics of breast infections with *Staph. aureus* phase type 80 have shown that if one baby in a nursery has the organism in its nose or mouth almost all the other babies will be similarly affected within 2 or 3 days. These infected babies, who may be thriving and not ill, are a dangerous source of infection to their mothers.

There are two main types of mastitis; cellulitis when the infection enters a crack in the nipple and spreads to the interlobular connective tissue, and adenitis when the infection is primarily in the lactiferous system, there being no break in the surface epithelium of the nipple. The second type is seen in epidemics and is confined to hospital practice.

Acute mastitis may arise at any time in the puerperium. The onset is rapid, with pain in the breast and fever which may rise as high as 40.5°C (105°F) within a few hours. In both types the clinical picture is the same, the infection being limited at first to one lobe. A wedge-shaped area of cutaneous hyperaemia is seen, and the affected lobe is tense and tender. There may be general malaise. Unless early treatment is successful the condition will progress to a breast abscess.

Treatment

Prophylaxis consists in scrupulous attention to aseptic technique. Any mother or baby with an infection must be removed from the ward or nursery and isolated. Ideally mother and baby should always be kept together and the mother should, as far as possible, attend to her baby's needs herself, thus reducing to a minimum the risk of cross-infection from handling by other persons.

As soon as mastitis occurs breast feeding on the affected side is suspended and the breast is emptied by gentle expression or with an electric breast pump. It is firmly supported over a large pad of cotton wool. A sample of milk is sent to the laboratory for culture and sensitivity tests; it is almost always possible to grow the infecting organism from the milk. If antibiotic treatment is going to prevent an abscess forming it must be started at once. Most of the infecting organisms in hospital are likely to be penicillin-resistant, but the prevalent strain may be known so that an appropriate antibiotic can be given. If the likely strain is not known treatment with flucloxacillin (Floxapen) may be given.

Abscess of the breast

A mammary abscess follows acute mastitis. A segment of the breast becomes painful and tender, with oedema and usually redness of the overlying skin. The temperature is raised and the axillary glands become tender and enlarged. The abscess may form near the surface or in the substance of the breast. If it is neglected a deep abscess may burrow in several directions and lead to almost total disorganization of the breast.

Treatment

Breast feeding and proper treatment of the abscess are incompatible. The baby must be taken from the breast, alternative feeding must be arranged, and lactation suppressed by bromocriptine 2.5 mg twice daily for 14 days. As soon as an abscess forms it should be drained. To wait for fluctuation is to wait too long; the presence of brawny oedema of the skin makes the diagnosis certain. The incision should radiate from the nipple to avoid cutting the ducts. Since these abscesses have loculi running in different directions, and not infrequently have superficial and deep portions connected by a narrow tract, the incision should be adequate and a finger inserted into the abscess to break down any septa or loculi. A drainage tube is inserted, and it is sometimes necessary to make a counter-incision to obtain dependent drainage. Antibiotic treatment is given.

Inhibition of lactation

Although oestrogens will inhibit lactation they are not now used because of the risk of venous thrombosis. Bromocriptine 2.5 mg twice daily for 14 days effectively inhibits lactation, but it is expensive. In many cases all that is required is to support the breasts firmly and to await the cessation of activity. Limitation of fluid intake, but not to a degree which causes severe thirst, may assist.

If lactation is already established weaning is achieved by omitting successive feeds, and only if there is an urgent need to suppress lactation, as in a case of breast abscess, should bromocriptine be used.

Galactocele

A galactocele is a retention cyst of one of the larger mammary ducts. Its content is chiefly milk. It is probable that most of these swellings occur because the lumen of the duct is blocked by inflammatory changes; as a result the retained milk may be mixed with pus. A local fluctuating swelling is felt, and the skin over it may be reddened, but there is not severe pain and no constitutional disturbance. A galactocele that is small and deeply situated may be mistaken for a carcinoma in the breast. The cyst should be excised.

Carcinoma of the lactating breast

When carcinoma occurs in the lactating breast it develops with great rapidity and is very malignant. The affected breast is larger than the other, the nipple is flattened or retracted and more or less fixed, and the skin over the tumour is oedematous—the so-called pig-skin thickening. There may be redness if the growth is close to the surface.

Immediate recognition is of the utmost importance. The rapidity with which the enlargement appears and the reddening of the skin suggest mastitis, but the lack of pain and the fact that the tumour is scarcely tender to palpation should give a clue to the correct diagnosis. This must be confirmed by biopsy, and the treatment will then often be by irradiation.

39

Coagulation disorders and thrombosis

The terminology of the factors concerned in blood clotting and in the lysis of clot is so complex that all except haematologists find it bewildering. This chapter is an attempt to summarize present opinions about these processes and in particular their obstetric applications. The life or health of the pregnant woman may occasionally be threatened by haemorrhage due to failure of coagulation of the blood or, more commonly, by the effects of local or widespread intravascular thrombosis.

The obvious purpose of the coagulation mechanism is to arrest bleeding from any breach of the vascular system. Throughout life damage to small capillaries and vessels frequently occurs. In response to such an injury histamine, 5-hydroxy-tryptamine and polypeptide kinins are released locally and cause strong contraction of the capillaries and arterioles. Even if the blood is totally incoagulable (for example after heparinization) haemorrhage will not always follow injury because of this vascular mechanism. In the uterus there is in addition the strong action of the myometrium; when the uterus contacts the large sinuses in its wall are compressed by the interlacing muscle bundles.

Yet in the normal course of events blood in contact with tissue or damaged endothelium coagulates, so that when the initial vascular compression or spasm relaxes the clot forms an effective plug. This local coagulation must obviously not be allowed to extend to the blood in the rest of the circulation. To prevent this the blood contains enzymes such as antithrombin; if thrombin reaches the general circulation it is greatly diluted, and enough antithrombin is usually present to prevent widespread coagulation.

If a vessel is blocked with clot this must be removed when healing occurs and the circulation to the tissues is restored. Fibrinolysis is a normal physiological mechanism for this, which is invoked by factors in the clot itself and in the damaged tissues. Local coagulation is always followed by fibrinolysis. The two processes are complementary and serve to keep the vascular compartment intact and patent. Coagulation seals any gaps with fibrin and this is removed by fibrinolysis after it has served its purpose.

If there is a failure of coagulation bleeding may occur, but this is usually easy to treat by simple replacement of blood, or sometimes by giving the substance, such as fibrinogen, which is deficient in the particular case. On

427

the other hand, if widespread intravascular coagulation occurs, not only will substances such as fibrinogen be depleted, so that postpartum or postoperative haemorrhage may occur but, what is far more important, a shock-like syndrome may arise from blockage of the pulmonary circulation by multiple small thrombi. For such pulmonary obstruction active lysis of the minute clots is beneficial, and it has come to be realized that attempts to inhibit it by giving such substances as ϵ-aminocaproic acid are misguided.

Coagulation

The normal clotting mechanism may now be outlined. When blood comes in contact with damaged endothelium or is shed on to surfaces other than endothelium clotting occurs. The synctiotrophoblast that lines the intervillous spaces of the placenta must have similar properties to maternal endothelium; otherwise intervillous thrombosis would always occur. In essence coagulation consists of the conversion of a soluble protein in the blood plasma, *fibrinogen*, to an insoluble protein *fibrin*, which polymerizes in adhesive strands. The plasma normally contains about 300 mg of fibrinogen per 100 ml. This fibrinogen-fibrin conversion is effected by *thrombin*, which is formed from an inactive globulin precursor *prothrombin*, normally present in plasma in a concentration of about 40 mg per 100 ml.

For the conversion of prothrombin to thrombin a combination of calcium ions, phospholipids (from platelets or damaged tissues), activated factor V and activated factor X is required. This combination (formerly described as thromboplastin) is generated by a sequence of enzyme reactions. There is (1) an intrinsic mechanism, in which all the factors required for coagulation come from the blood plasma or platelets, and (2) an extrinsic mechanism in which factors from damaged tissues play a part. Scheme I illustrates opinions at present held, but is only included here to allow identification of the various factors.

Fibrinolysis

Coagulation cannot be considered separately from fibrinolysis; blood clot contains factors which lead to its removal (Scheme II). Plasma contains an inert β-globulin *plasminogen*, which may be activated to become a proteolytic enzyme *plasmin* that will break down fibrin to polypeptide degradation products. This conversion of plasminogen to plasmin is controlled by a balance of activators and inhibitors in the blood. At the time of clotting plasminogen adheres to fibrin, and the clot therefore holds the agent of its

Scheme I

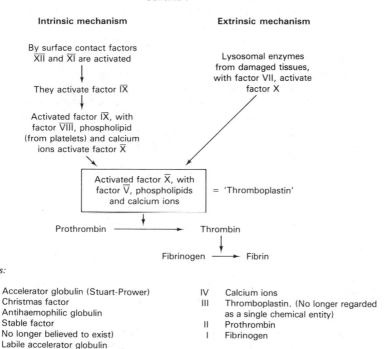

Intrinsic mechanism

Extrinsic mechanism

By surface contact factors $\overline{XII}$ and $\overline{XI}$ are activated

↓

They activate factor $\overline{IX}$

↓

Activated factor $\overline{IX}$, with factor $\overline{VIII}$, phospholipid (from platelets) and calcium ions activate factor $\overline{X}$

Lysosomal enzymes from damaged tissues, with factor VII, activate factor X

Activated factor $\overline{X}$, with factor $\overline{V}$, phospholipids and calcium ions = 'Thromboplastin'

Prothrombin ⟶ Thrombin

Fibrinogen ⟶ Fibrin

Factors:

X	Accelerator globulin (Stuart-Prower)	IV	Calcium ions
IX	Christmas factor	III	Thromboplastin. (No longer regarded as a single chemical entity)
VIII	Antihaemophilic globulin		
VII	Stable factor	II	Prothrombin
(VI	No longer believed to exist)	I	Fibrinogen
V	Labile accelerator globulin		

Scheme II

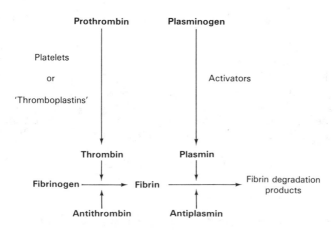

Prothrombin   Plasminogen

Platelets

or

'Thromboplastins'

Activators

Thrombin   Plasmin

Fibrinogen ⟶ Fibrin ⟶ Fibrin degradation products

Antithrombin   Antiplasmin

(Inhibitors in the plasma of the general circulation)

own destruction, which begins when activators diffuse into the clot from plasma or the adjacent tissues. The uterus is a potent source of plasminogen activator.

Plasmin can digest a variety of proteins, including fibrinogen, but any plasmin which enters the general circulation is inhibited by α-globulin *antiplasmins*. Although in theory this protective mechanism could be overwhelmed by an excess of plasmin, it is unlikely that this ever occurs to a degree that causes fibrinogen depletion. However, circulating plasmin may break down some of the fibrinogen to peptides of low molecular weight (fibrinogen degradation products) which may themselves interfere with haemostasis by blocking the action of platelets, coagulation enzymes and the polymerization of fibrin. Fibrinolysis also produces kinins which have a variety of physiological actions, including vasodilatation and hypotension.

Changes in the coagulation system in normal pregnancy

During pregnancy there is a progressive increase in the plasma fibrinogen concentration from about 300 to about 500 mg per 100 ml. In late pregnancy there is at the same time a decrease in the circulating plasminogen activator.

Most authorities state that there is no change in the platelet count during pregnancy, but the count rises by about 30 per cent during the puerperium, reaching a maximum of about 450,000 per cubic millimetre on the 10th day.

The concentrations of factors VII, VIII and IX are increased in late pregnancy.

The total effect of these changes is to increase the ease of clotting and to reduce clot-destroying activity. This may be regarded as a defence mechanism against bleeding after placental separation, but it has the disadvantage that the risk of maternal intravascular thrombosis during pregnancy is increased. Although it is fortunately still an uncommon event, the incidence of deep venous thrombosis in the leg during pregnancy is increased, and cerebral thrombosis is a rare complication of pregnancy.

The placenta contains large amounts of 'thromboplastins', which may enter the circulation in cases of abruptio placentae.

Coagulation disorders in pregnancy and labour

Coagulation disorders occur in some cases of:
1. Abruptio placentae.
2. Retention of a dead fetus in the uterus.

3. Amniotic fluid embolism.
4. Septic abortion.

Abruptio placentae. In cases of accidental haemorrhage (usually of the concealed variety) the escaping blood may not clot, venous puncture sites may continue to ooze, and there may be persistent haemorrhage from the uterus. It is suggested that this is because 'thromboplastin' from the placental site enters the general circulation and that intravascular conversion of fibrinogen to fibrin occurs. The platelet count usually falls because the platelets are aggregated in the fibrin deposits. The blood fibrinogen is depleted, and secondary fibrinolysis causes the release of fibrin degradation products.

If multiple small clots form in the pulmonary capillaries these cause circulatory obstruction, and a shock-like syndrome develops. Small fibrin deposits in the afferent glomerular vessels of the kidney may account for acute renal failure in these cases, and adrenal failure may result from obstruction to the adrenal vessels. Secondary fibrinolysis is usually beneficial as it removes these clots, but breakdown of fibrinogen and fibrin will release degradation products which interfere with coagulation. Some of the degradation products also cause vasodilatation and a fall in blood pressure.

Retention of a dead fetus in the uterus. No disturbance of the coagulation mechanism occurs until the fetus has been retained for about 4 weeks, and in fact spontaneous delivery of a dead fetus usually occurs before this time, and even after 4 weeks coagulation failure occurs in only a few of the patients. The failure develops much more slowly than in cases of abruptio placentae, but it appears to be of the same nature.

Amniotic fluid embolism. In very rare instances some liquor amnii may enter the maternal circulation with a uterine contraction during labour. Sudden severe shock, with respiratory distress and cyanosis occurs. A radiograph of the chest shows widespread mottled opacities, the central venous pressure is raised, and an electrocardiograph gives evidence of right-sided heart failure. Death frequently occurs, and at autopsy fetal squames from the liquor may be found in the pulmonary capillaries.

The mechanism is uncertain; there is an element of anaphylactoid shock, but also evidence of a widespread acute fibrinogen-fibrin conversion.

Septic abortion. Coagulation failure is sometimes seen with circulatory collapse in cases of septicaemia, usually those caused by Gram-negative organism.

Investigation and treatment

Except in cases of retention of a dead fetus in the uterus these coagulation disorders occur so quickly, and often with so little warning, that laboratory investigation is difficult or inadequate.

Hitherto far too much attention has been paid to the plasma level of fibrinogen. Fibrinogen levels will fall if there is a massive formation of blood clot in the uterus in a case of concealed accidental haemorrhage, but also if there are multiple small clots in the pulmonary capillaries and other parts of the vascular system. The obstructive effects of these clots on the pulmonary circulation are more important than haemorrhage from coagulation failure. A low fibrinogen level may even be advantageous if it restricts further clot formation in the lungs.

The usual method of estimating the plasma fibrinogen concentration is to incubate the plasma with an excess of thrombin and to observe the amount of fibrin formed. In an emergency it is doubtful whether elaborate laboratory tests add much to simple observation of the complete absence of clotting of a sample blood in a test-tube, but a fall in the platelet count suggests that active clot formation is occurring somewhere.

Although the clinician has at his disposal for purposes of treatment fibrinogen, drugs which inhibit fibrinolysis, substances which activate fibrinolysis, and drugs which inhibit coagulation, his difficulty is to know which process is at fault. Hitherto any patient with a low plasma fibrinogen concentration has usually been treated with this substance, but a low plasma fibrinogen level is not always associated with bleeding, and to give fibrinogen may make matters worse if there is obstruction of the pulmonary capillaries with clot. Unless it is certain whether coagulation should be encouraged or discouraged in the particular case it is often wisest to attempt neither form of treatment, but to concentrate on the circulatory state rather than the coagulation disorder. Fibrinogen depletion will usually undergo rapid spontaneous correction as soon as the phase of intravascular clotting or blood loss ceases, as it will when the uterus is emptied.

In cases of *abruptio placentae* early rupture of the membranes will reduce the amount of 'thromboplastin' entering the maternal blood, and administration of oxytocin will expedite delivery and reduce bleeding, whatever the state of the blood, by causing strong myometrial contraction. Blood transfusion will supply fibrinogen, and is essential from the circulatory point of view, but it may increase clot formation, and if there is evidence of pulmonary or renal obstruction heparin may be given as well. In cases of coagulation failure severe haemorrhage seldom follows vaginal delivery, but Caesarean section may be dangerous as uncontrolled bleeding may occur from surgical incisions.

In cases of *amniotic fluid embolism* the chief danger is of obstruction of pulmonary capillaries, and heparin is given to arrest this. Although the blood shows defective coagulation and excessive fibrinolysis, attempts to inhibit fibrinolysis are misguided.

With *retention of a dead fetus* in the uterus, even if the fibrinogen level is low haemorrhage seldom occurs. If the level is found to be low, injudicious methods of evacuating the uterus which carry other risks, such as sepsis, are unjustified. Induction with oxytocins, or by intra-amniotic injection of saline, may be considered, but if labour does not follow it is probably best to await events, holding fibrinogen available for administration at the time of labour.

With coagulation failure in cases of *septic abortion* the essential treatment is to limit the production of bacterial endotoxins by the control of the infection with antibiotics, and to treat the capillary vasoconstriction which is reducing the venous return with vasodilators such as propanolol.

Intravascular thrombosis

Intravascular thrombosis may be defined as a process of deposition of clot during life in the blood stream. It differs in several respects from extra-vascular clotting, or clotting of blood after death. In thrombosis platelets first adhere to the vascular endothelium and aggregate. A lattice of fused and disintegrating platelets forms, to which leucocytes become adherent. Thromboplastin is released by the platelets and filaments of sticky fibrin form and entangle red cells, which break down, so that the clot, which was red at first, gradually becomes greyish-yellow. There is often, but not always, an inflammatory reaction in the wall of the vein.

The local physical signs depend on two factors, the degree of obstruction to the circulation, and the degree of phlebitis. The obstructive effects will be slight if there is an adequate collateral circulation, but this may be reduced by reflex spasm of other vessels. Swelling, venous distention and local increase of temperature result from venous obstruction. Pain is the result of phlebitis, but this may be slight, even with extensive thrombosis. It must be stressed that there may be neither pain nor swelling with thrombosis of deep veins, and in most cases the clot is silently removed by fibrinolysis.

In a few cases the clot extends upwards progressively, and then there is danger of detachment of part of the clot, causing pulmonary embolism. If there is much local phlebitis the clot tends to be more adherent, and the 'silent' thrombus is perhaps the most dangerous.

The factors causing thrombosis in leg veins after operation or delivery are only partly understood. Recent investigation by phlebography with radio-opaque substances, or by injection of ^{125}I labelled fibrinogen which becomes aggregated in clot and can then be detected with an external counter, have shown that silent thrombosis of some of the deep veins of the leg may follow Caesarean section (or other operations of comparable sever-ity) in as many as one third of the cases. Blood flow in the large veins can also be investigated with ultrasound by using the Doppler principle; the frequency of the reflected ultrasound waves is altered if the blood is flow-ing, and unchanged if the blood is static.

Damage to the endothelium will cause clotting, but small particles of coagulum are usually washed away as they form and do not extend, and they are also attacked by fibrinolysins.

If a section of undamaged normal vein is doubly ligatured the blood within it will not clot, so that stasis alone will not explain thrombosis, yet slowing of the blood stream will allow aggregation of the clot, which would otherwise be washed away in small fragments. Thrombosis often extends upwards in an occluded vein until it reaches the next main junction.

The patient who is lying in bed or, to an even greater degree, the patient who is unconscious on the operating table, has pressure on the calf veins, and may have slowing of the general circulation as well. In late pregnancy the large uterus will impede the venous return in the iliac veins. If the leg muscles are inactive their pumping action, on which the venous return so largely depends, is not effective.

The vascular endothelium may be damaged by bacterial infection in adjacent structures, particularly by *Staphylococcus aureus*, and pelvic infection after delivery or abortion may cause thrombosis, but this is usually in the pelvic veins and differs from the postoperative thrombosis of the veins of the calf. Such pelvic thrombi may also be invaded by anaerobic streptococci.

Apart from endothelial damage of slowing of the circulation, changes in the coagulability of the blood may also increase the risk of thrombosis. During pregnancy the concentration of fibrinogen in the blood rises. The concentrations of factors VII and VIII are also increased during pregnancy, and in late pregnancy the amount of fibrinolytic activator in the blood is reduced. The total effect of these changes is to increase the coagulability of the blood. This may be a protective mechanism designed to counter the risk of haemorrhage after placental separation, and possibly also to maintain the integrity and separation of the maternal and fetal circulations, but it increases the risk of maternal venous thrombosis during pregnancy. The same risk arises in the case of women taking oral contraceptives, and in them the degree of risk is related to the oestrogen content of the pills. Oestrogens are not now used to inhibit lactation because of this danger.

The placenta contains large quantities of substances with thromboplastic activity, which may enter the general circulation at the same time of placental separation. These may account for the rare coagulation disorders already mentioned, but there is no evidence that they play a part in the more common cases of puerperal thrombosis.

During the first ten days of the puerperium the fibrinogen level is still high, and at this time the platelet count rises. Particularly after Caesarean section, these factors and the mechanical factors already mentioned are associated with an increased incidence of thrombosis in the deep veins of the legs.

Deep venous thrombosis of the lower limb

Isotopic studies have shown that deep venous thrombosis in the leg may occur without any symptoms or signs, and in most cases the clot is uneventfully removed by fibrinolysis. The usual initial site of thrombosis is in the venous sinuses within the soleus muscle. It may spread to the tibial, popliteal, femoral or iliac veins. In a few cases the primary thrombus may be in one of these veins, or in pelvic veins.

Some patients complain of pain in the calf, and on examination there may be tenderness over the soleus and pain on dorsiflexion of the foot. If the thrombosis spreads to the popliteal vein that will be tender and there may be oedema of the ankle. If the femoral or iliac veins are occluded the whole limb will be grossly swollen with tenderness in the line of the femoral vein, and in these severe cases there is often fever. The leg may be bluish in colour or, more commonly, white (*phlegmasia alba dolens*). Fortunately, since the introduction of anticoagulant treatment these severe cases, which often resulted in permanent disability with a swollen and painful leg, have become uncommon.

With deep venous thrombosis there is always a risk of pulmonary embolism, and this seems to be more common with unsuspected deep thrombosis than in the cases with evident physical signs. Probably this is the reason why anticoagulant treatment, which is usually only given to obstetric patients after thrombosis has been recognized, has reduced the duration and extent of venous occlusion but has not altered the incidence of pulmonary embolism.

Treatment. Preventative measures such as dextran infusion or administration of subcutaneous heparin that may be used in surgical practice could seldom be applied in obstetrics, except possibly for Caesarean section. Prevention of anaemia during pregnancy, transfusion in cases of haemorrhage during labour, careful delivery to avoid tissue trauma, prevention of puerperal sepsis and, above all, early ambulation will help to reduce the incidence of thrombosis in the deep veins of the legs, and therefore of pulmonary embolism.

Unfortunately investigation by injection of ^{125}I labelled fibrinogen is unsuitable during pregnancy because the isotope crosses the placental barrier, and also in the puerperium if the mother is breast feeding because it passes into the milk. Ultrasound can be used, and phlebograms can be performed. If deep venous thrombosis is suspected treatment often has to rest on clinical judgment, and the advice of a surgeon with experience of vascular problems is often helpful.

Anticoagulant treatment will not dissolve a thrombus, but will prevent its extension. The alternative policy of using fibrinolytic agents such as streptokinase is not in general use for puerperal cases. Two types of anticoagulants are in use: (1) heparin, which is injected intravenously and acts immediately and (2) oral anticoagulants, which are only effective after 36 to 48 hours.

Heparin is a polysaccharide formed from glucosamine and glycuronic acid, and it contains sulphate groups which give it a strong electronegative charge. It is present in many normal tissues, where it originates in mast cells, which are often found in proximity to the walls of small blood vessels. Its chief action is to inhibit the action of thrombin on fibrinogen. Heparin is best administered by continuous intravenous infusion through a Gordt needle. After an initial priming dose of 5000 units, it is given at a rate of 1500 units per hour. If it is given for more than 48 hours the dose must be adjusted so that the coagulation time is doubled (normal 4 to 8 minutes). Uterine bleeding is unlikely to occur during treatment with heparin, but protamine sulphate, 15 mg intravenously per 1000 units of heparin, is an effective antagonist. Heparin does not cross the placental barrier.

Oral anticoagulants are related to the naphthquinone derivatives which are necessary (as vitamin K) for the formation of prothrombin in the liver. Because of chemical similarity they replace vitamin K at the site of formation of prothrombin, and the production of prothrombin falls. They also reduce the activity of factors VII, IX and X. Oral antibiotics only become effective after 36 to 48 hours, so it is usual to give intravenous heparin during that time. The dose of oral anticoagulant is adjusted according to the effect on the prothrombin time, which is tested daily at first and twice weekly later. The prothrombin time should be increased by three times the control time. Aspirin and other salicylates make patients more sensitive to oral anticoagulants, and barbiturates may reduce their effect. Oral anticoagulants cross the placental barrier and are also excreted in breast milk.

This group of drugs includes dicoumarol, phenindione and warfarin sodium. Warfarin is now the preferred drug as the others may cause sensitivity reactions. An initial dose of 30 to 50 mg is followed by a maintenance dose, which usually lies between 3 to 10 mg daily in divided doses. The anticoagulant treatment is continued for at least a month. Occasionally bleeding may occur from a wound or the placental site; in that case the anticoagulant is stopped and the patient is given a blood transfusion and phytomenadione (vitamin K) 10 mg intravenously 6-hourly.

The pain and pyrexia generally subside quickly on anticoagulant therapy. Leg exercises are encouraged in bed, and once the pain has subsided the patient should be up and about, with temporary support for the leg with a crepe bandage or elastic stocking. If the oedema persists the stocking may be required for some time.

Superficial thrombophlebitis

This is common, especially in varicose veins. The skin over the thrombosed vein is reddened, and the clot can easily be felt. The tenderness soon passes, and there is very little fear of embolism. Anticoagulants are not used and the patient is encouraged to use the leg.

Pulmonary embolism

In the Report on Confidential Enquiries into Maternal Deaths for 1973−75 pulmonary embolism accounted for just under 10 per cent of the deaths. About a third of the deaths from pulmonary embolism occurred during pregnancy in undelivered patients. Among the other two-thirds the incidence of fatal embolism was 1 in 100 000 after vaginal delivery and 7 in 100 000 after Caesarean section; there were a few cases after abortion.

In only 21 per cent of all these cases were there warning signs of thrombophlebitis, and a few of the deaths occurred after the patients had left hospital.

With a massive embolus sudden death may occur without warning, except that there is sometimes an urgent desire to defaecate, so that death on the bed-pan or in the lavatory may occur. More often the embolus is not fatal, and there is pain in the chest with dyspnoea and shock. At first there may be no clinical signs in the chest or in a radiograph. Later a pleuritic rub may appear, and blood-stained sputum. Any sudden chest pain in a pregnant or puerperal patient should be attributed to this cause, for in such women coronary disease is extremely unlikely.

Anticoagulant treatment is immediately started with large doses of heparin (e.g. 15 000 units 4-hourly intravenously for 24 hours). Morphine for the pain and to relieve anxiety, and oxygen may be required. If heparin is given at once the mortality is about 5 per cent.

Some authorities advocate streptokinase for severe cases, and there is an occasional place for pulmonary embolectomy.

Haemorrhagic disease of the newborn

Fibrinogen and prothrombin are probably exclusively formed in the liver. For the formation of prothrombin a complex derivative of napthoquinone is essential (Vitamin K). Any ordinary diet contains adequate amounts of vitamin K, and it is easily synthesized by bacterial action in the bowel. The fetus *in utero* depends on the mother for a supply of vitamin K, and for 10 to 14 days after birth the infant's prothrombin level may fall until it starts to absorb the vitamin from its bowel.

With such prothrombin deficiency haemorrhage from mucosae, or from the skin or umbilical stump may occur. (See p. 496.)

40

Psychiatric disorder in pregnancy and the puerperium

Psychiatric disorder associated with childbearing is a particular instance of the way in which psychiatric symptoms and illnesses are provoked or exacerbated at certain times in life. A 'life event' which may be clearly stressful, such as a bereavement, or one that is outwardly more neutral or even beneficial, such as moving house or being promoted, challenges the individual's ability for psychological adaptation; and the meaning of the event for the individual is more important than its simple outward form. In the case of severe mental illness, which is sometimes called endogenous, a presumed biochemical predisposition is a major factor, but even in these cases some 'life event' is a precipitant or a trigger. Childbearing is a 'life event' with a profound physical as well as psychological change, but the effects of the physical changes on brain function and the psychological state are not yet fully understood. However, there are many sources of psychological stress, including concern about the health of the baby, the labour, changes in sexual interest, loss of attractiveness, incipient change of rôle, and about symptoms such as nausea, sickness, heartburn and backache. The impact of these on the individual will be determined by her personality, her attitudes and beliefs about childbearing, her social circumstances, and also by any inherited predisposition to psychiatric illness.

There are at present many gaps in our knowledge of the psychiatric problems of childbearing, but a general picture can be pieced together. What is clear is that the management of pregnancy and the puerperium will be mechanical and incomplete unless attention is paid to the patient's psychological state.

Pregnancy

Minor psychological problems

The most prominent of these minor problems is *anxiety*, which affects most women at some point. Minor degrees of anxiety do not indicate psychiatric illness, and indeed are part of the normal process of adapting to change. This is not to say that the resolution of anxiety should not be assisted, because if it persists it may lead on to significant distress and more serious problems during pregnancy and the puerperium. The usual source is one of the factors already mentioned, but before the doctor can help he must realize that anxiety is present. This demands not only that his mind must be open to the psychological state of his patient but also the realization that while some patients may present their worries in a straightforward way, many do not.

First, and particularly if the doctor manages to convey the impression of being both Olympian and busy, a fairly major worry may only be mentioned diffidently, apparently in passing and perhaps as the patient is leaving. The doctor should develop the habit of asking, and in a way that conveys willingness to listen to an answer, if the patient has any worries. Secondly it is necessary to be aware that anxiety involves physiological arousal of the cerebral cortex and the autonomic system. There may be one or more signs of this, the commonest of which are increased muscular tension producing headache in frontal and occipital regions, or sometimes over the whole head, and described as 'pressing' or 'band-like', tremor, increased sweating, raised heart rate perhaps experienced as 'palpitations', raised systolic blood pressure, epigastric discomfort sometimes with nausea, dry mouth, frequency of micturition or defaecation, and difficulty in falling asleep. Patients from other cultures or those of lower intelligence may present their anxiety with a complaint of one or more of these physical symptoms, and the doctor must then make a differential diagnosis. Finally, the patient may find it easier to express a worry to another member of the team, perhaps a midwife. It is, therefore, part of the doctor's duty to ensure that his colleagues share an interest in the psychological state of the patients, which is probably best achieved by setting an example. He will sometimes find that his colleagues are already far ahead of him in this respect.

Having made a diagnosis of anxiety, the next stage is to discover what it is about. This can only be achieved by helping the patient to talk. It will often be found that the worry that is presented is only an indicator of others that the patient is too embarrassed to mention. Once this is discovered the doctor can make it clear by his sympathy that the problem has been understood. In many cases the patient needs information expressed in terms she can grasp. This process of clarifying the problem and giving appropriate information is what 'reassurance' is. It is not the giving of rapid instructions to stop worrying, or off-the-cuff explanations which neither the patient nor the doctor can believe. Good reassurance is usually all that is needed to deal with the minor psychological problems of pregnancy.

If social problems are prominent the help of a social worker should be sought.

Neurotic disorders

A brief description of neurosis is that it is an exaggerated response to stress in a person of vulnerable disposition. The symptoms of anxiety neurosis are the same as those of normal anxiety but are more severe and persistent and apparently out of proportion to the provoking stress. The distinction between normal anxiety and 'neurosis' is largely arbitrary, although it is clear enough in severe cases.

During pregnancy the neurosis most commonly encountered will be anxiety, already described, and depressive neurosis. The latter is best thought of as an exaggeration of ordinary misery, with tearfulness, resentment and possibly difficulty in sleeping. The mood is not constant and the patient can be cheered up by pleasant experiences; her main preoccupations will centre on the external events and inner concerns that have provoked the depression. Furthermore, these neuroses shade into each other so that as a rule there is some anxiety associated with the depression, and vice versa.

The prevalence rate of neurosis for all women of childbearing age is between 10 and 15 per cent, but in the first trimester of pregnancy the rate is higher than this, while it is probably lower in the rest of pregnancy. Women who develop a neurotic illness during pregnancy are more likely to have a previous history of psychological problems, to admit to marital tension, to have had a previous termination of pregnancy, or to entertain transient thoughts of seeking termination of the existing pregnancy.

The mainstay of the management of neurotic disorder is the same process of reassurance that has already been described. It is more likely that the help of others such as the general practitioner, the social worker and occasionally the psychiatrist will be needed. Drug treatment may be required, but should not be the first line of management. None of the drugs about to be mentioned have known adverse effects on the fetus, but on general grounds they should be avoided if possible during the period of high risk in early pregnancy. For difficulty in sleeping a non-barbiturate benzodiazepine such as nitrazepam (Mogadon) 10 mg may be used, and for daytime anxiety diazepam (Valium) 5 mg three times daily.

In more severe cases of neurotic depression anti-depressants may be used, although their value in treating neurotic states is less well established than it is for more severe illnesses. There are two main types of these:

1. Tricyclics such as imipramine (Tofranil) or amitryptyline (Triptizol) are drugs that are thought to act by preventing the re-uptake of transmitters released at synaptic clefts in the brain. The daily dose varies between 75 and 150 mg and little benefit is obtained in less than 10 to 14 days. Common side effects are drowsiness and autonomic disturbances such as dry mouth, constipation and partial paralysis of visual accommodation. They should be used with caution in cases of heart disease. There are many new drugs in this class, but the list is too long to be considered here.

2. Monoamine oxidase inhibitors (MAOI) such as phenelzine (Nardil) are thought to act by increasing the concentration of neurotransmitters in the presynaptic neurone. A typical regime would be phenelzine 15 mg three times daily and, as with tricyclics, there is a delay of about 10 days

before any benefit is obtained. Although MAOI are called antidepressants they also have a strong effect on anxiety. Direct side-effects include dizziness, drowsiness, weakness, gastrointestinal disturbances and postural hypotension. More serious interactions with other drugs and certain foods (e.g. cheese) may occur, and patients are given a standard warning card. MAOI can be used during pregnancy but in most cases the advantages are outweighed by the disadvantages. If any drugs incompatible with MAOI are to be used in labour, the latter must be stopped 3 weeks beforehand, a strategy which may call for a degree of clairvoyance.

Psychoses

Psychoses are about 50 times less common than neuroses. They are more severe psychiatric disturbances with a more clearly demarcated clinical picture. In a proportion of cases there is a family history of similar disorders, and although an illness may be precipitated or exacerbated by a 'life event' the link between the event and the subsequent illness is less clear. Drug or other physical treatments are usually necessary. The incidence of psychoses is not increased during pregnancy but the obstetrician may see patients who become pregnant while they are already psychotic or rarely those who coincidentally develop such an illness during pregnancy. In such cases joint management with a psychiatrist is essential.

There are two main types of psychotic illness, affective illness and schizophrenia.

Affective illness. In affective illness the main disturbance is of the mood. The commonest affective disorder is *depressive illness*. The patient is deeply depressed, and she may say that the feeling is different from misery, having a quality of bleak emptiness. The mood is not relieved by pleasant experiences, but is at its worst in the early morning and lifts towards evening.

There is a gloomy and self-blaming view of the past and present and a hopeless view of the future; nearly everything is seen in this dismal light. There are disturbances of appetite and sleep, with waking in the early morning hours. Interest in life is lost and concentration is impaired. Speech, thought and movement may all be very slow. In extreme cases the guilty ideas take on the form of accusing hallucinatory voices. There is a high risk of suicide. Episodes of illness last about 6 months to a year and are followed by spontaneous recovery, but there is a risk of recurrence. The drug treatment of choice is with tricyclic antidepressants, and they usually produce a remission. They must be continued for about 6 months to minimize the risk of relapse.

When distress is extreme or drugs have been ineffective and the risk of suicide is high, electroconvulsive therapy (ECT) may be needed and will produce a rapid response. Electroconvulsive therapy is very rarely used during pregnancy but, provided that the indications for it are there, it is less hazardous than continuing drug treatment. The anaesthetic used, and the treatment itself, are both brief and safe. Some of the public disquiet about ECT derives from misunderstanding of the treatment and from its undoubtedly excessive use without proper indication.

The second affective disorder is *hypomania*. It is much less common than depressive illness, and in many ways is the opposite of it. The patient is elated, over-confident and even grandiose. Speech and thought are speeded up to the point of incoherence, and there is tiresome overactivity. Interest in life and concentration are subjectively heightened to a brilliant level, but objectively this is dissipated by extreme distractibility. Appetite is increased, but early morning waking and diurnal variation of mood are present as in depressive illness.

The immediate management is with phenothiazine drugs such as chlorpromazine (Largactil) or a butyrophenone such as haliperidol (Serenace). These may have many side effects, of which the most alarming is the production of extrapyramidal syndromes, including Parkinsonism and dyskinesia due to dopamine block. These drugs are not known to have adverse effects on the fetus, but the same general caveat must apply to the high-risk period in early pregnancy.

The obstetrician may encounter patients who have had a number of episodes of depressive illness, with or without attacks of hypomania as well, who are taking lithium carbonate as a long-term prophylactic. So far no adverse effect on the fetus has been established, but the dosage must be carefully controlled by regular blood level estimations. The first evidence of excessive dosage may be nausea and diarrhoea, but unless this is corrected serious brain and kidney damage may occur. If relative sodium depletion occurs in a patient on lithium the blood level rises with the risk of toxicity, and this may happen if there is vomiting or if diuretics are given. Any pregnant patient on lithium demands the closest liaison between obstetrician and psychiatrist.

Schizophrenia.   The other main psychosis is schizophrenia. Only a brief description can be given here, the central feature being the development of abnormal perceptual experiences. The most common of these is the hearing of hallucinatory voices which are often heard discussing the patient's thoughts and actions. As well as 'voices' the patient may experience interference with her thoughts which seem to be suddenly stolen away; she may also say that alien thoughts are inserted into her mind by some telepathic process. From these experiences spring delusional beliefs and unpredictable emotional reactions. About a third of the patients recover completely, but the remainder show varying degrees of chronic illness and social decline.

The main drug treatment is with oral phenothiazines, but more chronic patients may be on regular depot injections of fluphenazine enanthate (Modecate) or some similar drug. These patients may be receiving a wide range of social services in an attempt to prevent relapse. Again, very close liaison between obstetrician and psychiatrist is essential.

Drug abuse

This problem must be briefly mentioned. A patient who is dependent on opiates will present difficult problems in management, not only because of the drugs themselves and the risk of the baby being born physically dependent on opiates, but also because the patient's general health may be poor, as also may be her cooperation in antenatal care.

There is a danger that less attention will be paid to the more common and equally serious problem of the alcoholic mother, with the consequent risks of the fetal alcoholic syndrome.

Some registered addicts will be attending a Drug Dependency Clinic and psychiatric assistance will be available for them, but in the case of other addicts and untreated alcoholics an attempt must be made to persuade the patient to see a psychiatrist.

The puerperium

In the puerperium there is a sharper increase in psychiatric morbidity than at any time in pregnancy. A striking feature is that the majority of these disturbances begin on the second or third day after delivery, and they are often preceded by relative well-being. The period of increased incidence is over by 6 to 8 weeks after delivery. Disorders starting within this period may last beyond it, but after the 8th postpartum week the incidence of new cases is no higher than in the general population. There is some evidence that the morbidity may rise again slightly in the second postpartum year, and this will be mentioned again later.

Minor psychological problems

At least 50 per cent of women suffer from fleeting and mild degrees of depression in the sense that they are miserable and tearful, an occurrence sometimes called 'the maternity blues'. Perhaps surprisingly there is no correlation between this condition and the mental state during pregnancy. It is more frequent in primiparae and in those with a past history of premenstrual tension.

During pregnancy some women have idealized their baby and their relationship with it. They may be disappointed to find after delivery that they have lost the imagined baby and given birth to a stranger they must get to know. The reality of caring for another human being may strike them for the first time, and panic and feelings of inadequacy may follow this disillusion.

Others may have enjoyed the 'irresponsibility' of pregnancy when they may have received extra care and attention from their husband and parents and resent the loss of childhood, which on becoming a mother can no longer be denied.

The management of these minor disturbances is by the simple measures of sympathetic support and reassurance outlined earlier. However, the emotionally immature mother needs the insight of her obstetrician as much as his support, in understanding her distress.

Neurotic illness

About 10 per cent of women develop more severe and persistent neurotic depression with a strong admixture of anxiety, usually arising as a deepening and prolongation of the 'blues'. Prominent in the clinical picture is excessive anxiety about the baby and its feeding, and fatigue and difficulty in falling asleep are also common. This neurosis is sometimes called 'atypical depression'. The patient should always be asked about such symptoms at postnatal visits. Many patients do not recover for several months. The management is the same as for neurotic illness during pregnancy.

It is almost impossible to predict which patients will develop puerperal neurosis, but neurosis in the first trimester of pregnancy, marital tension during pregnancy and doubts about going through with the pregnancy are associated with a higher risk of puerperal neurosis. It is more common in women over 30 and in those who have been trying to conceive for 2 or more years. Late marriage or late pregnancy may indicate that these have been postponed because of conflict about them. It can be said that the greater a woman's ambivalence about becoming a mother the greater will be her anxiety over the fait accompli. On the other hand the relatively infertile woman has had her doubts hidden by the difficulty in becoming pregnant, and may face them for the first time with the birth of her longed-for baby.

Psychoses

The incidence of psychotic illness is increased in the puerperium in contrast to that in pregnancy. The problem of puerperal psychosis has changed greatly in the last 50 years. At the beginning of that period organic delerious states, often with a fatal outcome, were quite common and mainly related to puerperal infection. Since the introduction of antibiotics, and with higher standards of obstetric care, psychoses of this type have virtually disappeared. It is now recognized that there is no specific 'puerperal psychosis' but that illnesses developing at this time are usually of the affective or schizophrenic type which have already been described.

The total incidence of psychosis in the puerperium severe enough to require admission to a psychiatric unit is 1 in 1000 births. Depressive illness is three times more frequent than schizophrenia, but hypomania is rare. The family histories and subsequent psychiatric histories of women with puerperal psychoses are not more abnormal than those of women with non-puerperal psychoses; the puerperium is in some way particularly liable to provoke psychoses in those who are predisposed. In both puerperal depression and schizophrenia there is concern about the baby, but it is in the cases of severe depression that the rare instances of infanticide may occur.

In all psychoses expert psychiatric care is essential and admission to a psychiatric hospital may be necessary. This may be to a special 'mother and baby unit' if one is available, but there is nothing magical about such units; their main advantage is that the mother can begin to look after the baby under supervision directly her illness begins to improve.

Whether in or out of hospital, the physical treatments are those that have already been mentioned: tricyclic antidepressants or ECT for depressive illnesses, and phenothiazine or butyrophenone drugs for hypomania and schizophrenia. All the drugs are excreted in breast milk in small quantities, and although no adverse effects on babies have been reported, this fact must be taken into account in deciding whether to continue breast feeding.

Termination of pregnancy

Since the passage of the Abortion Act (1967) the number of patients requesting termination of pregnancy referred to psychiatrists has declined sharply. This is because the patient's social circumstances can now be taken into account in making decisions about termination, and there is less emphasis on psychiatric considerations. It strengthens the suspicion that before the 1967 Act many patients exaggerated their misery and made threats of suicide simply to get what they wanted.

If there has been a previous puerperal psychosis the risk of a recurrence is 20 per cent, and in making a decision the severity of the previous illness must also be taken into acccount. Unfortunately the risk of recurrence may be nearly as high after termination. A patient who is in doubt about termination is particularly likely to have unpleasant psychiatric sequelae if she has the operation done. Thus for every apparent psychiatric indication for termination there is a nearly balancing contraindication, which has led some to argue that there are no purely psychiatric indications for termination. When termination is requested on psychiatric grounds an assessment should be made of the true wishes of the patient herself, her social circumstances, her ability to cope with other children, and her present psychiatric state and past history. The decision, which is never easy, is made on the balance of these factors. One of the lessons of this dilemma is that particular efforts should be made to ensure that all women who have had psychiatric disturbances related to childbearing receive appropriate and effective contraceptive advice, or sometimes sterilization.

Beyond the puerperium

The members of the obstetric team have a good opportunity to assess their patients during antenatal care, childbirth and the postnatal period and to learn something about their personalities and their social circumstances. Some thought should be given to the future beyond the postnatal visit, and there are two specific matters to be considered.

First, there appears to be a small peak of psychiatric illness during the second postpartum year. Women who have three or more children aged under 14, an unsupportive husband and no job outside the home are particularly at risk for episodes of depression. The risk is greater if the patient lost her own mother by death or separation before the age of 11. Where a situation of this kind appears likely to develop care should be taken to offer contraceptive advice and possibly social-work support before there is another pregnancy.

Secondly, where there is a relatively immature young mother who has been brought up in a home where there has been much physical violence, who is impulsive, tense and uncertain of her capacity to care for a baby, who has unrealistic ideas about motherhood, and whose husband is also immature, there is a risk of child abuse. If some supportive discussion, centred on the anxieties about looking after the child can be tactfully started in hospital and then carried on by the social worker, health visitor or general practitioner after the mother has gone home, this may reduce the risk of child abuse happening, and also provide an early warning system if it does.

41

Haemolytic disease

It is at present unexplained why the maternal immunity mechanisms do not reject the fetus, whose tissues must contain many factors inherited from the father which could excite these mechanisms. The placental barrier is far from perfect, as fetal trophoblast can be found in the maternal lungs, and fetal red cells may enter the maternal blood, particularly at the time of labour.

In the case of the rhesus factor, which is carried on the fetal red cells, immunity reactions between mother and fetus may occur.

In 1940 Landsteiner and Weiner showed that the red cells of 85 per cent of Caucasians contain a substance which they named the rhesus factor because of the similarity to an antigen found in the red cells of the *Rhesus macacus* monkey. Individuals possessing this factor are called Rh-positive and the remainder Rh-negative.

Transfusion of Rh-positive blood to an Rh-negative recipient stimulates the production of an agglutinin in the recipient's serum called the anti-Rh antibody. This is a true agglutinin, and if a second transfusion of Rh-positive blood is given to a sensitized individual the agglutinin already present in the patient's serum causes agglutination and haemolysis of the transfused cells. Such transfusion reactions are severe and often fatal.

The condition of erythroblastosis fetalis, in which severe haemolysis occurs in the fetus or newborn child, had previously been recognized, and Levine showed that most mothers of erythroblastotic fetuses were Rh-negative, while the fetuses were Rh positive, and that the maternal blood contained antibodies which caused agglutination and haemolysis of the fetal cells.

The rhesus antigens

Five other antigens related to the rhesus system were subsequently found, some of which are very rare, and for a time nomenclature was confused.

Fisher suggested that each of the six antigens was carried by a single gene, and that these genes were transmitted in groups of three on a single chromosome (triple allelomorphic system). As the chromosomes are in pairs, any person will carry six genes linked in three pairs. The genes are designated C, D, E, c, d, e, and any one chromosome will carry C or c, D or d, E or e. Some examples of the patterns found on pairs of chromosomes are: CDe/cde, CDe/CDe, cde/cde, cDE/cde, CDe/cDE. These are in fact the five commonest genotypes found in London.

The gene that makes a person Rh-positive is D. This is inherited as a Mendelian dominant, and if it is found on either or both of the pair of chromosomes the individual is Rh-positive (e.g. CDe/cde, or CDe/CDe). If it is on neither (e.g. cde/cde) then the individual is Rh-negative.

For practical purposes this complexity may be ignored and individuals classified as Rh-positive or negative, according to whether their cells contain the D antigen or not, as D is the offending antigen in almost every case.

An additional complication exists in the occurrence of homozygous and heterozygous Rh-positive individuals. The homozygous Rh-positive father (DD) will pass on the D gene to all his offspring, whereas the heterozygous Rh-positive father (Dd) will have an equal chance of having a Rh-positive or a Rh-negative baby by a Rh-negative woman. In European communities 15 per cent of individuals are Rh-negative, 38 per cent homozygous positive and 47 per cent heterozygous positive.

Feto-maternal transfusion

Fetal red cells contain haemoglobin which is more resistant to denaturation with acid than adult haemoglobin. If a film of maternal blood is treated with acid and then stained any fetal cells which have entered the maternal circulation can be distinguished and counted (Kleihauer and Betke test). By using this test it can be shown that it is uncommon for any significant feto-maternal transfusion to occur during pregnancy, but that it is a common event during labour, and especially in the third stage. Manual removal of the placenta or Caesarean section will increase the risk. Immunization is uncommon after spontaneous abortion, but the risk is much increased after surgical procedures for termination of pregnancy. If the placenta is punctured by amniocentesis during pregnancy fetal blood may enter the maternal circulation, and manipulations such as external version may have the same effect.

It is probable that transfusion of as little as 0.1 ml of fetal blood is sufficient to cause the initial sensitization, but the maternal response varies considerably. It has also been found that if the Rh-positive fetal cells are ABO incompatible with those of the Rh-negative mother rhesus antibodies are less often produced.

There are two types of Rh antibodies. The antibodies which cross the placenta and damage the fetal red cells are IgG gamma-globulins which sensitize and coat the red cells. They only agglutinate the cells in a relatively concentrated protein medium. They are detected by Coombs' antiglobulin test.

The other antibodies cause agglutination of red cells suspended in saline, but are of little clinical importance. They are IgM gamma-globulins of larger molecular size, and do not cross the placenta.

Because feto-maternal transfusion does not usually occur until labour antibodies are rarely produced during a first pregnancy, but if the mother is sensitized she will show a rapid increase in antibody titre during any subsequent pregnancy in which the fetus is Rh positive, presumably because of passage of minute amounts of fetal blood into her circulation.

Since there are now effective methods of preventing sensitization against rhesus positive red cells (see below) haemolytic disease from this cause ought to disappear, but because of the rare cases in which the fetal red cells enter the maternal circulation before labour, and of cases in which preventative injections are not given because of human error, haemolytic disease continues to exist on a small scale.

Clinical features of haemolytic disease

The basic process in haemolytic disease is agglutination and haemolysis of the fetal cells by the antibody passed across the placenta from the maternal serum. This blood destruction is balanced by hyperplasia of erythropoietic tissue in the fetus, both medullary and extra-medullary, in an attempt to maintain a normal cell count. The outcome depends on whether the production of cells can keep pace with the destruction, and on the severity of the haemolytic process.

In the most severe cases the fetus may die *in utero* or at birth. Intrauterine death only rarely occurs before the 28th week from this cause. There is generalized oedema of the fetus (*hydrops fetalis*) with pleural, pericardial and peritoneal effusions. All the tissues are stained yellow with bilirubin. The primitive areas of red cell formation in the liver, spleen and lymphatic structures show activity (*erythroblastosis*). The placenta is enlarged and oedematous, and microscopical examination shows abnormal persistence of the cytotrophoblastic layer. The liquor and membranes are coloured with bile. Death may occur from cardiac failure soon after delivery.

In slightly less severe cases anaemia and jaundice appear almost at once after birth, because the placenta is no longer able to remove the bile pigments, and the liver of the newborn child cannot easily deal with these (see p. 497). The liver and spleen are enlarged.

If the serum bilirubin persists at levels above about 340 mmol/l (20 mg/100 ml) *kernicterus* may occur. In this condition the basal ganglia of the brain are deeply bile-stained, and microscopical examination will show that there is necrosis of nerve cells. If the infant survives there will be extrapyramidal rigidity, spasticity, deafness and often mental retardation.

The early clinical signs of kernicterus include reluctance to feed, lethargy, increased muscular tone with a tendency to opisthotonus, and bulging of the fontanelle.

In the very slightest cases there may only be transient anaemia, which is associated with the presence of nucleated red cells in the blood.

Diagnosis

The Rh group of every pregnant woman must be determined early in pregnancy, and a test for Rh antibodies made in all those who are found to be Rh-negative. Even if the test then shows no antibodies it should be repeated at the 28th and 36th weeks.

The obstetric history and that of the outcome to the children is of the utmost importance, and will give some indication of the severity of the disease and whether the inheritance is heterozygous. Whenever the history is suspicious, or Rh antibodies are found, the genotype of the father should be determined, and information sought about the blood groups of any children.

The tests for antibodies are repeated from time to time during pregnancy. Although less attention is now given to changes in titre than formerly, very high titres or a sudden rapid rise suggest severe disease.

Amniocentesis.   The amount of bilirubin in the liquor amnii is a useful indication of the severity of the disease, and in many centres amniocentesis is repeatedly performed. There is a small risk of damaging the placenta and causing the entry of fetal blood into the maternal circulation, but this risk can be reduced by ultrasonic localization of the placenta and careful technique. The amount of bilirubin in the liquor is determined by spectrophotometry, and in assessment a chart is used which makes allowance for the normal change in bilirubin level according to the duration of gestation.

Tests after birth.   Immediately after birth the following tests should be carried out on cord blood to confirm the diagnosis and indicate the severity of the haemolytic process:

1. Rh grouping.   Grouping of the cells of the infant will show whether Rh incompatibility is possible. If the infant is Rh-negative (cde/cde) incompatibility cannot exist.

2. *Coombs' test.*   The direct Coombs' test will show whether the red cells have been sensitized by absorption of globulin (i.e. antibody). A suspension of the red cells in saline is mixed with rabbit antiglobulin; agglutination occurs if the cells are coated with globulin.

3. *Haemoglobin concentration.*   In some mildly affected babies the cord blood haemoglobin concentration at birth may be normal, with levels of 15 g per 100 ml or more, and yet the infant may develop anaemia and jaundice after an interval of some hours. In more severely affected infants

the haemoglobin level at birth is low, and values at any level down to 3 g per 100 ml may be found.

4. *Serum bilirubin level.* Repeated estimations are made, as the level may rise rapidly after birth, with a risk of kernicterus.

5. *Nucleated red cell count.* A high erythroblast count indicates that there is considerable hyperplasia of the bone marrow and that severe intra-uterine haemolysis has occurred. A low erythroblast count with severe anaemia at birth suggests marrow exhaustion.

Prevention

It has been known for many years that if Rh-positive fetal cells are introduced into the circulation of a Rh-negative mother, and if there is ABO incompatibility between mother and fetus, the fetal cells quickly disappear from the circulation and Rh immunization only occurs infrequently.

In 1960 Finn suggested that Rh-positive cells in the circulation of a Rh-negative mother could also be removed by injection of a small dose of anti-D gamma globulin. Clarke, Freda and others soon proved that IgG anti-D gamma globulin effectively prevented immunization if it was injected within 24 hours of delivery. Obviously the treatment is of no value if the mother is already immunized by a previous pregnancy or blood transfusion.

Because of shortage of gamma-globulin the treatment was at first restricted to mothers who were shown to have a significant number of fetal cells in their blood by the Kleihauer test, and whose blood was also ABO compatible with that of the fetus.

Since the Kleihauer test is not totally reliable and some women with no evidence of feto-maternal transfusion later developed antibodies, and since ABO incompatibility does not give complete protection, gamma-globulin should be given to all Rh-negative women (who are not already immunized) within 48 hours of the birth of a RH-positive infant, and supplies are now adequate for this. The dose now used is 100 μg of gamma-globulin, given by intramuscular injection. This dose may not be enough for protection against exceptionally large feto-maternal transfusion, and if the Kleihauer test shows many fetal cells in the maternal blood larger doses are given. A dose of 50 μg is given to Rh-negative patients who have spontaneous or therapeutic abortion.

Treatment

In any pregnancy in which antibodies are present delivery must be conducted in hospital and preparations to treat an affected baby must be made in advance.

Induction of premature labour

If the infant is Rh-positive there is a risk of intrauterine death, and the longer the fetus remains in the uterus the greater is the risk in severe cases. For this reason labour may be induced before term. The time at which this is done depends on the prognosis, judged from the obstetric history and fetal outcome in previous pregnancies and may be at the 35th week or even earlier in severely affected cases. The need for, and timing of, induction will often rest on repeated observation of the bilirubin content of the liquor and of changes in the antibody titre.

Treatment of the infant after delivery

The affected baby at birth has a proportion of his red cells already sensitized by antibodies and destined for destruction. His serum contains a certain quantity of antibodies which will destroy further red cells and this process will continue until all antibodies have been absorbed or eliminated. The destruction of the red cells causes an anaemia which overproduction by the marrow attempts to restore, and the survival of the infant is dependent on whether destruction or production is the greater. At the same time the haemolysis of the erythrocytes causes progressive jaundice which can itself be lethal.

The treatment of the affected baby depends on the severity of the condition. The clinical state of the infant at birth, the cord blood level of haemoglobin and bilirubin, the strength of the Coombs' test and the previous obstetric history of the mother are the factors which must be considered.

When the disease is mild many infants require no treatment at all, while others slowly become anaemic, without showing jaundice and require a simple transfusion with Rh negative blood to correct the anaemia.

The infant who is moderately or severely affected at birth is usually pale, with enlargement of the liver and spleen. Jaundice develops within a short interval after birth and rapidly deepens. It is for these infants that exchange transfusion is essential.

Exchange transfusion

Exchange transfusion:
1. removes bilirubin from the serum, and
2. replaces Rh-positive cells with Rh-negative cells which are unaffected by circulating antibodies, and
3. removes antibodies by replacement of the serum, and
4. corrects anaemia.

The indications for exchange transfusion immediately after birth have been variously stated. A rather conservative view suggests that replacement transfusion is indicated at that time if:

1. The cord blood haemoglobin level is below 14 g per 100 ml.
2. The cord blood bilirubin concentration is greater than 51 mmol/l (3 mg/100 ml).
3. The Coombs' test is strongly positive.
4. The infant is affected and there is also a history of a previous badly affected baby.

If exchange transfusion is not indicated immediately after birth the serum bilirubin is estimated 6 hours later and then at intervals. A rate of rise that seems likely to bring the bilirubin level to the danger point of 342 mmol/l (20 mg/100 ml) strongly indicates the need for exchange transfusion.

Technique of exchange transfusion. With careful aseptic technique a polyvinyl catheter is introduced into the umbilical vein and passed so that the tip reaches the portal sinus. By means of a system which includes a three-way tap and a syringe blood is withdrawn from the vein in volumes of 10 to 20 ml, and replaced with equal volumes of Rh-negative blood. The exchange is continued until a total volume of 160 ml of blood per kg body weight has been removed and replaced. This will effect a 90 to 95 per cent exchange of the infant's cells.

Exchange transfusion is a dangerous and potentially lethal operation in unskilled hands, and should only be carried out by those with special experience. The pulse rate, respiration rate and activity of the baby must be carefully monitored throughout the procedure, and the temperature maintained. After the transfusion serial estimations of bilirubin and haemoglobin are carried out over the ensuing 5 days. Repeated exchange transfusions are often necessary, because bilirubin enters the circulation from the tissues and may reach dangerous levels.

Intrauterine transfusion of the fetal peritoneal cavity

Exchange transfusion has lowered the mortality in haemolytic disease but not completely eliminated it. Some infants are so severely affected that they die in utero before term from hydrops fetalis. Observation of the antibody levels and of liquor bilirubin levels may predict these severe cases, and if the fetus is not mature enough for premature delivery then intrauterine transfusion may be indicated.

After accurate determination of the position of the fetus by radiology or ultrasound, a long needle is passed through the maternal abdominal and uterine walls into the peritoneal cavity of the fetus. Fresh Rh-negative blood, with partially packed cells, is given slowly in volumes related to the weight of the fetus, e.g. 85 ml/kg. The red cells are absorbed from the fetal peritoneal cavity by the lymphatics. The transfusion is repeated at 1 to 2 weekly intervals until the fetus is mature enough for delivery. The technique carries a mortality of up to 50 per cent, and it should only be undertaken by those with special experience of it.

Incidence and prognosis

The incidence of haemolytic disease has been dramatically reduced since the introduction of anti-D γ-globulin.

Because 85 per cent of people in this country are Rh-positive a Rh-negative woman has an 85 per cent expectation that her husband will be Rh-positive. If allowance is made for the fact that more than half of the husbands will be heterozygous, it can be calculated that the possibility of haemolytic disease arises in about 8 per cent of pregnancies. The actual incidence is only about 0.5 per cent because the volume of fetal cells and the maternal response to the antigen vary greatly, and also because any Rh-positive cells which are ABO incompatible are agglutinated and may not produce antibody reaction. Mismatched blood transfusion with Rh-positive blood will produce antibodies in about 50 per cent of Rh-negative women.

The first baby produced by the mating of a Rh-negative woman and a Rh-positive man very rarely suffers from haemolytic disease unless sensitization has been caused by a previous transfusion or a miscarriage. If Rh antibodies are present in a woman's serum all subsequent Rh-positive fetuses are likely to suffer from haemolytic disease. It used to be said that the severity of the disease increased in successive pregnancies, but there is no evidence for this.

Haemolytic disease due to factors other than D

Rare cases of maternal immunization to one of the other antigens of the Rh group (with the exception of d) have been described, but such cases are rare because these are 'weak' antigens.

It might be expected that immunization of a mother of blood group O to an A or B factor inherited by the fetus from the father would be common, and this does occur if the child is a 'secretor', which means that his A or B group specific substances are water-soluble and are therefore in the plasma and other tissue fluids. This type of haemolytic disease may occur in a first pregnancy as it does not depend on feto-maternal transfusion of red cells.

Fortunately this type of haemolytic disease is usually mild, probably because anti-A or B antibodies do not easily pass the placenta, and if they do they are absorbed on to many fetal tissues besides the red cells. The child rarely requires treatment except in cases of high bilirubin levels in premature infants. There will be anti-A or B antibodies in the maternal blood, but the Coombs' test is unreliable in these cases.

Exceedingly rare cases of maternal immunization to other blood factors have been described.

42

Care of the newborn infant

At the moment of delivery the integrity of the placental circulation is lost and the infant is launched on an independent existence and must assume the vital function of respiration or die. The fetal circulation must quickly adjust to the needs of pulmonary gas exchange. Later, heat regulation, assimilation and digestion of food and excretion must be achieved. Thus, immediately after the traumatic experience of birth the infant must undergo profound physiological changes.

Changes in the respiratory system. The fetus *in utero* rehearses the movements of respiration to a point just short of expansion of the chest and lungs. These respiratory movements are phasic and are interrupted by long periods of rest. Amniotic fluid is drawn in and out of the nasopharynx, the bronchial tree and the alveolar spaces during intrauterine respiratory movements, and this may be of importance when extrauterine respiration is initiated. Although inhaled liquor may be drained from the bronchial tree by postural drainage and suction after birth, some of the fluid in the alveoli is absorbed into the pulmonary capillaries. Meconium residues in the liquor may be left in the alveoli and cause irritation.

The moderate degree of hypoxia produced in the fetus during the course of labour, with a slight fall in arterial oxygen tension (Pa_{O_2}) and a rise in arterial carbon dioxide tension (Pa_{CO_2}) heightens the responsiveness of the newborn infant's respiratory centre to a variety of stimuli. With increasing hypoxia the centre becomes depressed, leading to primary apnoea followed by release of the primitive gasping reflex as a means of initiating respiration.

The thorax is squeezed as the body passes through the birth canal, and fluid is expelled from the chest, which is then replaced by air during the elastic recoil after completion of delivery of the trunk. Once the baby is born its body extends from the fetal position, and the straightening of the spine and change in shape of the chest and descent of the diaphragm facilitate respiration.

The fall in the environmental temperature after delivery is an added stimulus to respiration, particularly if a draught of cool air impinges on the sensitive area around the mouth and nose. A combination of these factors is thought to be responsible for the establishment of full respiration. It must be remembered that any anaesthetic or sedative administered to the mother is shared by the fetus, and may depress the respiratory centre.

In normal circumstances the first breath draws air into the bronchial tree, unless there is obstruction from inhaled liquor amnii or mucus. With successive respiratory movements the thoracic cage expands and a negative intrapleural pressure is created. The difference between this negative pressure and the atmospheric pressure of the air in the bronchial tree causes the solid fetal lung to expand by entry of air into the alveoli. The walls of the unexpanded alveoli are held together by a thin layer of fluid, and the surface tension between the walls must be overcome before full expansion can be achieved.

The maturing lung is able to produce *surfactant* from special cells (type 2 pneumocytes) in the alveolar wall from about 32 to 34 weeks gestation. The main constituent is a phospholipid, lecithin, and its function is to reduce the surface tension within the alveoli and so to permit easy and equal expansion throughout the lungs. If the production of surfactant is diminished by prematurity or hypoxia, or both, there is incomplete expansion of the lungs which may be the starting point of the respiratory distress syndrome (hyaline membrane disease, see p. 466). Normal alveolar expansion is at first rapid, but several hours elapse before complete expansion of the lungs occurs, especially of the lower lobes.

Although the first breath is usually taken immediately after birth, respiration may be suspended for many minutes. The newborn infant appears to be less susceptible to the ill effects of prolonged hypoxia than the adult, but nevertheless deep hypoxia lasting for only a few minutes may cause bradycardia with falling blood pressure leading to impaired cerebral circulation, and result in subsequent cerebral palsy or mental retardation.

Changes in the fetal circulation at birth.   The fetal circulation has already been described on p. 29. Remarkable changes occur soon after birth. The infant's first breaths expand the lungs and open up the pulmonary vascular bed. This produces a sharp fall in the pulmonary vascular resistance and a considerably increased flow of blood to the lungs, where it is oxygenated. Immediately afterwards there is contraction of the ductus arteriosus to about half its original diameter, and complete contraction of the umbilical arteries. It is thought that the ductus arteriosus and umbilical arteries have a natural tendency to contract but are prevented from doing so by prostaglandins which are circulating at high concentrations in the fetus. It is suggested that there are enzyme systems in the lungs which break down the prostaglandins once the pulmonary blood flow is established after birth. The fall in the level of circulating prostaglandins, along with the rise in the arterial oxygen saturation, allows these vessels to contract. It is possible that the use of prostaglandin inhibitors to suppress premature labour might lead to premature closure of the ductus in the fetus.

The systemic arterial pressure rises as the low resistance of the placenta is replaced by the high resistance of the peripheral circulation in the baby, and with the concomitant fall in the pulmonary artery pressure the pressure gradient across the ductus is reversed. This permits blood to flow in the opposite direction through the partially closed ductus to augment the pulmonary blood flow at this critical time. The fall in pulmonary vascular resistance produces a fall in right sided pressures, and the increase in systemic resistance a rise in left sided pressures. These changes, together with the increased pulmonary venous return, lead to a rise in left atrial pressure over and above that in the right atrium and consequent functional closure of the foramen ovale.

Ultimately, but not for several days or weeks, the ductus becomes obliterated by endarteritis, and the final transition from fetal to adult circulation is complete. The umbilical cord desiccates and separates, leaving a raw area which heals by granulation and is then covered by epithelium. The umbilical vein is now a redundant vessel and closes by aseptic thrombosis. The ductus venosus atrophies and disappears, while the umbilical vein remains as the ligamentum teres. The umbilical arteries show retrograde closure as far as the hypogastric arteries and persist as sclerosed remnants.

Changes in the gastro-intestinal tract. Although the placenta digests and excretes for the fetus, the gastro-intestinal tract is active during intrauterine life. During the later months of pregnancy liquor amnii containing desquamated epithelial cells is swallowed by the fetus. Mucus and debrided intestinal epithelial cells are added to the gut content and, with the swallowed liquor, are digested by intestinal ferments to form *meconium*. This is coloured greenish-black by bile pigments. By late pregnancy the meconium has traversed the gut as far as the rectum, and if strong intestinal contractions are stimulated during labour by fetal distress, and the sphincters are atonic or paralysed, meconium may be voided into the amniotic fluid. If premature respiration is also induced, meconium-stained liquor may be inhaled into the bronchial tree, and this may cause respiratory difficulties after delivery.

With the first inspiration air enters the stomach and rapidly traverses the gut, reaching the ascending colon within 3 hours.

Hydrochloric acid is present in the stomach in relatively high concentration on the first day of life, but in only moderate amounts during early infancy. Amylases from saliva and from the pancreas are at a low level during the early weeks of life, and this explains the difficulty in digesting starch shown by some infants. The trypsin and lipase of pancreatic secretion are present in good concentration, even during intrauterine life, and are responsible for the digestion of meconium.

The genito-urinary tract. There may be delay in passing urine after birth for up to 24 hours, but this is usually not of pathological significance. Suprapubic pressure often results in passage of urine. The first specimen may have a pinkish colour from a high concentration of urates.

Regulation of body temperature. The fetal temperature is dictated by the surrounding maternal environment and the fetal heat-regulating centre is probably dormant. After birth, unless special precautions are taken, the infant's temperature falls by 1 to 3°C and external heat must be supplied. After a few days the temperature-regulating centre becomes effective and the infant's temperature is kept normal despite environmental variations. Brown adipose tissue has an important rôle in maintenance of body temperature in the newborn, and deficiency of this tissue in pre-term and small-for-dates babies contributes to their thermoregulatory difficulties.

Defences against infection. Placental transmission of antibodies from maternal serum affords the infant a non-specific passive immunity against certain diseases. This immunity wanes after a short time, and the infant is at risk from common infections until an acquired immunity is developed. Immunity acquired from the mother may be specific for diseases against which she has developed an active immunity, such as diphtheria, tetanus, measles, mumps, smallpox and poliomyelitis. The infant begins to develop his own IgG at about 2 or 3 months of age. The newborn infant's ability to form IgA is suppressed. Instead, the infant should be receiving IgA from the mother's breast; it is in high concentration in colostrum but continues to be secreted in mature milk. This immunoglobulin plays an important part in protecting the baby against infections acquired through the alimentary tract, and possibly also against the development of hypersensitivity.

The immediate care of the healthy infant

When the infant is delivered it may be limp, with only moderate muscle tone, and there is a purplish-blue cyanosis of general distribution. Liquor drains from the nose and mouth, and to assist this drainage the infant should be inclined head downwards with the arms extended above the head. The mouth should **not** be cleaned with gauze swabs, as this will damage the delicate buccal mucosa.

The nasopharynx should be cleared of fluid with a sterile disposable mucus extractor. A mechanical sucker regulated to avoid a negative pressure of more than 50 cm of water may also be employed. Whichever method is used the procedure must be carried out with the utmost gentleness to avoid damage to the mucous membranes or the production of laryngeal spasm.

The stomach of the newborn infant, especially when delivered by Caesarean section, contains large quantities of amniotic fluid which may possibly be regurgitated later and inhaled. Unless the infant is crying lustily the stomach should also be aspirated after the nasopharynx has been cleared. This can be done by passing the soft tubing of the disposable mucus extractor gently down the oesophagus into the stomach. This tubing is sufficiently firm to permit immediate diagnosis of oesophageal atresia should this be present (see p. 490).

As soon as the nasopharynx has been cleared the infant will normally take a breath and give a cry and, as respiration begins, the colour of the skin rapidly changes to pink. Cyanosis of the extremities may persist for a time, but this is not usually of pathological significance.

Care of the eyes. In the past it was the practice to instil one drop of 1 per cent silver nitrate solution into each eye immediately after delivery as a prophylactic against gonococcal infection. Most institutions have abandoned this because the silver nitrate solution itself often caused conjunctivitis and because antibiotics now offer effective treatment if infection should occur. Penicillin eye drops (2500 units per ml) were also used.

Because there is now effective treatment, the use of prophylactic eye drops is not advised unless there are special indications, except in countries where antenatal and postnatal supervision are lacking. Daily wiping of the eyes with cotton wool moistened with saline is a common but undesirable practice, the only result of which may be to produce pyogenic conjunctivitis.

Care of the umbilical cord. The time and method of clamping the cord is discussed on p. 123. Afterwards the cord is kept dry and clean until it shrivels and comes away leaving a small area of granulation tissue, which heals over after a few days. Daily application of 0.5 per cent chlorhexidine in 70 per cent spirit is a good way to keep the umbilicus clean and dry.

General care of the baby. After ensuring that respiration is well established and the Apgar score (see p. 463) has been checked, the infant is inspected rapidly to note whether there are any obvious abnormalities before being wrapped in a warm towel and handed to the mother to be cuddled and put to the breast to suckle the colostrum. It is essential to protect the baby from cold, but if the delivery room is sufficiently warm it should be possible to have naked 'skin to skin' contact between mother and baby, although it is a wise precaution for the baby to be under the cover of a towel. This natural procedure has been neglected in recent years but now maternity units are appreciating once again its value in helping to give the mother and baby the best possible start to a close relationship.

After this initial period of close contact, the baby is wrapped firmly in warm towels and laid prone in its cot alongside the mother with head turned to one side and facing her. Unless there is need for special care, it is important that the baby should not be removed from close proximity to the mother. Even if she falls asleep from exhaustion it is reassuring for her to find her baby beside her when she wakes.

During this initial period it is important to check the baby's temperature. Because of the risk of rectal injury from broken thermometers some centres have abandoned rectal in favour of axillary temperatures (remembering that the latter will give a slightly lower reading). Alternatively the rectal temperature can be recorded electrically with a plastic covered probe; this has the advantage that it gives an immediate reading so that prolonged exposure of the infant is not required, and it would immediately reveal an imperforate anus.

Details of a more complete physical examination are given below.

Identification.   In institutions the infant must be identified in such a way that confusion between babies cannot arise. A plastic wrist band or a piece of tape sewn round the infant's wrist with the name marked in indelible ink are commonly used.

The baby's bath.   At birth the infant is covered with greasy vernix caseosa and blood. For aesthetic reasons it has been traditional to bathe the baby immediately after birth, but it is sufficient to clean the baby's face with sterile moistened swabs before presenting it to the mother. Vernix is acid and greasy and provides a natural barrier to infection. Although its main function is to protect the baby's skin from the effects of prolonged immersion in liquor, excess of it left in the neck folds, axillae and groins may cause irritation of the skin. The use of diluted hexachlorophane solution for skin cleansing is effective in reducing sepsis but has been generally condemned because of fears of harmful effects when it is absorbed. Its occasional use in a talcum powder is harmless, since it forms an outer 'skin' which is not absorbed.

Most maternity units now agree that just one bath given by the mother, under instruction, on the day before discharge is all that is required. Daily inspection of the skin, the eyes, the mouth and most particularly the umbilicus, should be carried out by experienced nursing staff. The stump of the cord desiccates and separates between the 4th and 11th days, usually on the 7th day. Until healing of the moist raw area has occurred it provides an ideal site for growth of pathogenic bacteria.

Examination of the newborn infant.   At the earliest convenient time after the birth of the infant a systematic physical examination should be made. External examination is of great importance, and attention should be paid to any minor congenital defects. Skin naevi, pre-auricular sinuses, branchial fistulae, supernumary digits or nipples should be noted. Defects such as cleft lip or palate, spina bifida and club feet may escape notice if of minor degree, and especial attention should be given to possible omphalocele, penile abnormalities, cryptorchidism and imperforate anus.

The skull should be palpated and the state of the sutures noted. The circumference of the skull should be recorded. Careful examination of the skull soon after birth may yield information of which the importance is only apparent later. Widening of the sutures and an increase in the circumference of the skull may be found in cases of subdural haematoma or hydrocephalus, and an early diagnosis may only be possible because the state of the skull at birth has been recorded. Areas of softening or lacunae in the parietal bones may be found, or an encephalocele.

The baby should be handled and the limbs moved to ensure that no fracture or paralysis is present. The hips should be examined for undue mobility or the presence of a click which will suggest a congenital dislocation. The range of movement of the ankles must be tested to detect minor degrees of talipes.

Examination of the heart should be carried out with care, and the presence of any bruits noted. The significance of any murmur may only become apparent after observation for several days. Palpation of the femoral pulses should always be carried out.

The chest may show signs of incomplete expansion or the persistence of moist sounds from inhaled liquor. These conditions are discussed on p. 465.

On examination of the abdomen the liver edge can usually be felt just below the costal margin, and the tip of the spleen is often palpable. In a well-relaxed abdomen the lower poles of the kidneys may be easily felt.

Normal reflexes. Certain reflexes are normally only present in the newborn infant. The Moro reflex is a startle or concussion reflex elicited by banging the table on which the infant is lying, by letting the head drop backwards or by flexing the head on the trunk. Abduction and extension of the arms is followed by adduction of the arms like an embrace, and the legs are extended. The infant may cry. This reflex is usually symmetrical and indicates normal neuromuscular coordination. Variations from the normal response are seen when there is a nerve palsy, a fractured clavicle or long bone, or an intracranial lesion.

If the infant is touched on the area near the mouth he will turn his head and try to suck the object which touches him. This rooting reflex is followed by the sucking reflex which seems to be designed to enable the baby to draw the nipple well back into the mouth so that the gums can gently massage the milk sinuses just below the surface of the areola and stimulate milk ejection.

A grasp reflex is seen when the palm of the hand or the sole of the foot is touched and is normal in the newborn infant. A 'walking' reflex is also usually seen in the normal infant.

Normal progress of the full term infant. During the first week of life the baby continues to adjust himself to the extrauterine environment.

Traumatic lesions such as a caput succedaneum, a 'chignon' after vacuum extraction, petechiae or oedema disappear rapidly. The baby begins to assume an infantile position instead of that of intrauterine folding. The feet are less dorsiflexed and the hands less firmly clenched. The chest becomes less flattened and the head is moved freely. The cry is definite and begins to assume characteristics for hunger and pain.

Weight gain. There is loss of weight from the first 2 or 3 days of up to 10 per cent of the birth weight. After feeding is established the weight increases and will usually return to birth level by the 7th to the 10th day. If this is not achieved it may indicate inadequate feeding, or some condition which is preventing normal progress, but some breast feeding mothers take longer than others to establish lactation, and their babies may take up to 3 weeks to regain their birth weight without any harmful effects.

Temperature. At birth the infant is thermolabile, and the temperature may fall below 36°C, but it is unwise to allow the rectal temperature to fall below this. The infant responds quickly to the application of external heat, and in a few hours the full term infant stabilizes his temperature regulation. The rectal temperature shows a normal daily variation from 36 to 37.2°C.

Normal stools. Meconium is normally passed within a few hours of birth, but may be delayed for 12 or even 24 hours. Although this is not necessarily pathological it demands observation, as it may indicate intestinal obstruction. The first meconium stool is often preceded by a plug of whitish mucus, and if this plug is large the appearance of meconium may be delayed for 24 hours and the abdomen may show some distention.

In the next 2 or 3 days meconium is passed several times a day. Normal meconium is sticky, odourless and greenish-black in colour. After a few days 'changing stools' are passed, and these are non-homogenous, thin, sour, slimy and yellowish-brown in colour. Undigested milk elements can often be seen in the stool.

Towards the end of the first week 'milk stools' are seen. The stool of the breast-fed infant is smooth, pasty, slightly sour, acid, and mustard or golden-brown in colour. The motion of the artificially fed infant is paler in colour, alkaline, pasty and non-homogeneous.

The breast-fed baby may have the bowels open only once in the day, or have any number of stools up to 5 or 6 in the 24 hours and yet be normal. When the stools are frequent they may be green and this should not lead to a hasty diagnosis of gastro-enteritis in a baby who is otherwise well. It is usually due to a temporary excess of lactation when the milk 'comes in' and it is important to leave the baby to continue to feed normally and maintain the stimulus to lactation. Later, the maternal diet may affect the baby's bowel habit as many aperient substances are secreted in the milk.

Micturition. The baby usually passes urine shortly after delivery, but micturition may not occur until 24 hours have elapsed, especially if the infant has voided urine just before or during delivery. The bladder may then become palpable, and the genitalia must be examined to ensure that there is no evident congenital defect. Pressure on the abdomen will often stimulate micturition.

The urine may at first be dark in colour, but rapidly becomes colourless and of low specific gravity. During the first day or two the napkin may be stained pink from the deposit of urates.

Breast engorgement. The breasts of infants of either sex may swell and become engorged during the first week of life. Milk ('witch's milk') may be secreted and the female may bleed from the uterus. These effects are due to transfer of maternal hormone and require no treatment. On no account should the engorged breasts be handled or squeezed as they readily become infected to produce neonatal mastitis or breast abscess.

Skin. In Caucasian infants the colour of the skin soon changes from the ruddiness seen after birth to a paler hue. The skin may become dry and scaly as it dries out after the long intrauterine immersion. Fissures and cracks may appear in the folds of the ankles and wrists, but heal quite quickly. Milia or various non-specific rashes may be seen. It is common to observe blotchy erythematous rashes on the trunk, limbs and face. No treatment is required.

Sleep. After delivery the baby usually settles to sleep and for the next week or so falls asleep after feeds, waking up only to protest with hunger, discomfort or thirst.

Variations from the normal

Asphyxia neonatorum (failure to establish respiration)

If the infant fails to respond to nasopharyngeal aspiration, and the onset of respiration is delayed, prompt action is required. In the majority of these babies the heart rate is normal, limb tone is present, and the failure to breathe is due to liquor or mucus blocking the respiratory tract, the respiratory centre being normally responsive. In other infants limb tone is poor or absent, the heart rate is slow or absent, and the respiratory centre is depressed by trauma sustained during delivery or by analgesics administered to the mother.

The Apgar score is often used to evaluate the physical status of the infant at one minute after delivery and to estimate any improvement in the subsequent few minutes. An Apgar score of 10 represents the infant in an ideal physical state. The lower the score the worse is the condition of the baby, and the greater the urgency of resuscitation.

Apgar score

Sign	0	1	2
Heart rate	absent	less than 100	more than 100
Respiratory effort	absent	slow, irregular	good, crying
Muscle tone	limp	some limb flexion	active
Response to stimulus (nasal catheter)	nil	grimace	vigorous cry
Colour	blue, pale	body pink limbs blue	pink

When the Apgar score is more than 5 (and in practice this will be a baby with a heart rate of more than 100 per minute) the infant will be in good condition, and provided that the airways are clear respiration is likely to begin within 1 minute. This is what used to be called *asphyxia livida* or *blue asphyxia*, but is now often referred to as *primary apnoea* or *pre-gasping apnoea*. All that is usually necessary is to watch the clock and keep a check on the heart rate, but directing a stream of oxygen towards the baby's nose and mouth can do no harm and will ensure that the first breaths take in oxygen-enriched air. Drugs have no place in treatment with the exception of naloxone hydrochloride which is given if the mother has received morphine or pethidine within 4 hours of delivery. The recommended dose is 0.01 mg per kg, but the drug has a short half-life and may have to be repeated. It does not have any depressant effect (unlike N-allyl morphine which was previously used).

However, if the baby remains unresponsive at the end of 1 minute or if the heart rate begins to fall, a laryngoscope must be passed and the larynx and trachea aspirated through a catheter. This will often remove the liquor or mucus obstructing the respiratory tract and the infant will gasp, breathe and cry and rapidly become pink. Intranasal oxygen should be continued until regular respiration and strong crying have become established.

If tracheal aspiration is unsuccessful in initiating respiration a plastic endotracheal tube is inserted in the trachea and oxygen administered in short puffs through a T tube, by means of a bag connected to a manometer which ensures that the pressure in the bag is kept below 30 cm of water. This will often improve the oxygenation of the baby and start respiration after a short time. When spontaneous respiration is seen the endotracheal tube is removed and nasal oxygen continued until the condition of the infant is completely satisfactory. Sometimes, especially with an initially low Apgar score, or when the infant has been narcotized, it may be necessary to continue assisted respiration through the endotracheal tube for long periods. The technique of endotracheal intubation should be learned by all doctors and senior nursing staff who are likely to attend deliveries because it is the only sure way to resuscitate the baby. Artificial respiration or mouth-to-mouth insufflation may be dangerous measures if performed too vigorously, and can cause a pneumothorax.

If the Apgar score is below 5 (and certainly if it is 3 or under) the baby will be pale and limp with a heart rate of less than 100 per minute. This is the condition formerly called *asphyxia pallida* or *white asphyxia*, but which is now generally referred to as *secondary apnoea* or *post-gasping apnoea*. Such a baby is in a state of shock with falling blood pressure, and is likely to die if nothing is done or, if he should recover, to be left with varying degrees of cerebral damage. Such a baby must be resuscitated with endotracheal intubation *without delay*, assisted by cardiac massage performed by gentle compression of the chest with two fingers placed in the 3rd and 4th interspaces to the left of the sternum. In these infants intermittent positive pressure ventilation at 15 to 30 puffs per minute may need to be continued for some time. Babies with severe intracranial haemorrhage may present a similar clinical picture, and the diagnosis does not become clear until resuscitation has been carried out.

The severely asphyxiated infant becomes acidotic, and when recovery is unduly delayed 5 ml of 8.4 per cent sodium bicarbonate solution may be injected slowly into the umbilical vein. It is also suggested that 2 to 4 ml of 20 per cent glucose solution may be given by this route, but the injection of hyperosmolar solutions is dangerous; in particular there is a possibility of portal thrombosis. If the injection is made in error into the umbilical artery this may cause spasm and subsequent thrombosis of the vessel, which may spread to involve the internal or common iliac arteries with a risk of gangrene of the legs or sciatic nerve palsy by interference with the blood supply to the nerve.

The baby with secondary apnoea may have aspirated meconium into the lungs. In such circumstances gentle bronchial lavage may be performed by instilling small amounts of normal saline through the endotracheal tube and sucking it back with a mechanical sucker, making sure that the negative pressure never exceeds 50 cm water.

After resuscitation the severely asphyxiated baby is kept in an incubator under close observation until fully recovered.

Persistence of cyanosis despite establishment of respiration

Generalized cyanosis which includes cyanosis of the tongue indicates a significantly low arterial oxygen tension. Observation of the baby during episodes of crying is helpful in differentiating the cause. Cyanosis which deepens with crying suggests a congenital cardiac lesion with a right to left shunt, or intracranial damage. Cyanosis which is lessened by crying and which returns with shallower respiration suggests a respiratory cause such as atelectasis or secretion remaining in the respiratory passages. Alternatively a short exposure to 100 per cent oxygen through a mask applied gently to the face will provide the same information, cases from cardiac and cerebral causes usually remaining unchanged.

Respiratory causes of cyanosis

Atelectasis. As previously indicated the fetal lung contains fluid which has to be replaced by air as soon as the infant is born. This is mainly achieved by absorption of fluid into the lymphatics, but is assisted by the squeezing of the chest in passing through the birth canal followed by its elastic recoil, and by shallow respiratory movements. These convert a chest full of liquid into a chest full of air without any change in volume. Then follows a rapid increase in the volume of the chest as the alveoli are fully expanded by the powerful initial inspiratory movements; but once expanded, further relaxation and re-expansion of the alveoli during respiratory movements is achieved effortlessly because of the presence of surfactant. Although the initial expansion of the lung progresses rapidly with successive respiratory efforts, total expansion may not be attained for some hours, especially in the premature infant. The tissues round the lung roots and the posterior parts of the lower lobes are the last to expand. When the process is particularly slow the infant may develop worrying symptoms. Some babies born by Caesarean section, for example, may take some time to clear the lungs of fluid, and auscultation of the lung bases posteriorly may reveal fine crepitant râles. Such babies have rapid shallow respirations, often associated with an expiratory grunt, and periods of apnoea and cyanosis may be present. It has become fashionable to refer to this as *transient tachypnoea of the newborn* (Avery's syndrome). A radiograph of the chest will usually reveal the atelectasis by the presence of an 'air bronchogram' in some part of the lung fields and perhaps some hazy or streaky shadowing.

As a rule the only treatment necessary is to increase the ambient oxygen until cyanosis is relieved, and then to diminish the oxygen concentration as the condition improves. These babies should be nursed on an apnoea alarm, so that apnoeic attacks can be treated by immediate stimulation. Rarely does the condition deteriorate to such an extent that intubation and assisted ventilation is required for a time. In some cases differentiation from neonatal pneumonia is not possible and antibiotics are given. In view of the possibility of infection by the Group B haemolytic streptococcus high dosage of penicillin, preferably combined with gentamycin, is recommended pending the result of bacteriological reports. (See p. 509.)

Respiratory distress syndrome (hyaline membrane disease). This condition is most commonly found in small pre-term babies, but it also occurs in the infants of diabetic or pre-diabetic mothers; it is rare in term infants. Perinatal hypoxia is a predisposing factor. Caesarean section should not be associated with an increased incidence if care is taken to avoid hypoxia. With increasing skill in the management of pre-term deliveries and early and effective resuscitation, the incidence of this disorder has fallen dramatically in recent years.

The syndrome occurs when there is deficiency of surfactant, either because of the immaturity of the lungs or because the function of the pneumocytes which produce it is temporarily depressed by hypoxia. After about 34 weeks gestation surfactant is normally produced in adequate quantities, and premature delivery should be delayed beyond this time if possible. Before any decision to effect delivery before term is taken the level of surfactant production can be checked by amniocentesis and measurement of the lecithin content of the amniotic fluid. Since absolute measurements will be dependent on the degree of dilution by amniotic fluid this is commonly expressed as a ratio of lecithin to sphingomyelin. When the LS ratio is 2:1 or greater all should be well, but a ratio of under 1.5:1 means that there is a high risk of hyaline membrane disease. There is some evidence that when the fetus has been subjected to stress, including that of labour, the LS ratio is increased. There is also evidence that administration of corticosteroids to the mother will facilitate the production of surfactant if the steroids are given for 48 hours before delivery.

Dexamethasone 2 mg 6-hourly is often prescribed. Prolonged steroid therapy is, however, undesirable, and the difficulty in predicting the time of delivery limits the use of this treatment in practice.

The diagnosis is suspected when respiratory distress develops within 3 or 4 hours of birth with an expiratory grunt, increased respiratory rate to more than 60 per minute, indrawing of the lower chest and intercostal recession. In room air there is cyanosis, and on auscultation there are usually diminished breath sounds and fine crepitant râles throughout the chest. Generalized oedema is often present and signs of cerebral irritation may appear. A radiograph of the chest has a ground-glass appearance or a reticular pattern, with an 'air-bronchogram' where the air in the bronchi contrasts with the surrounding opaque lung fields. In fatal cases autopsy reveals almost airless lungs and a hyaline membrane lining the terminal air passages which takes up eosinophilic stains. Intraventricular haemorrhage is not uncommonly found.

As a result of the pulmonary disorder the Pa_{O_2} falls and the Pa_{CO_2} rises. The pH falls from respiratory acidosis, which leads on to metabolic acidosis and hyperkalaemia.

Mildly affected infants recover with no more than good nursing care, graduated oxygen therapy and minimal handling, but the mortality overall may reach 20 per cent. With modern intensive care even severely ill infants can be saved, and since it is difficult to predict the course of the disease from the outset all affected babies should be transferred at an early stage to a centre with facilities for expert care.

Since it will be necessary to monitor the arterial oxygen tension it is advisable to introduce an arterial umbilical catheter at an early stage. (It is possible that transcutaneous arterial monitoring will eventually do away with the need for this). These babies tolerate oral fluids well, especially if given by continuous intragastric infusion. For this to be given safely it is necessary to nurse the baby prone and, fortunately, it has been shown that pulmonary ventilation is increased in this position. Milk is given through a naso-gastric tube at 60 ml per kg. The metabolic acidosis is rapidly alleviated when adequate oxygenation is achieved, and the administration of sodium bicarbonate intravenously is no longer regarded as essential; it may contribute to the complication of intraventricular haemorrhage. Oxygen is given in high concentration in a Perspex Gairdner head-box, the concentration being carefully monitored and adjusted according to the arterial P_{O_2}. This should be kept between 7 and 12 kPa (50 and 90 mm Hg). If 60 per cent oxygen in the head-box does not achieve satisfactory oxygenation it will be necessary to resort to other methods. Various methods of maintaining continuous positive airways pressure have been tried with apparent success, the aim being to maintain a low pressure in the alveoli during expiration, thus preventing their collapse. The pressure required as measured at the mouth is 0.3 to 0.8 kPa (2 to 6 mm Hg). If this fails to maintain an adequate Pa_{O_2} it will be necessary to resort to intermittent positive pressure ventilation, for which an experienced team of doctors and nurses is essential.

If the infant survives the first week of the illness there is every chance of total recovery.

Pneumothorax.   Forceful attempts to expand the lungs may rupture overdistended bullae to produce interstitial emphysema and pneumomediastinum or pneumothorax. There is a risk of this during artificial inflation of the lungs if insufficient care is taken to keep the inflating pressure within safe limits. However, the baby's own respiratory efforts may occasionally cause this complication, especially when attempting to overcome some obstruction in the airway. Pneumomediastinum is a common complication in cases of renal agenesis (p. 503) and this possibility should be borne in mind.

Provided that the lesion is unilateral there may be obvious physical signs—relative immobility and overdistention of the affected side, with hyper-resonance and reduced breath sounds. When the pneumothorax is under tension and the baby is cyanosed and distressed immediate relief can be obtained by inserting a needle into the pleural cavity through the 3rd intercostal space in the midclavicular line. The needle is connected to a length of tubing, the other end of which is placed under water so that the air bubbling out can be seen.

Asymptomatic pneumothorax which is a chance finding on x-ray examination needs no treatment as it will quickly absorb.

Nasal obstruction.   The newborn infant breathes through the nose by instinct, but has to learn mouth breathing. Nasal obstruction by secretion, oedema or congenital atresia of the nares may cause cyanosis and asphyxial attacks which are only relieved by insertion of an airway or by holding the tongue forward with the mouth open. Relief of obstruction from infection or oedema may be given by the use of nasal drops of ephedrine 0.25 per cent in saline before feeds. The drops should not be used for more than 48 hours, as they can produce local irritation if continued for too long.

Cardiovascular causes of cyanosis

Reference to the description of the circulatory adjustments which take place at birth (p. 456) shows that the haemodynamic factors are in a delicate equilibrium which is easily disturbed if respiratory difficulties arise. For example, extensive atelectasis may result from meconium aspiration in an asphyxiated baby, and the hypoxia resulting from inadequate ventilation and from perfusion of unaerated segments of lung prevents the normal fall in pulmonary vascular resistance, so that the right atrial pressure remains elevated. The reduced pulmonary venous return diminishes the left atrial pressure and the foramen ovale is opened, permitting right-to-left shunting and a fall in arterial PO_2. The hypoxaemia leads to a fall in the systemic arterial pressure, the ductus arteriosus opens widely and right-to-left shunting through the ductus is favoured by the change in pressure gradient. If this reversion to fetal pulmonary hypertension persists, the baby will develop cyanosis, cardiac enlargement and heart failure. The reversed flow through the ductus may produce a harsh systolic murmur down the left sternal border and the diagnosis of cyanotic congenital heart disease is suspected.

The advice of a paediatric cardiologist is invaluable, because it is imperative to make an accurate diagnosis of the cause of cyanotic heart disease at an early stage, so that surgical treatment can be given if necessary. Congenital heart lesions which cause cyanosis in the newborn are usually complex and severe anomalies, some of which do not produce cardiac murmurs. Expert investigation is likely to be required.

Other causes of cyanosis

Cyanosis may also be due to intracranial injuries, chilling, abdominal distension, and the delayed effect of anaesthetics and analgesics given to the mother.

Polycythaemia will allow the baby to become cyanosed easily since a relatively slight fall in oxygen saturation will produce the 5 g of reduced haemoglobin which is necessary to show cyanosis. Congenital methaemoglobinaemia is a rare cause of a slaty blue cyanosis in a baby with no cardiac or respiratory embarrassment; spectroscopic examination of the blood provides the diagnosis. Acquired methaemoglobinaemia can occur if artificial feeds happen to be made up with water containing an excess of nitrites.

43

Infant feeding

The rate of growth during the first year is greater than at any other stage of life after birth. The normal baby doubles his weight in 5 months, trebles it in 12 months and quadruples it in 24 months. To achieve this the intake of food must be relatively great and of a quality that allows easy digestion. It must contain in liquid form a reasonably balanced mixture of protein, fat, carbohydrate, minerals and vitamins.

Discussion of infant feeding is beset with difficulties that are largely created by the use of fixed systems. No system will ever meet the needs of every infant, for each baby is an individual with his own idiosyncrasies from the moment of birth; if a baby does not thrive it may be that the error lies in the system rather than the infant. However, some rules can be stated as to the quantity and quality of food needed, and these rules can do no harm so long as they are adjusted to meet the requirements of each baby. These rules apply after the age of 7 days and are appropriately modified during the first 7 days.

Although the metric system is now in use in hospitals some mothers still do not understand it and some avoirdupois measurements are *given in italics*.

Daily fluid requirement. The infant needs water in relatively greater amounts than at any other period of life. The infant's kidneys are not as capable of concentrating urine as those of the adult, and to remove the waste products of metabolism the urinary output must amount to nearly half the total fluid intake. The losses of fluid from the skin, lungs and faeces are proportionately greater than in adult life. The infant needs approximately 150 ml of fluid per kg of body weight (*2½ ounces per pound*) during 24 hours. Infants below normal birth weight require even more; a baby of 2.5 kg would need 220 ml per kg (*3½ ounces per pound*) in 24 hours.

Calorie requirement. The diet should provide 110 calories per kg in 24 hours. This calls for 70 calories per 100 ml of feed (*20 calories per ounce*). Smaller infants require more calories per kg—up to 150 calories per kg in 24 hours.

Protein, fat and carbohydrate. Sufficient of these are supplied in a diet of breast milk or some reasonable dilution of cow's milk.

Minerals. The only mineral which may be inadequately provided by a milk diet is iron, an element which is always jealously conserved in

470

nature. At birth the baby has only small iron reserves. During the period of intensely rapid growth in early infancy there is a corresponding increase in the total number of red cells. The reserve stores of iron are soon exhausted in forming haemoglobin for the additional red cells, and unless adequate supplies of iron are available in the diet the infant will develop hypochromic anaemia. Breast milk supplies enough iron during the first 6 months, particularly as the lactoferrin content ensures rapid and complete absorption. Unmodified cow's milk contains insufficient iron, and it is desirable to supplement the diet with additional iron after the second month of life, and earlier in the premature infant. Ferrous sulphate mixture for infants (BPC) may be given in doses of 5 ml daily.

Vitamins. The vitamin content of breast milk is adequate, but cow's milk which has been heated may not contain enough. The optimal daily intake of vitamin C for an infant is 50 mg. The recommended intake of vitamin D to prevent rickets is 800 i.u. daily, and any natural source of vitamin D which yields this will also provide enough vitamin A. Milk usually contains sufficient vitamin B.

Vitamin D should be given to babies who are artificially fed, especially during the winter when they receive little exposure to ultraviolet light. One or 2 drops of National Health Service 'A and D drops' of vitaminized oil may be given daily, gradually increasing the dose to 7 drops daily.

Vitamin C is usually given as the juice of half an orange diluted with water and sweetened with a little sugar as an extra drink. If the infant cannot tolerate this, which sometimes causes colic, rose hip syrup, black currant puree or ascorbic acid may be added to the feeds.

Breast or bottle feeding

The fact that artificial feeding has become so widespread throughout the world is perhaps an indictment of the apathy of doctors, nurses and others who are in a position to give advice and education to future parents, in the face of the immense power of commerce and advertising. The trend is encouraged by the changes in society and our way of life which seem to make artificial feeding more convenient. The general public knows that when care is taken with bottle feeding the babies seem to thrive well, and the mother who is repeatedly given information on how much feed her baby should have is more content when she can see 'the correct quantity' in the bottle.

In almost all discussions about infant feeding it is assumed that the process is solely concerned with supplying the infant with adequate nutrition, whereas anyone who has watched a successful and contented breast-feeding couple will have appreciated that it is a two-way process which was intended to provide a pleasurable experience for both parties. This 'feedback' to the mother can make the feed time something to look forward to, rather than a routine duty whose sole purpose is to make her baby grow bigger. An important part of the process is to help the mother fall in love with her baby. In this way the mother—infant attachment is made secure so that she will not wish to be parted from her baby in the early months, and her continuous presence will give the baby security and the mother a proper understanding of his needs throughout his early development. Certainly a mother who is bottle feeding will need to work harder to establish a good relationship with her baby, especially as there is a tendency for other well-meaning helpers to interfere. Indeed, there is a widely held belief, fostered by some psychiatrists, that one of the advantages of bottle feeding is that it enables the father (or other relatives) to take part in the 'mothering', thereby giving the mother more freedom and providing the baby with additional stimulation. However, experience suggests that the closest relationship is achieved by one 'mother' receiving maximal stimulation from the baby; and the natural mother is best equipped for this purpose. Failure to recognize the importance of good mothering is undoubtedly a contributory factor in child abuse and later delinquency.

Unfortunately not all mothers enjoy breast feeding, and for some the process is painful or distasteful. For them, as well as for the small number of women who are incapable of providing adequate lactation, it is important to provide sympathy and understanding so that they are not left with feelings of guilt, but are helped to concentrate upon making a success of bottle feeding.

Modern research reveals more and more reasons why the milk from his own mother provides the baby with the best form of nutrition and the best protection against infections, especially enteric infections, and against the development of hypersensitivity. Several mechanisms are involved in protection against infections. These include maternal secretory IgA and lysozymes which either kill organisms or prevent their adherence to the intestinal wall, lactoferrin which ensures rapid absorption of iron so that it is not available for the essential needs of replicating organisms, and encouragement of the growth of *Lactobacillus bifidus* to the exclusion of other pathogenic organisms which flourish in the more alkaline intestinal environment provided by the ingestion of cow's milk. While secretory IgA is thought to be an important factor against the development of hypersensitivity, avoidance of the powerful antigenic effect of cow's milk protein is equally important.

There is also cumulative evidence that the health of the breasts is best preserved when they are allowed to fulfil their physiological function. When the reasons for breast feeding are fully explained to them, most mothers become its strong advocates. As a result of concerted efforts by many people there is at present an encouraging resurgence of enthusiasm.

Anatomy and physiology of the breast

Anatomy and maturation.   The breast is composed of about 20 segments arranged radially from the nipple, the glandular tissue being mainly peripheral. The branching duct system from each segment unites to form a single duct which opens on the nipple. Immediately before opening on the nipple each duct has a dilatation called a lactiferous sinus. This lies immediately below the areola of the nipple and is a thin-walled part of the duct which can be dilated by milk to a calibre of 0.5 to 1 cm. The ducts and alveoli of the glandular tissue are surrounded by myo-epithelial contractile cells, and there are smooth muscle cells under the areola. The pectoral fascia ensheathes the whole breast and sends laminae between the lobes and alveoli. There are many fat cells and a rich supply of blood vessels.

Before puberty the nipple is flat, and the duct system is rudimentary with little glandular tissue. In the female as puberty approaches the nipple becomes prominent and fat is deposited. With successive menstrual cycles oestrogens cause development of the duct system, but active development of the secreting tissue does not occur until pregnancy under the influence of oestrogens and progesterone. During pregnancy the enlargement of the breast is mainly due to hyperplasia of the glandular tissue from the 12th week onwards. From the end of the 24th week the breast is capable of secreting milk and during the last 12 weeks colostrum can be expressed from the breast, although active lactation is dormant.

Physiology of lactation. It is convenient to discuss the processes of secretion, or formation of milk, and of excretion separately.

Secretion of milk is the transformation of amnio acids, glucose, lipids and minerals present in the blood plasma into caseinogen, lactalbumin, lactose and milk fats which are secreted into the alveoli by the activity of the alveolar epithelial cells. Only a portion of the milk yielded at a feed is preformed; the major portion is secreted during the time of feeding.

Prolactin is mainly responsible for the secretion by the alveolar cells. This pituitary hormone is secreted by cells of the anterior lobe of the pituitary gland (*lactotrophs*). Oestrogens cause hyperplasia of the lactotrophs during pregnancy and prolactin levels in the blood rise. Milk secretion does not occur at this time because high levels of oestrogen also inhibit the responses of the alveolar cells to prolactin. The release of prolactin is normally held in check by a hypothalamic inhibitory factor which is probably dopamine.

After delivery the oestrogen level falls so that the alveolar cells become responsive. The basal prolactin level is lower than that of late pregnancy, but in response to stimulation of the nipple by suckling there is a surge or release of prolactin which lasts for about 30 minutes, presumably because discharge of prolactin inhibiting factor is inhibited. Prolactin release is also stimulated by thyroid releasing hormone, but this is not thought to be part of the normal mechanism.

After delivery colostrum is secreted for about 48 hours and then the breasts become engorged and milk is secreted.

Excretion of milk. The baby is often said to suck milk. Sucking is a relatively unimportant part of the complex process, and the word wrongly suggests that suckling is entirely dependent on an activity of the baby. When lactation is well established, if a sucking infant is removed from the breast milk will continue to spurt or flow from the nipple, indicating active excretion by the breast apart from any activity of the infant.

When the baby takes the breast the nipple is drawn into the arch of the hard palate and held there by the tongue to be exposed to suction, which clears the milk to the back of the mouth to be swallowed. The lips form a seal on the nipple and areola and the gums champ on the areola to compress the lactiferous sinuses and propel their contents into the infant's mouth.

The active excretion of the breast is due to the contractile myo-epithelial network of cells which invest the alveoli and ducts. Stimulation of the nerve endings in the nipple initiates impulses which reach the posterior lobe of the pituitary gland and provoke a release of oxytocin into the blood stream. The oxytocin causes contraction of the myo-epithelial cells and propulsion of the milk along the ducts. In veterinary circles this is termed the 'let down reflex'. The reflex can be interrupted or inhibited psychologically with failure of excretion of milk. The let down reflex is known to parous women as 'the draught' and is noted as a prickly sensation in the breast after the baby has begun to feed. The practical importance of these physiological responses is considered in more detail on p. 475 under 'frequency of feeding'.

Composition of colostrum and breast milk.   For the first 2 days colostrum is secreted, and on the 3rd and 4th days the secretion changes to normal breast milk. Colostrum is a yellow fluid containing large fat globules, the colostrum corpuscles, and it has a high mineral, moderate protein and low sugar content. Colostrum has a high content of antibodies, especially secretory IgA, which play an important part in protection against infection. Colostrum may help to sterilize the small intestine if that becomes contaminated by infected material swallowed during the birth process. Colostrum is said to possess laxative qualities, but no laxative constituent has ever been demonstrated.

When the secretion changes from colostrum to milk its colour changes to bluish-white. With successful lactation the amount of milk increases daily, reaching 300 ml (*10 ounces*) on the 5th day and over 480 ml (*16 ounces*) on the 10th day.

Table 43.1   Composition of breast milk

	Protein per cent	Fat per cent	Carbohydrate per cent
Colostrum	2.25	3.15	4.00
Milk	1.25	3.50	7.25

Breast milk protein contains three fractions: caseinogen, lactalbumin and lactglobulin. The latter is present only in small amounts and the proportion of lactalbumin to caseinogen is 2 to 1. The calorie value of breast milk is 70 calories per 100 ml. (*20 calories per ounce*).

Preparation for lactation.   See p. 59.

Management of breast feeding

The essence of the initial management of breast feeding is a gradual increase in the time at the breast and the amount which the infant is allowed to take or can obtain. The objects of this gradual approach are to stimulate lactation, to encourage the baby to suck without allowing him to become discouraged by failure to obtain milk, and to accustom the nipples to the mild trauma of sucking. The following points should be considered:

Interval after birth when first feeding is permitted.   It is to be hoped that whenever possible the mother will be encouraged to handle her baby soon after birth and that she can put the infant to the breast for a short time. This will enable the baby to obtain the valuable colostrum while starting the stimulus to lactation. After this initial contact both mother and baby may require rest for a few hours before further feeding is attempted. Only if the infant is ill, or has suffered a difficult delivery, should he be kept from the breast and rested for 24 hours or longer.

Frequency of feeding.   In the past maternity hospitals have tended to rather strict regimentation of baby care. Because most babies ultimately settle down to an approximate 4 hour interval between feeds, it has been customary to establish babies on a 4-hourly regime as soon as possible. This policy was not always successful, and seldom so without recourse to a night supplement. Where there has been complete acceptance of a policy of 'rooming in' with freedom for the mother to feed her baby on demand it has been found that there is a wide range in the frequency with which healthy babies demand feeds during the early stages of lactation. In one investigation this varied from a minimum of 6 feeds per day up to a maximum of 24, with a mean of 11. It may take 2 or 3 weeks before the baby settles down to 4-hourly feeds, and a further 2 or 3 weeks before the night feed is willingly foregone. The probable physiological basis for this is shown by a recent study of the frequency of spontaneous milk ejections. These were found to occur at precise and regular intervals, short at first but lengthening over the passage of days. The intervals were almost 35 minutes on day 14, 45 minutes on day 28, 90 minutes on day 56, and 120 minutes on day 112. Animal experiments have shown that in addition to oxytocin release in response to stimulation of the nipple during suckling, oxytocin release occurs spontaneously at precise intervals independently of any suckling stimulus, and suckling young who are attached to the nipples are seen to suckle only after spontaneous milk ejection has occurred. The sucking reflex then stimulates further milk secretion by release of prolactin. If, as seems likely, a similar mechanism operates in women, there are sound physiological reasons for allowing the baby to be attached to the nipple frequently during the early days to take advantage of the frequent spontaneous milk ejections as a stimulus to suckling, which in turn will increase lactation by stimulating release of prolactin.

Oxytocin release occurs not only in response to stimulation of the nipple during suckling, but also to other factors such as the cry of the baby. However, it is inhibited by maternal anxiety, especially anxiety engendered by fear of being unable to feed the baby, so that encouragement and some simple explanation of these automatic responses may be helpful in some cases.

Despite fears, the completely flexible demand-feeding schedule has not been associated with an increased incidence of cracked nipples, possibly because the baby is only actively suckling when the milk is flowing freely. On the contrary, establishment of lactation is easier and engorgement of the breasts is rarely seen.

Time at the breast. Strict adherence to times is not necessary as babies tend to regulate their own time of feeding. During the first week the frequency may be increased but the time at the breast is short. Short frequent feeds of the more dilute milk which is yielded in the early part of a feed will provide the baby with a reasonable quantity of water, while the breasts are receiving the maximum stimulus to lactate. The time at each breast increases gradually as the frequency of feeds declines.

Alternation of breasts. It is customary to start feeding on the breast which was taken last at the previous feed. This is based on the idea that 'rich milk' may be left in the second breast with loss of valuable calories, since it is known that the fat content of milk increases towards the end of a feed. It was also argued that the first breast should be emptied completely to stimulate lactation. Efforts to persuade the baby to empty one breast completely are wrong, because it has been shown that the increase in fat content provides the baby with a self-regulating mechanism; if he is thirsty he will wish to stop feeding at each breast while the milk is still dilute, perhaps after only 5 minutes each side, but he will demand more frequent feeds.

Amount taken from the breast. As already indicated, it is best to allow the baby to regulate the supply of milk and its character according to his needs and his mother's milk yield. The time taken for a full feed may be anything between 3 minutes each side to nearly 15 minutes each side. The commonest mistake is to leave the baby on each breast for too long as this may make him progressively more tired, so that he does not demand feeds as he should and he becomes underfed, especially if his tiredness is misinterpreted as contentedness.

Position during feeding. The infant is usually nursed by the mother propped up in bed or sitting in a low-armed chair. The infant is held in the crook of the arm on the same side as the breast which is to be given, with the weight of the baby supported on the forearm. The head should be allowed to extend beyond the bend of the elbow as most infants feed better with the neck extended. With the baby in this position the mother should bend forward slightly and allow the nipple to fall into the baby's mouth. If the breast is large the redundant tissue can be restrained with the fingers of the other hand and the nipple allowed to protrude between the extended fingers.

Air swallowing. During a feed the infant must alternate between swallowing and breathing. The ability of different babies to achieve this varies greatly, and inhalation of milk during respiration causes choking and the expulsion of the milk from the air passages by coughing. However, most babies swallow air with the milk. If the air remains in the stomach and the pylorus remains closed the stomach becomes distended to capacity before an adequate amount of milk is taken, and the infant refuses to feed any longer. If he is replaced in his cot the air may be expelled and carry milk with it as vomit. Although some infants do not appear to suffer discomfort from considerable gastric and intestinal distention with air, the majority are inconvenienced by this, and it is therefore desirable to bring up the wind one or more times during a feed. To do this without spilling out the milk as well calls for a certain degree of practice on the part of both the mother and the infant. The infant is sat upright to bring the air bubble to the fundus of the stomach. The mother places one hand across the upper abdomen with the baby leaning forward against this hand. With her free hand the mother rubs or pats the back of the baby; after an interval the baby will bring up wind with a loud noise. Alternatively the baby may be held face downwards against the mother's shoulder or lying across her knee. The wind should also be brought up at the end of the feed.

Difficulties in breast feeding

Difficulties may arise from causes in the infant or in the mother.

Causes in the infant. Reluctance to feed will often indicate that the baby is ill. A healthy baby will sometimes refuse to take one breast, but will feed if the other breast is offered first. In other cases the infant refuses to 'get on' the breast, but may be encouraged if a few drops of milk are expressed and allowed to fall on his lips.

If the baby is suffering from an infection, cerebral trauma or a congenital heart lesion he may be too weak to take the breast or may tire before a sufficient amount of milk is taken. In such cases the infant must be fed with a spoon or tube for a time.

When the baby is very small there may be disproportion between the size of the nipple and the baby's mouth, but this will be remedied as the baby grows. Cleft lip and cleft palate cause less difficulty in feeding than might be expected. Micrognathos is a much more important cause of difficulty. Difficulty will also arise if there is obstruction to nose breathing (see p. 468).

Causes in the mother.   *Anatomical.*   When the nipples are poorly developed or retracted the infant cannot draw them into the correct position in the mouth for satisfactory feeding. This should be detected during antenatal examination and corrected by wearing nipple shells. Sometimes the condition may improve under the stimulus of the infant's attempts to feed, or may be overcome by feeding through nipple shells, but in many cases inadequate development of the nipples proves to be an insuperable barrier to satisfactory feeding.

Engorgement.   On the 3rd or 4th day after delivery the breasts may become engorged and painful so that milk cannot be taken and the mother is not able to tolerate the infant at the breast. This condition may develop very rapidly, and it should be recognized before it is fully established, when it may be relieved by allowing the baby to suckle frequently. Manual expression may give relief, but often the breasts are too tender for the patient to tolerate this. Some midwives become very expert at expression of the breasts by hand, and in some centres women are taught to express their breasts daily during the last few weeks of pregnancy and it is claimed that this reduces the frequency and severity of congestion of the breasts in the puerperium. The breasts may also be emptied by a breast pump. The old-fashioned glass and rubber pump is ineffective and may traumatize the nipple, but modern electric pumps which provide rhythmical negative pressure in a soft rubber breast cup are effective.

Cracked nipple.   See p. 422.

Acute mastitis and breast abscess.   See p. 423.

Deficient lactation.   Adequate lactation has been defined as secretion of 300 ml (*10 ounces*) daily by the 5th day and 480 ml (*16 ounces*) by the 10th day. If these amounts are not achieved a baby of normal weight will not be adequately fed. Failure of lactation may occasionally be due to inadequate development of gland tissue, although this has nothing to do with the size of the breasts. Some women with small breasts with little fat produce large quantities of milk, while large fat breasts may contain little secreting tissue. There is no treatment which will produce lactation if the glandular tissue is deficient.

Lactation is sometimes delayed. In most instances this is due to withholding for longer than usual the natural stimulus of the baby sucking at the nipple, but there are some women in whom lactation is slow to appear. They need reassurance, and to be told that if food and fluid intake is adequate lactation will eventually be established. There is a danger that they will be wrongly advised to drink large quantities of fluid, which has been shown to *reduce* the milk yield. This may be related to inhibition of the release of antidiuretic hormone and possibly of oxytocin at the same time. Breast feeding women should drink enough to satisfy thirst and not more. Attempts to increase lactation by injection of prolactin have been disappointing, while milky drinks such as Lactogol are probably only effective by their psychological effect. The best stimulus for a mother with delayed lactation is to allow the baby to suckle more frequently.

Contraindications to breast feeding

Breast feeding may be contraindicated in cases of severe heart or kidney disease or of active tuberculosis in the mother. The risk to the infant if the mother has active tuberculosis is of the same degree whether the mother gives him feeds by bottle or at the breast (see p. 223).

Excretion of drugs in breast milk

No drug should be given to a lactating mother unless there is some definite clinical indication for its use, because some of the drug or its degradation products are likely to be excreted in the milk, but many drugs which are essential for the mother are only excreted in small amounts, so that breast feeding need not be discontinued except in the case of a few drugs. Cytotoxic drugs and radioactive iodine are positive contraindications. If a thyrotoxic mother is receiving carbimazole it is necessary to monitor the baby's thyroid function and discontinue breast feeding if it is impaired. Warfarin, senna, phenobarbitone, phenytoin, digoxin and steroids pass into the milk in harmless amounts. Antibiotics are excreted in extremely small amounts, but there is a theoretical possibility of sensitization of the infant.

Artificial feeding

When breast milk is not available the infant is usually fed on cow's milk, nowadays almost invariably in modified form. In rare cases of intolerance to cow's milk other mammalian milks have been used, such as those from the ass, the mare or the goat, but there are now several artificial preparations which are preferred, such as hydrolysed amino acid preparations, or vegetable milks made from soya bean. Milk allergy causes colic and frequent loose stools. Because of the risk of allergy of even minor degree there is an increasing tendency to use such 'non-allergenic' preparations when complements or supplements to feeds have to be introduced. Unfortunately some babies have been known to develop sensitivity to soya bean preparations.

    In comparing human milk and cow's milk it has been customary to concentrate on the differences in the fat and protein content and their respective digestibility, and to suggest that all that was necessary was to modify these constituents and to add some sugar to make the cow's milk preparation a satisfactory nutritional substitute.

Table 43.2   Comparison of the composition of human and cow's milk

	Protein per cent	Proportion of caseinogen to lactalbumin	Fat per cent	Carbohydrate per cent
Human milk	1.25	1 to 2	3.5	7.25
Cow's milk	3.5	4 to 1	3.5	4.75

Calorie value of milk: 70 calories per 100 ml (*20 calories per ounce*)

The increased risk of enteric infections in artificially fed babies has been attributed to lack of sterility in the preparation and administration of the feeds. Certainly there is much to be said for this argument, but important new discoveries about the way in which raw human milk actively maintains the sterility of the small intestine, whilst cow's milk preparations have a tendency to encourage bacterial colonization, have suggested that this difference is the basic reason why cow's milk is suitable for the calf and human milk for the baby. Because the cow is a ruminant the calf requires a type of feed which encourages the formation of a rumen, which has been described as a vat full of bacterial ferments which enables the cow to subsist on a vegetable diet. Human beings are not ruminants, and healthy babies have a relatively sterile upper gastro-intestinal tract. This fundamental difference in the character of the intestinal contents makes considerable differences in the availability of most of the nutrients. For example, the availability of calcium depends upon the lactose content, which is high in human milk; iron is bound to lactoferrin in human milk and to transferrin in cow's milk; zinc absorption is assisted by a prostaglandin in human which is absent from cow's milk. The high lactose content of human milk, by increasing the availability of calcium, makes it possible for the level of calcium and phosphate to be relatively low, thus giving human milk a lower buffering capacity so that the bactericidal action of the more acid intestinal contents is maintained. By ensuring rapid and complete absorption of iron, the lactoferrin deprives the intestinal bacteria of iron needed for their replication. Other factors which inhibit bacterial growth which are present in human milk include specific IgA, maternal lymphocytes, lysozyme and copper.

The tremendous efforts which have been made to 'humanize' cow's milk have been doomed to failure, although a crude approximation to human milk has been obtained.

General principles of artificial feeding

Whatever the choice of feed the principles for feeding are the same. After the 7th day of life the infant takes an average of 150 ml of fluid per kg of body weight daily (*2½ fluid ounces per pound*). Since the amount of milk provided by a lactating mother is at first quite small and gradually increases, the same principle is applied for artificial feeding. It is convenient to start with 30 ml per kg of the milk preparation on the first day, and thereafter to increase the total quantity by 20 ml per kg each day until the baby is receiving 150 ml per kg. The fully constituted artificial feed should provide 65 to 70 calories per 100 ml (*20 calories per ounce*). If the baby seems thirsty during the early days additional water may be given, either separately or by diluting the feeds slightly.

Although there is no need to keep rigidly to a strict time schedule for bottle feeding, and a certain amount of flexibility is appropriate for most babies, the same frequency of feeds is not required as in the early days when lactation is being established. Babies tend to settle down to a 3 or 4-hourly rhythm, and some flexibility enables each baby to show his own preference. Once full feeds are established the amount offered at each feed will be 25 or 30 ml per kg of body weight, depending on whether there are 5 or 6 feeds in the 24 hours.

The cow is a most unsuitable mammal to choose for the provision of a milk substitute for the human infant, but it was originally chosen because domestic cattle had been around for centuries as milk providers in the Western world, where the habit of artificial feeding was first popularized, and so the routinely used artificial milk preparations are made from cow's milk which is modified in one way or another. These preparations are now available in hospitals as pre-packed sterilized feeds, which only require the application of a sterile teat to the bottle before being given to the baby. However, these pre-packed feeds are not yet available for home use, where feeds are still in the form of dried milk powders or evaporated milks which need to be reconstituted by the addition of water. The dilution required for each preparation is different, and the instructions on the packet or tin must be followed carefully. Included with the powdered milk preparations are special scoops, and it is important that the powder and the water are measured accurately. The scoop should not be heaped or packed tightly as this can make up to 20 per cent difference in the composition of the feed. Some mothers find it convenient to make up all the feeds for 24 hours in a batch, and if this is done the feeds must be stored in a refrigerator. Bottles and teats are carefully washed and sterilized in dilute hypochlorite solution (Milton). In hospital bottles are usually sterilized by autoclaving.

Preparations available. The use of undiluted cow's milk ('doorstep milk') is not recommended until the baby reaches the age of 6 months.

Both dried milk powders and evaporated milks are available as full-cream and low-solute preparations.

Full-cream preparations have the same fat content as the raw milk from which they are prepared, although the character of the fat may be slightly altered during the manufacturing process. This process also causes some degree of breakdown of the protein of the milk into simpler compounds. It also destroys vitamins to some extent, especially vitamin C, and the manufacturers add vitamins and iron to their preparations.

Low-solute preparations. In the past half-cream preparations made from partly skimmed milk were widely used because it was believed that the fat in cow's milk was poorly digested and absorbed, so that a great deal of it was wasted in the stools, carrying with it valuable calcium and thereby increasing the risk of neonatal tetany. The high osmolality of these preparations increased the risk of hypertonic dehydration in sick infants. They had a lower calorific value, and sugar was usually added by the manufacturer to make up for this. Half-cream preparations are no longer so widely used, as it is held that feeding should begin with a low-solute modified milk which has protein, fat and mineral content close to that of human milk, and which is therefore less likely to be associated with hypernatraemia, hypocalcaemia or obesity.

Cow's milk not only contains more protein than human milk, but the protein in it is predominantly curd protein (casein), whereas breast milk protein consists of about equal parts of casein and whey protein (mainly lactalbumin). The fat content of breast milk is approximately equal to that of cow's milk, but the fat is of a different quality; it is more easily absorbed and it contains more polyunsaturated fatty acids, which are probably essential for man.

In making a low-solute preparation some manufacturers reduce the milk to a demineralized whey, containing whey protein and a low content of minerals, and then add a small amount of skim milk to provide some casein, further lactose, and some minerals in their naturally occurring forms, while other minerals such as iron, copper, zinc and manganese may be added. The fat which is added consists of a mixture of animal and vegetable fats, the composition of which approximates to that of the fat of breast milk. Examples of this type of low-solute milk are SMA Gold Cap and Cow and Gate Premium.

Alternatively the relative concentration of protein and minerals can be reduced by simply adding carbohydrate. This must be carefully chosen to avoid the risk of fermentation diarrhoea. Examples of such preparations are Cow and Gate Baby Milk Plus and Ostermilk Complete Formula.

In the demineralized whey products there has been anxiety about the completeness of the additions, and it has also been found that the infant's requirement for vitamin E is increased when preparations rich in polyunsaturated fats are given. There is also a suspicion that whey proteins are more immunogenic than casein.

After an episode of gastro-enteritis it may be found that babies on prepacked low-solute feeds have a recurrence of diarrhoea, and this may be due to the presence of small amounts of lactulose in the feeds, which result from the method of manufacture. A change to one of the powdered preparations will then effectively stop the diarrhoea.

Complementary and supplementary feeds. A complementary feed is one which is given to augment a feed from the breast; a supplementary feed is one which replaces a breast feed. Complementary feeding is sometimes necessary when lactation is only slowly established. It is unnecessary before the 5th day as the baby can be given water if he is thirsty. If the weight is still falling or is stationary, or the baby seems very hungry, test weighing may be carried out to determine exactly how much milk the baby is obtaining from the breast. The baby is weighed fully clothed before the feed and again after the feed, without changing soiled napkins. If the milk yield is insufficient the baby may be offered a complement after each feed to make up the deficit. The amount which is required may be determined by test weighing at each feed, but it is probably better to offer a standard amount after each feed and to let the baby take as much or as little as he wants.

The occasional use of a cow's milk preparation for complementary feeding may destroy the protective effect of maternal secretory IgA in breast milk against hypersensitivity. It is to be hoped that some expressed breast milk will be available in most maternity units, but if this is not so and the baby has a family history of atopy it would be best to use a soya bean preparation (Prosobee or Velactin) if complementary feeding is unavoidable.

44

Diseases of the newborn

Birth trauma

Birth injuries vary from minor skin abrasions to severe internal haemorrhage. Their prevention depends on the art of obstetrics, and a balance must be struck between the safety of the mother and that of the child in difficult labour. It is a reflection of the improvement in antenatal and perinatal care in recent years that serious birth trauma is now uncommon.

Birth injuries to the scalp and skull

Caput succedaneum. This is caused by oedema of the subcutaneous layers of the scalp (Fig. 44.1). It lies over whatever part of the head presents through the cervical opening. The swelling is maximal at birth and resolves within a few days. A localized caput, referred to as the 'chignon' is produced by the vacuum extractor. (ventouse)

Cephalhaematoma. This is a subperiosteal haematoma which most commonly lies over one of the parietal bones (Fig. 44.2). It never extends

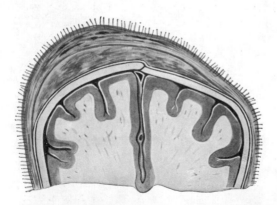

Fig. 44.1 Caput succedaneum. The swelling is formed by oedema of the structures lying superficial to the pericranium. Note that it is not limited to one bone. Compare with Fig. 44.2.

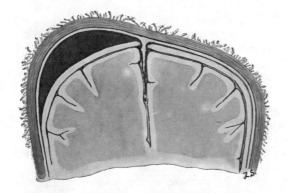

Fig. 44.2 Cephalhaematoma. The swelling is seen to consist of blood lying between the pericranium and the skull and limited to the bone on which it started by the attachment of the pericranium to the suture.

beyond the limits of a single bone, and it is fluctuant but incompressible. It never varies in tension with crying, thus differing from the less common encephalocele. Spontaneous absorption occurs, but this may take several weeks. Ossification may take place round the periphery and create a raised rim which can be mistaken for a depressed fracture.

No treatment is necessary; aspiration invites infection. There may be asymmetry of the skull which persists for many months, but ultimately this resolves completely.

Subaponeurotic haematoma. After vacuum extraction a few cases of subaponeurotic haematoma have occurred. The blood lies in the loose areolar layer between the aponeurosis and the periosteum. The haematoma is not limited to a single bone, and a large collection of blood may even extend as far as the cervical region. Slow absorption takes place.

Sometimes an extremely large cephalhaematoma or subaponeurotic haematoma may cause anaemia or moderately severe jaundice.

Skull fractures. These are now rarely seen. They may be depressed, linear or stellate. They usually occur over a parietal or frontal bone as a result of difficult forceps delivery. Often there are no symptoms and even depressed fractures may resolve spontaneously. If there are signs suspicious of underlying haemorrhage or pressure on the brain a neurosurgical opinion should be obtained, in case elevation of a depressed fracture is required.

Craniotabes. Although it is not caused by injury this condition is mentioned here for convenience. The skull may show areas of softening near the suture lines, especially in the parietal region, and the bone in these areas can be indented like a table tennis ball. Craniotabes is of no significance, and the bones develop and thicken normally as the infant grows. Upper beaten skull

Intracranial injuries

Intracranial haemorrhage, especially when it is combined with hypoxia, causes a number of stillbirths and neonatal deaths. Such haemorrhage may occur in any difficult, instrumental or breech delivery, and especially with premature birth. It may even occur occasionally during normal delivery or Caesarean section.

The cerebrospinal fluid acts as a cushion to the brain and permits some mobility of the intracranial contents, but injury occurs when excessive moulding or sudden changes in pressure occur during delivery. The site of the haemorrhage may be extradural, subdural, subarachnoid, intraventricular or intracerebral.

Extradural haemorrhage caused by rupture of the middle meningeal artery or the veins near the sigmoid sinus is rare in the newborn infant. It may occur with a fracture through the middle temporal fossa or from forcible separation of cranial sutures. In cases of tearing of the tentorium cerebelli or falx cerebri there may be extradural bleeding, but the blood also escapes into the subarachnoid space, and the symptoms produced are chiefly due to this.

Subdural haemorrhage takes the form of slow bleeding into the space between the dura and the pia-arachnoid, and is due to rupture of small veins crossing this space. A haematoma usually forms slowly over a period of some days, but may develop more quickly. See below p. 488.

Subarachnoid haemorrhage is most commonly seen in association with prolonged or traumatic delivery, but hypoxia plays a part in causing it. It can arise from a tear of the tentorium or falx, with rupture of small vessels or of a dural sinus. With gross tentorial tearing there may be fatal rupture of the great cerebral vein of Galen.

Intraventricular haemorrhage occurs most frequently in premature babies and is the result of anoxia. The bleeding may follow venous stasis and rupture of poorly-supported blood vessels in the highly vascular germinal layers of the brain close to the ventricles. The blood then breaks through into the ventricle. Massive intraventricular haemorrhage may also come from the choroid plexus. Intraventricular haemorrhage is usually fatal, but if survival occurs the infant usually has irreversible brain damage.

Intracerebral haemorrhages are often only petechial but they are distributed throughout the substance of the brain. Such haemorrhages are usually the result of severe asphyxial episodes. Although the haemorrhages may be small and not fatal they may be associated with cerebral palsy, mental retardation and a high incidence of morbidity.

Clinical signs. Minor intracranial haemorrhages must often escape recognition, while massive haemorrhages cause stillbirth or almost immediate death. Lesions of intermediate severity create intricate diagnostic problems, in which physical signs are often misleading or difficult.

General signs and symptoms may occur, including convulsions, asphyxia pallida, depression of respiration and heart rate, associated with alterations in muscular tone. Cyanosis or unusual pallor, fever, a shrill cry, excessive restlessness or somnolence may all occur. An anxious facial expression, adder-like movements of the tongue and unusual yawning may suggest the diagnosis. With an extensive haemorrhage the fontanelle may become tense or even bulge.

The clinical picture may be differentiated according to the site of the bleeding:

Supratentorial bleeding usually affects the surface of the hemisphere and the basal ganglia. The picture is one of irritation, with fullness of the fontanelle, convulsions which may be unilateral, and excessive response to stimuli of sound, light and touch. The eyes may roll upwards and the face twitch during the clonic contractions, and adductor spasm may be demonstrated. The vital centres are involved in the terminal stages.

Infratentorial bleeding is often associated with early neck rigidity, opisthotonus, and alteration in the rate and depth of respiration. Cyanosis is common. The baby tends to be limp and toneless, and the vital centres are affected early.

Treatment. The infant must be kept quiet and warm and sheltered from any noise or disturbance which might induce further restlessness or convulsions. Unnecessary handling is avoided. Respiration and oxygenation must be maintained. These conditions are achieved by nursing the baby in an incubator in which optimal conditions of warmth, humidity and oxygen concentration can be provided. The infant can be unclothed and need only be placed on a napkin to collect the excreta. It has been claimed that the tendency to further bleeding is reduced if the infant is propped upright on pillows, but the greater comfort to the baby of lying flat outweighs other possible advantages. The infant can be fed in the incubator and need not be removed for any nursing services. If the baby sucks badly or refuses to feed, tube feeding is given at intervals of 4 to 6 hours.

Phytomenadione (vitamin K_1) 1 mg should be given by intramuscular injection to prevent the risk of any further bleeding from haemorrhagic disease (see p. 496).

An infant who has convulsions should be given sedatives until these are controlled, as they may provoke further bleeding. First, paraldehyde 0.15 ml per kg is given by intramuscular injection. The addition of hyaluronidase, made up in water and well shaken, increases the rate of absorption. Afterwards an intravenous infusion is started, and 2 hours after the fit occurred phenytoin 8 mg per kg is given intravenously over 15 minutes to prevent recurrence of the fits. Twenty-four hours later a maintenance dose of phenytoin is started; 3 mg per kg is given 12-hourly for 48 hours.

Lumbar puncture will prove the diagnosis by demonstrating blood in the cerebrospinal fluid, and it will also exclude a diagnosis of meningitis.

The prognosis in cases of cerebral haemorrhage is always in doubt and is usually poor. The infant may survive to show cerebral palsy, convulsions or mental retardation; but complete recovery may follow a subarachnoid haemorrhage.

Subdural haematoma. These cases may be described separately as the clinical signs often develop more slowly. There is slow bleeding into the space between the dura and the pia-arachnoid. The haematoma increases in size because of further small haemorrhages or because of lysis of the clot and accumulation of serum.

Symptoms may occur soon after birth or may be delayed for 24 hours or more. Early symptoms are those of supratentorial irritation (see above) but more delayed symptoms are failure to gain weight, irregular fever, vomiting and irritability. Coma or convulsions may occur at this stage, but it is more common to find fits with enlargement of the skull simulating hydrocephalus during the first few months of life. The diagnosis is made by needling the subdural space through the lateral angles of the fontanelle when blood-stained or xanthochromic fluid may be found. Repeated aspiration is performed until the cavity is emptied. Surgery is rarely indicated, and has not been found to reduce the occurrence of sequelae due to cortical atrophy, namely convulsions, spasticity and mental retardation.

Real-time ultrasonic scanning and CAT scanning may prove to be helpful in the diagnosis of intracranial conditions in the newborn.

Fractures of the long bones

These are now uncommon. They were more often seen when breech extraction was practised more frequently.

Clavicle. This is the bone which is most frequently broken during delivery. The injury is usually detected when the infant fails to raise his arm above his head, or there is an absent Moro reflex (p. 461) in one arm, or callus formation is noticed. X-ray shows an oblique fracture. Healing occurs without treatment.

Humerus. Epiphyseal detachment or fracture of the shaft may occur. The injury is often difficult to detect clinically. The usual symptom is failure to move the arm. Bandaging the arm to the trunk gives sufficient fixation.

Femur. Fractures have occurred in breech extraction.

In nearly all fractures of the long bones healing is rapid, and subsequent growth of the bone corrects any angulation and deformity.

Visceral injuries

Rupture of the liver, spleen or kidney may occur in difficult deliveries, especially breech extraction. There will be signs of shock, and enlargement of the viscus may be observed. The diagnosis is difficult, but ultrasonic or

CAT scanning may make this easier in the future. If the diagnosis is made the infant is given a blood transfusion and laparotomy is performed to try to repair the injury. The mortality is high.

Haemorhage may also occur into the adrenal glands. The infant may be stillborn or die soon after birth with severe shock and cyanosis. If the enlarged adrenal is palpable the diagnosis may be made, and treatment consists of blood transfusion and administration of hydrocortisone

Peripheral nerve injuries

Facial nerve. The nerve may be damaged by pressure of a blade of the forceps, but palsy has also occurred after normal delivery. Very rarely the nerve is involved in a basal fracture affecting the temporal bone.

On the affected side the eye does not shut, the corner of the mouth drops and the naso-labial fold is less marked than on the other side. When the child cries the mouth is drawn to the normal side. In the vast majority of cases recovery occurs spontaneously within a few days.

Brachial palsy. This may occur from overstretching or tearing of the nerves by lateral traction on the neck, usually during a difficult extraction of the shoulders. The clinical picture depends on the nerve roots involved. If the roots of C5 and C6 are damaged (Erb's palsy) the arm lies at the side of the trunk with internal rotation at the shoulder, inability to bend the elbow, and clenched fingers. If the roots C7, C8 and D1 are involved there is paralysis of the muscles of the forearm with wrist drop and flaccid digits (Klumpke's palsy). In fact Klumpke's palsy is very rare and most cases of wrist drop are caused by compression of the radial nerve against the humerus during labour. In such cases the discovery of a nodule of fat necrosis at the site of compression is diagnostic.

If the nerves have merely been compressed or stretched recovery occurs, but if rupture of a nerve has taken place spontaneous recovery will not occur. If there is no indication of early recovery the arm must be placed in the position which avoids stretching the paralysed muscles. For Erb's palsy first aid treatment is to fasten the back of the hand to the top of the head, but for all the injuries plastic splints can be devised with orthopaedic advice. In a few cases that do not improve surgical exploration of the plexus may be advised, but the prognosis is not good.

Digestive disturbances during the neonatal period

Vomiting

Vomiting is a relatively frequent symptom during the neonatal period. While most cases are not serious, this symptom sometimes has grave significance and it must never be treated lightly.

Vomiting of mucus. Many infants vomit mucus, which may be blood-stained, during the first few hours after delivery. This may persist after feeding has started, and the probable explanation is that the gastric mucosa has been irritated by material swallowed during delivery, with the production of gastritis. If the vomiting is severe or persistent lavage with normal saline is performed until the wash-out is clean. This may require to be repeated.

Overfeeding. Vomiting is sometimes due to the taking of more food than can be retained in the stomach, and the excess is regurgitated. Failure to help the baby bring up wind after feeds often causes vomiting as the milk is brought up with the swallowed air after the baby is laid in the cot. In both instances the treatment is obvious.

Obstructive vomiting. Vomiting which begins shortly after birth and is persistent raises the possibility of an obstructive lesion of the gastro-intestinal tract. The vomiting is frequent, non-projectile, copious and usually bile-stained, unless the obstruction is above the level of the ampulla of Vater. Bile-stained vomit (which is grass-green in colour) always demands consideration as a symptom of an obstructive lesion. Abdominal distention, visible abdominal peristalsis and failure to pass meconium are usually present, and are associated with a progressive loss of weight and deterioration in the general condition. These symptoms demand immediate radiological investigation and surgical consultation. A plain radiograph of the abdomen should be taken. If the infant is unwell, a lateral film taken with the infant lying supine in the incubator will usually give all the information required, and it has the advantage of showing whether there is gas in the rectum. The films will show dilatation of the gut, with fluid levels that are characteristic if there is obstruction. It is neither necessary nor desirable to use barium contrast media as these may complicate surgical treatment. Possible causes of obstruction include oesophageal atresia, duodenal stenosis or atresia, jejunal or ileal atresia and meconium ileus.

Tracheo-oesophageal fistula or atresia

Oesophageal atresia, with or without tracheal fistula, occurs relatively infrequently, but delay in diagnosis reduces the chances of survival. The possibility must be borne in mind with every infant who shows difficulty with the first feeds. Because of the association with hydramnios in every instance of this condition the baby must be investigated soon after birth to exclude atresia.

Atresia occurs just above the level of the bifurcation of the trachea. There is usually an associated tracheal fistula which may arise from the upper or lower oesophageal segment. The initial symptom is invariably difficulty with the first feed. Regurgitation of the fluid taken and inability to keep the mother clear of saliva should raise suspicion. When the upper segment communicates with the trachea through a fistula, the first feed causes choking and cyanosis, and immediate clearing of the oro-pharynx is required. (Similar symptoms occur if there is a tracheo-oesophageal fistula, even if there is no oesophageal atresia). If the lower segment communicates with the trachea, regurgitation of acid secretion from the stomach into the respiratory tract causes pneumonia.

Any suspicion that swallowing is not normal should lead to prompt investigation by attempting to pass a moderately stiff catheter through the oesophagus into the stomach. A soft catheter may coil up in the segment above the atresia and delude the observer into believing that it has passed into the stomach. The aspiration of acid secretion and the emptying of the stomach of air provide proof that the oesophagus is patent. Failure to pass the catheter more than half way down the oesophagus proves the presence of atresia. The catheter should be radio-opaque so that its position can be confirmed with x-rays. Directly the diagnosis is established the infant is transferred to a paediatric surgical unit with frequent suction during the journey. Surgery in specialized units offers a good chance of survival.

Abnormalities of the diaphragm

Diaphragmatic hernia. Congenital failure of development of one side of the diaphragm presents a difficult diagnostic problem. Persistence of the posteriorly situated pleuro-peritoneal sinus on either side allows the abdominal contents to herniate into the pleural cavity. This occurs more commonly on the left side, and at an early stage of fetal life when there is still a universal mesentery, so that almost all the intestine can enter the thorax. Such herniae cause cyanotic attacks and vomiting. The diagnosis may be suspected if heart sounds are heard on the right and gut sounds in the chest, and it is proven by x-ray examination. During transfer to surgical care assisted respiration may be necessary with an endotracheal tube, and the stomach and gut should be kept deflated with another tube.

Eventration of the diaphragm. Occasionally the diaphragm fails to develop the normal musculature and is a non-contractile fibrous septum which is pushed up high into the chest. Gut sounds are heard in the chest, the lungs are poorly expanded, and the infant is cyanosed. X-ray examination shows the abnormal position of the diaphragm. Some infants succumb, and survivors may have frequent chest infections. An operation to plicate the diaphragm may be necessary.

Hiatus hernia. Herniation of the cardiac end of the stomach through the oesophageal hiatus may cause vomiting. The infant regurgitates small amounts between feeds and fails to thrive. The condition is demonstrated by a barium swallow. Sometimes no hiatus hernia can be found, and the diagnosis of gastro-oesophageal reflux or lax cardia is made. When regurgitation of gastric acid occurs there is likely to be oesophagitis, with blood or altered blood in the vomit.

Thickening the feeds and posturing the infant are usually sufficient to relieve the symptoms. The infant is placed in the prone position on a firm mattress which is elevated to an angle of 30°. Thickening of the feeds can be achieved without the addition of salt or increasing the calorie content by adding small amounts of powdered carob bean (Nestargel, Carobol), starting with one scoop to 150 ml of feed. For a breast-fed baby the powder is mixed with a little water and given before the feed.

Congenital atresia of the gut

Duodenal atresia or stenosis.   This causes vomiting, failure to void meconium and upper abdominal distention. The vomit is usually heavily bile-stained. A radiograph of the abdomen in the erect position shows a double bubble of gas from the stomach and proximal duodenum, with empty gut beyond. The lesion is frequently associated with Down's syndrome. Treatment is surgical.

Jejunal and ileal atresia.   Single or multiple atresic lesions of the small bowel can cause vomiting, abdominal distention and failure to pass meconium. A radiograph shows gaseous distention of bowel loops above the lesion with fluid levels. Surgical exploration is urgent.

Meconium ileus

The infant suffers from cystic fibrosis, in which there is lack of pancreatic secretion into the bowel. During intrauterine life the meconium is not normally digested and it becomes packed into the lower ileum, forming a mass of putty-like consistence and appearance. Vomiting and abdominal distention occur, and x-ray examination shows gaseous distention and fluid levels in the small bowel, with lack of gas and a finely mottled opacity in the right lower quadrant of the abdomen. Surgical treatment often involves resection of bowel and in most cases an enterostomy, which is left open until the bowel is functioning normally. If a sweat test confirms the diagnosis of cystic fibrosis the infant will need subsequent care for this disease.

Congenital hypertrophic pyloric stenosis

Symptoms arising from the obstruction caused by hypertrophy of the circular muscle of the pylorus are uncommon before the 2nd week of life. The condition occurs five times more often in male than in female infants. The symptoms are projectile vomiting, failure to gain weight and constipation. The infant usually feeds eagerly despite the vomiting which occurs at the end of feeds, and will accept re-feeding immediately after having vomited. As a rule the vomit does not contain bile.

With continued vomiting the condition of the infant deteriorates and he become dehydrated with loss of skin turgor, depression of the fontanelle and dryness of the mouth. The loss of chloride in the vomit causes a low plasma chloride level and compensatory alkalosis. Careful examination, with the baby relaxed during a feed, reveals gastric peristaltic waves and a pyloric tumour is felt.

The condition may be treated medically or by operation. Surgical treatment by Ramstedt's pyloroplasty gives excellent results provided that dehydration and chloride deficiency are first corrected. Medical treatment consists of the initial use of gastric washouts, and the administration of drugs to relax the pylorus. Atropine methyl nitrate (Eumydrin) is given in a strength of 0.6 per cent w/v in ethyl alochol in doses of 1 to 3 drops 15 minutes before each feed. Medical treatment is suitable for mildly affected infants who develop symptoms after the age of 6 weeks, and is also employed for infants who are too ill to undergo surgery.

Other causes of vomiting

Vomiting may be a symptom of increased intracranial pressure or cerebral irritation. It may be the initial and sometimes the only sign of an infection in any system during the neonatal period, and is then often accompanied by diarrhoea. It cannot be too strongly emphasized that vomiting and reluctance to feed may be the earliest symptoms of pyelonephritis, meningitis and other severe illnesses, and such symptoms must never be lightly disregarded.

Diarrhoea

Diarrhoea is sometimes diagnosed without justification because of ignorance of the normal variation in bowel habit of healthy infants. Frequency of stool is not necessarily pathological.

The passage of frequent loose and watery stools, usually containing curds of undigested milk and often green in colour with unchanged bile, is evidence of hurry through the gut. The presence of mucus suggests irritation of the intestinal mucosa, and blood in the stool is suggestive of infection. Colic and screaming often accompany the diarrhoea, and signs of dehydration such as loss of skin turgor, loss of weight and sunken fontanelle occur early.

The most common causes of diarrhoea are:
(a) Errors in feeding, either in the quality of the food or in the amount.
(b) An excess of sugar in the feed causing fermentation in the gut.
(c) Infection of the gastro-intestinal tract by bacteria or viruses.

Feeding irregularities. In breast-fed babies there may be some intestinal hurry at the time when lactation is becoming established between the 3rd and 5th days. The stools are frequent and greenish in colour and may contain a moderate amount of mucus. No ill effects result, and after a few more days the stools become less frequent, and become pasty in consistency and yellow in colour. Sometimes in artificially fed babies there may be a similar hurried transit of gut contents if the amount of the feeds is increased too rapidly in the first few days. In them it is advisable to reduce the quantity of milk until the frequency of the stools diminishes, but it may be necessary to maintain the fluid intake by adding more water to the feeds for a day or two.

Excess of sugar in the feeds.   Adding sugar to some dried milks which already have a high carbohydrate content may induce looseness of the stools from fermentation in the gut. There is often frothy diarrhoea and the buttocks may be sore. The obvious remedy is to reduce the sugar content.

Infection of the gastro-intestinal tract.   Diarrhoea caused by the dysentery group of organisms is uncommon in the neonatal period. Occasionally infections with pathogenic coliforms and other organisms of relatively low pathogenicity may occur. Contamination of feeds with staphylococci is possible, and if fresh milk is not sterilized infection with a great variety of bacteria may occur. In nurseries epidemics of diarrhoea among newborn infants may be caused by virus infections (see below).

Bacterial infection is usually accompanied by vomiting, diarrhoea and failure to feed. The infant is usually, but not always, febrile; a few babies may be prostrated with subnormal temperatures. The stools are watery, loose and undigested. They may contain mucus, pus and red cells. The infant will fail to gain or will lose weight. In severe cases dehydration occurs rapidly and the condition of the infant is poor. Metabolic acidosis occurs.

Infants with these symptoms must be isolated from all other babies immediately, and in institutions they must be nursed with full barrier precautions. Milk feeding is stopped until the diarrhoea improves. Sodium chloride solution 0.18 per cent, with glucose 4 per cent, and with potassium chloride 2 g per litre, is given frequently in small amounts at intervals of 2 or 3 hours. The total daily intake should be approximately 175 ml per kg of body weight, the excess being necessary to make good the additional fluid loss caused by the diarrhoea. Should vomiting persist, or the baby become further dehydrated despite this treatment, it will be necessary to give fluid by intravenous infusion, the type of fluid being dictated by electrolyte estimations.

Stool cultures are taken at the onset to determine the infecting organism and its sensitivities to antibiotics. Antibiotic therapy will not usually influence the symptoms, but is sometimes advisable to reduce cross-infection. The prognosis must always be guarded until the reponse to treatment is seen.

Epidemic diarrhoea of the newborn.   In other cases a baby with symptoms of gastro-intestinal infection may fail to show pathogenic bacteria on stool culture, and a virus infection must be postulated. This can sometimes be confirmed by electron microscopy. The symptoms may not be severe, but the loose stools and low grade fever with failure to gain weight may persist for more than a week. The stools are voided in explosive fashion and tend to be watery, yellow and acid, but seldom contain mucus, pus or blood. The condition of the infant may deteriorate rapidly, and the need for rehydration may become urgent. The condition may improve but only to relapse during treatment, and the infant may develop intercurrent infections of the lungs, ears or septicaemia. The infectivity is high, and the disease may spread in nurseries in epidemic form.

Isolation and full barrier nursing is essential as soon as the diagnosis is suspected. The treatment consists of the cessation of milk feeding and oral or intravenous administration of electrolyte containing fluids to combat dehydration and acidosis.

Colic

Colic is manifest by screaming, flushing of the face, clenching of the fists, flexing of the arms and legs and tenseness of the abdominal wall. The common causes are distention of the gut with wind or spasmodic contractions of the gut due to some irritative stimulus. Swallowing of air and failure to help the baby bring it up is the most common cause, but improper feeding techniques may be responsible. When it is obvious that the colic is severe, or the baby has screaming attacks, the possibility of some mechanical obstruction such as volvulus or intussusception must be considered.

Elimination of the cause, whether it is aerophagy or improper feeding will relieve most cases.

Constipation

True constipation in the newborn infant is comparatively uncommon. Cases of obstruction such as gut atresia have already been mentioned. Hirschprung's disease does not usually give rise to marked symptoms in the neonatal period, although delay in the passage of the first meconium may be the earliest sign of this condition. Constipation in young infants is usually a variation in normal bowel habit, and the passage of hard motions at irregular intervals is most commonly the result of insufficient intake of food or fluid, or the use of artificial feeds which are too rich in protein or too low in sugar content. Treatment consists in correction of the dietetic error and giving extra water.

In breast-fed babies, once lactation is fully established the stools may be passed infrequently. It is not unusual for 3 or 4 days to elapse without a stool being passed, but when it appears it is yellow and pasty. Obviously no treatment is required.

Haemorrhagic states in the newborn

Haemorrhagic disease.   In this condition there is a tendency to spontaneous and prolonged bleeding in the first week of life, usually from the 2nd to the 5th day. The common site of bleeding is the gut, causing vomiting of blood or melaena, but the lungs, brain, skin or mucous membranes may be affected. The bleeding coincides with the period of low prothrombin level which occurs in the newborn infant from the 2nd to the 7th day, when the level may fall to 20 per cent of normal, but some other factor may also be involved. Bleeding and clotting times and the platelet count may be abnormal. The prothrombin level may be raised to normal by administration of vitamin K_1, but not every case responds to this treatment. In such instances injection of a small quantity of fresh-frozen plasma arrests the haemorrhage. Excessive administration of vitamin K_1 should be avoided, as it increases the risk of jaundice. An intramuscular injection of 1 mg of phytomenadione (vitamin K_1) is usually sufficient, although this may be repeated the next day.

Disseminated intravascular coagulation.   A more serious disorder may occur, especially in sick babies of low birth weight following asphyxia or as a complication of septicaemia. It is due to widespread intravascular coagulation and consumption of available clotting factors. Severe bleeding may occur from almost any site, and there is widespread purpura because of the low platelet count. There is an increase in fibrin degradation products, and blood films show numerous fragmented red cells. The only effective treatment is exchange transfusion; heparin is of little value as the coagulation has already occurred.

Umbilical bleeding.   This may occur from a slipped ligature in the first 24 hours, of from infection of the stump after the cord has separated. Life may be endangered as 30 ml of blood lost is equivalent to about 10 per cent of the baby's total blood volume. A fresh ligature must be applied, or if the cord has separated the bleeding point must be controlled by pressure or application of artery forceps. Blood transfusion may be urgently required.

Thrombocytopenic purpura.   Congenital thrombocytopenia may cause a petechial rash, ecchymoses and bleeding from various sites. It is to be distinguished from simple traumatic purpura of the head and neck from pressure; in the latter the platelet count is not reduced. The infant is frequently affected if the mother has had thrombocytopenic purpura during pregnancy. Most cases resolve quickly, but it may be necessary to treat the infant with steroids.

Anaemia.   The most common cause of anaemia at birth is haemolytic disease; otherwise it is usually the result of haemorrhage. Haemorrhage may occur from tearing of the cord during delivery, incision of the placenta during Caesarean section, or from bleeding from the fetal side of the placenta during delivery. The infant will be pale at birth with a low haemoglobin level. Immediate transfusion may be required.

Bleeding from the fetal into the maternal circulation may occur and can be proved by the demonstration of fetal cells in the mother's blood (see p. 448) but is hardly ever of such an amount as to cause fatal anaemia. Occasionally in twin pregnancies with a shared placenta one twin may lose blood into the circulation of the other. At birth one twin may be pale and anaemic, while the other is polycythaemic.

Vaginal bleeding. Slight bleeding from the endometrium occasionally occurs as a result of withdrawal of maternal oestrogens.

Jaundice in the newborn infant

Jaundice in the neonatal period may be due to a variety of causes. Breakdown of red blood cells results in the production of indirect, non-conjugated bilirubin, which is insoluble in water and is carried in the serum bound to albumin. Normally this type of bilirubin is conjugated in the liver to form water-soluble bilirubin glycuronide which is excreted in the bile. Conjugation is effected by the glucuronyl transferase system of enzymes. In the newborn infant this enzyme system is at first inadequate, and the concentration of unconjugated bilirubin may rise in the serum for a few days and cause 'physiological jaundice'. In cases of haemolytic disease and in some premature infants the serum albumin becomes saturated with bilirubin, leaving free bilirubin to cross the blood-brain barrier and damage the basal ganglia. See kernicterus, p. 449.

Physiological jaundice. This does not begin before the second day; it may last for only a few days or until the 10th day. The skin is lemon yellow in colour, but the conjunctivae are only jaundiced in a few severe cases. The liver and spleen are not increased in size and the stools remain normal in colour. There is no fever or constitutional upset, although the infant may be sleepy and less eager for food. No special treatment is required and the prognosis is entirely favourable, except in premature infants in whom kernicterus can occur if the bilirubin level rises above 340 mmol/l (20 mg per 100 ml). In such cases exchange transfusion (p. 453) is indicated.

Jaundice in the neonatal period may have many pathological causes:

Haemolytic disease (Icterus gravis neonatorum). See Chapter 41, p. 447.

ABO and other group incompatibilities. See p. 454.

Congenital spherocytosis (acholuric jaundice). This is a rare cause of haemolytic anaemia and jaundice.

Congenital atresia of the bile ducts. This rare anomaly may be partial or complete. Jaundice appears at the end of the first week of life or later. The liver progressively enlarges and becomes firm, the stools become white and the urine contains bile. Laparotomy should always be advised as 15 per cent of the infants have extrahepatic atresia which can be treated surgically.

Sepsis. Sepsis, especially when accompanied by septicaemia, may cause anaemia and jaundice after the first few days of life. A urinary tract infection may be associated with jaundice of hepatic origin.

Syphilis. Congenital infection may cause cirrhosis with jaundice.

Toxoplasmosis. Mothers who have suffered an occult infection with the protozoon *Toxoplasma gondii* may give birth to infants affected by the disease. Internal hydrocephalus, choroidoretinitis, fits and mental retardation may result. If infection occurs shortly before birth the infant may have hepatosplenomegaly and jaundice. Diagnosis is made by complement fixation tests and tests for dye-modifying antibodies. There is no effective treatment.

Viral infections. Intrauterine infection with *rubella virus* or *cytomegalic virus* may cause neonatal jaundice associated with thrombocytopenic purpura and hepatosplenomegaly. For rubella see p. 227. In both cases estimation of the titre of antibodies, especially specific IgM, will assist in the diagnosis. It is important to remember that affected infants excrete live virus.

Infection with *herpes virus* is another cause of neonatal hepatitis with jaundice. The infection is usually acquired from the mother during delivery. In severe cases signs of general infection usually appear during the 2nd week. The disease is often fatal.

There is no certain evidence that the virus of infective hepatitis is transmitted to the fetus during maternal infection, but neonatal infection which is thought to be caused by one of the *hepatitis viruses* may occur, with hepatic enlargement and jaundice, and often with splenomegaly. The jaundice may be prolonged, with obstructive features clinically indistinguishable from those of congenital atresia of the bile ducts.

Coxsackie B5 virus may cause generalized infection of the newborn, with myocarditis, encephalitis and hepatitis. There is a high mortality.

Glucose-6-phosphate dehyrogenase deficiency. The genetically determined deficiency of this enzyme, which is essential for the survival of erythrocytes, is not uncommon in Asiatic and Mediterranean races, and a less severe form occurs in Africa. Spontaneous destruction of red cells in the neonatal period may cause haemolytic jaundice, and this may be precipitated by various drugs.

Galactosaemia. This inherited metabolic disorder usually presents with jaundice and hepatomegaly (see p. 511).

Cretinism. Prolonged neonatal jaundice without any obvious cause, especially in an apathetic anorexic infant, should raise suspicion of cretinism.

Management of neonatal jaundice.

The most important question to ask is when the jaundice appeared. Icterus appearing within the first 24 hours of life is almost certainly pathological and due to rhesus or ABO incompatibility, or to glucose-6-dehydrogenase deficiency. A Coombs' test, ABO and rhesus grouping of the infant, and examination of a blood film for spherocytes are obligatory.

Jaundice appearing from the 2nd to the 5th days of life is usually physiological, whereas jaundice appearing for the first time after this is usually pathological, and careful consideration of all the possibilities mentioned above is required.

In cases of early jaundice caused by haemolysis, apart from exchange transfusion, the bilirubin level can be reduced by two other forms of treatment. Phenobarbitone given to the mother before labour results in a lower incidence of neonatal jaundice, because the drug facilitates the enzyme systems in the infant's liver. However, a more effective measure is to give the infant phototherapy with a specially constructed unit that avoids overheating. The baby's eyes must be covered to avoid conjunctival reaction. Blue light converts bilirubin in the skin to a colourless compound which is not harmful to the brain.

Congenital malformations

The cause of many congenital malformations is unknown. Some are genetically determined; others have been attributed to pressure effects related to the intrauterine posture of the fetus, to the adverse effects of drugs, radiation, fetal infections or metabolic disturbances. The fetal tissues which are most actively growing at the time when the adverse factor operates are most likely to show the defect.

The malformations which may occur are numerous and varied. Some are incompatible with life and no treatment is possible. The lesions which are especially important to recognize in the neonatal period are those which endanger life but which, with prompt intervention, can be treated. Other lesions can be treated later in infancy.

Rubella syndrome. See p. 227.

Congenital heart disease. Exact diagnosis is particularly difficult at this age but the presence of cardiac disease should be recognized in most cases by careful examination. During the routine examination the apex beat and femoral pulses should be palpated. Since it is not always easy to feel the apex beat in the newborn it is useful to place a finger just below the xiphisternum to assess the strength of epigastric pulsation; this will be increased if there is cardiac enlargement.

Absent or weak femoral pulses will suggest the diagnosis of coarctation of the aorta. The blood pressure in all four limbs should be measured by the 'flush' method. A cuff is inflated until the limb is blanched. As the pressure is slowly released the limb will suddenly flush. The pressure reading at that moment gives the mean systolic pressure. In coarctation the pressure is lower in the legs than in the arms.

If the pulses in all four limbs are easily felt and seem to be collapsing in quality the diagnosis of patent ductus arteriosus is suggested, and there may be a harsh systolic murmur in the second left interspace close to the sternum. The murmur may not be continuous at this age.

Soft basal murmurs come and go in the normal newborn infant, but harsh basal murmurs are likely to be due to aortic or pulmonary stenosis. The commonest form of congenital heart disease, ventricular septal defect, usually does not produce symptoms or signs in the immediate neonatal period. It may take four weeks for the pulmonary vascular resistance to fall sufficiently to allow a significant pressure gradient between the ventricles to develop, and there will be no appreciable left to right shunt until this happens.

Cyanotic heart lesions have been mentioned on p. 468.

Laryngeal stridor. This may accompany inspiration in some newborn babies. It is worse with crying and quietens when the baby is asleep. There is often indrawing of the lower ribs. The cause is debatable, but it is usually attributed to congenital softening of the cartilage of the larynx, with infolding of the epiglottis during inspiration. The condition usually resolves by the time the infant is 18 months old. Rarer and more severe stridor may be caused by congenital anomalies such as a laryngeal web or cyst.

Oesophageal atresia and tracheal fistula.   See p. 490.

Intestinal obstruction.   See p. 492.

Imperforate anus.   This abnormality must be looked for carefully at the first examination. The gap between the anal dimple and the blind rectal pouch may be only membrane thick or several centimetres wide. The rectal pouch may communicate with the vagina, urethra or bladder. The infant must be referred for surgical treatment at once.

Umbilical variations.   The skin of the abdominal wall normally invests the base of the umbilical cord for a short distance, and when the cord separates the skin dimples to form the navel. If the skin extends onto the cord further than usual, separation of the cord leaves a protruding cylinder of skin. Such a *cutis navel* needs no treatment and will be taken in to the abdominal wall with growth. When the skin does not reach the base of the cord a wide raw area is left which heals by granulation and fibrosis—the *amnion navel*.

Meckel's diverticulum may form an intestinal fistula at the umbilicus. A persistent urachus may form a urinary fistula or a cystic swelling deep to the navel.

A single umbilical artery is found in a small number of infants and may be associated with other congenital abnormalities, often of the genito-urinary tract or the cardiovascular system.

Umbilical hernia. The gap in the rectus sheath through which the components of the cord enter the abdominal cavity can be felt as a ring after separation of the cord. Normally this closes down, but sometimes an umbilical hernia forms. Although a few cases will require surgical treatment later in childhood, the use of trusses, binders or coins is never indicated.

Exomphalos. The infant is born with an extensive defect of the anterior abdominal wall and the intestines are extruded, usually covered by peritoneum. The condition looks very grave, but if no other gross congenital defect exists the viscera should be covered with sterile dressings and surgical advice immediately obtained. It is often possible to repair the defect if the operation is performed at once with full antibiotic cover.

Cleft lip and cleft palate. These lesions cause surprisingly little difficulty in feeding. Breast feeding can be successfully achieved but bottle feeding may be more difficult, and it may be necessary to resort to cup and spoon. A cleft palate may permit milk to enter the nose and cause choking. Early reference to a plastic surgeon is advisable so that treatment can be planned.

Congenital dislocation of the hip. In the newborn infant this is a potential rather than an actual dislocation. Examination of the hips of the newborn for excessive mobility or for a characteristic click felt on full abduction of the flexed thighs is suggestive of dislocation. Because congenital dislocation of the hip is almost entirely preventable, it is important that all doctors who are involved with routine examination of the newborn should learn the technique of examination of the hips from a senior colleague who is experienced in the method. Orthopaedic advice must be sought in any doubtful case, and early treatment in abduction splints may prevent trouble in later infancy.

Talipes equinovarus. The intrauterine position of the fetus tends to produce this deformity, which only seldom persists. When true adduction is present treatment by manipulation and splinting must be started at once.

Spina bifida and meningocele. Failure of fusion of the vertebral arches permits herniation of the meninges at any level in the spinal column, usually in the lumbar area. The herniation may be covered with skin or only by a bluish membranous roof, and the sac may include nerve roots or spinal cord (myelomeningocele), which can be recognized as a flat or raised neural plaque in the midline. The absence of the various coverings which protect the cord allows meningeal infection to occur early, but this can be prevented by immediate surgery to cover the defect. However, the overall prognosis is poor with the more severe lesions, with complete paralysis of the legs, incontinence of urine and faeces, and the probable association with hydrocephalus. It is important that babies with a relatively good prognosis should be sent to a special centre where appropriate surgery can be performed without delay. Only experience can decide whether it is justifiable to operate on very severe cases.

Neural tube defects can be diagnosed *in utero* by amniocentesis and testing the amniotic fluid for α-fetoprotein (see p. 370). Testing the maternal serum for fetoprotein may serve as a preliminary screening test, but the diagnosis must be confirmed by amniocentesis before termination of pregnancy is considered. The defect may also be demonstrated by ultrasonic examination.

Hydrocephalus. Hydrocephalus is caused by obstruction to the normal circulation of the cerebrospinal fluid, and this is often caused by a congenital abnormality of the brain. The head is large and the sutures and fontanelles are wide. The skull is globular and appears enormous in comparison with the small triangular face, with bulging of the forehead and above the ears. There is sometimes an associated myelomeningocele. The condition may be present before birth and obstruct labour (see p. 294), or the baby may show slight enlargement of the head after birth. If hydrocephalus is suspected the head circumference is measured and recorded every three days, and if the rate of growth is much faster than normal a neurosurgical opinion is sought, as it is possible to prevent progression of the hydrocephalus by insertion of a valve.

Down's syndrome. This is caused by a chromosomal abnormality. In about 95 per cent of cases there are 47 chromosomes instead of 46. The extra chromosome is present because of non-disjunction of chromosome 21 (trisomy 21). In a small proportion of affected infants there are 46 chromosomes, but one is abnormally large, probably number 15 which incorporates part of number 21 from a translocation.

The syndrome can often be diagnosed soon after birth. The infant has a flat face with slanting eyes ('mongolism'), epicanthic folds, a snub nose, a mouth like an inverted bow, and often a protruding tongue. The head is round with a poorly developed occiput and unusual ears. The posterior and third fontanelle are often easily palpable. The infant is hypotonic with over-extensible joints. The hands show a single transverse palmar crease, and there is a simian cleft between the great and the next toe. Congenital heart disease may be detected.

The incidence of the syndrome is about 1.5 per 1000 births. The incidence rises sharply with maternal age and reaches 1 in 50 when the mother's age is over 40. Chromosomal studies should be undertaken when a young mother gives birth to an affected infant. If the baby is found to have a translocation of chromosome 21, the discovery of translocation in either parent indicates a greatly increased risk of another affected child in any subsequent pregnancy. If it is found in the mother approximately 20 per cent of her later children may be affected; and if in the father the risk is about 6 per cent.

Down's syndrome may be diagnosed in utero by amniocentesis to obtain fetal amniotic cells for tissue culture and chromosomal study. If the abnormality is found to be present termination of pregnancy might be considered. Such a test should be offered to women over 40, to those who already have an affected child, and if either parent is known to have an abnormal chromosomal pattern, provided that they understand that the test carries some risk to the fetus and takes time, and that termination may not be possible until the pregnancy is at about 20 weeks.

Renal agenesis (Potter's syndrome). This condition is often associated with oligohydramnios. Both kidneys fail to develop. The infant looks prematurely senile, with wide set eyes, flattened nose, a receding chin, and low set ears with poorly formed cartilage. The infant dies within a few days.

Abnormalities of the male genito-urinary system. All degrees of hypospadias and epispadias may be met. In the milder degrees of hypospadias it may be thought that the meatal orifice is not patent, but careful search will reveal a minute orifice on the ventral surface of the corona or shaft of the penis. The meatus is sometimes stenosed and so it is important to see the urinary stream, as meatotomy is sometimes required. Coronal hypospadias is also sometimes associated with curvature of the penis (chordee). In such cases it is important to avoid circumcision, as the surgeon may wish to use preputial skin during corrective operation at a later date.

Hydrocele may occur in the neonatal period, but requires no treatment as it usually resolves spontaneously within a few weeks.

Circumcision. There are really no medical grounds for circumcision in infancy. Retraction of the foreskin may suggest the presence of phimosis, but if the prepuce is drawn gently forwards (as happens during micturition) it will be seen that it opens up to reveal an adequate channel. Indeed the foreskin should never be retracted in the baby, because this may lead to tearing and scarring and genuine phimosis as a result. The parents should be advised to leave the foreskin alone and allow it to retract normally as the boy grows. The presence of the preputial covering prevents meatal ulceration which could otherwise occur from the contact of wet napkins.

Ritual circumcision is practised in Jewish infants and is usually performed on the 8th day. It is sometimes necessary to advise that the operation should be postponed if the infant is ill, jaundiced or shows undue loss of weight. It is wise to maintain a close watch for haemorrhage for the 12 hours following the circumcision, which is not always performed by the usual surgical technique.

Abnormalities of the female genitalia. Pseudohermaphroditism is usually due to the adrenogenital syndrome. (See *Gynaecology by Ten Teachers* p. 73). Hypertrophy of the clitoris may occur if the mother has been given large doses of progestogens for habitual abortion.

Labial adhesions. The external genitalia may appear abnormal because adhesions between the labia minora obscure the urethral and vaginal orifices. The adhesions separate easily if the labia are drawn apart.

Infection in the newborn infant

The newborn infant has a low natural resistance to infection and may succumb to infections which are of low pathogenicity to adults, the organisms being carried by attendants who have themselves no symptoms. For this reason, carriers of streptococci in the throat or individuals suffering from low grade staphylococcal infections or head colds represent a great potential danger to infants in their care.

The response to infection shown by newborn infants is very different from that shown by older children. Symptoms which denote neonatal infection are seldom local, but are general and merely indicate a general deterioration in health. The onset of serious infection in the newborn infant is often insidious, and it may be well established before it is realized that the infant is gravely ill. Vomiting and diarrhoea are commonly seen in infants suffering from infection which appears to be remote from the gastro-intestinal tract. Refusal to feed, lethargy and sleepiness are common early symptoms in generalized infection.

The temperature response to infection is seldom marked, and quite a severe infection may cause fever of only 0.5°C. With very severe infections there may sometimes be a subnormal temperature, slow pulse rate, reduced respiration rate, sleepiness and collapse without localizing signs. The symptoms do not always point to the site of the infection and a careful clinical search for the site may be necessary. Frequently the help of the laboratory is required to localize the infective process. Examination of the urine, throat or umbilical swabs, blood culture and sometimes lumbar puncture may be necessary to determine the nature of the infection.

Respiratory tract. *Head cold and nasal catarrh.* When a young infant contracts a cold in the head, the nasal secretion may cause embarrassment during feeding and the infant may be fretful at this time. The real danger to the infant is in the supine position, when infected secretion drains down the back of the throat, and with the poor cough reflex of the infant may pass the barrier of the larynx and cause collapse and consolidation of part of the lungs by blocking a bronchus, especially the middle lobe bronchus. These infants are best nursed prone on a firm mattress which is raised at the head end to an angle of about 20°. Another possible hazard for a snuffly baby is apnoea during sleep when both nostrils are blocked, and this is one of the possible causes of sudden infant death. Nasal drops can perpetuate local irritation, but they may be beneficial for 1 or 2 days.

Otitis media. The relatively straight and wide Eustachian tube forms an easy channel for ascending infection, or the passage of infected secretions or vomited material. The symptoms are those of low grade fever, irritability and general malaise, and the site of infection is only discovered on full routine examination, which must always include examination of the tympanic membrane. Spread of infection to the meninges is a possible danger. Early diagnosis and antibiotic therapy are essential, with myringotomy when indicated.

Pneumonia. The infection is usually a descending infection from the upper respiratory tract to the lung which has already a lesion such as atelectasis or has been damaged by inhalation of mucus, food or vomitus. Cough is an uncommon symptom in infancy, and attention is usually drawn to the disease by a rising respiration rate, cyanosis, pallor or a slight rise in temperature, with anorexia and general malaise. Examination of the chest may show little that is abnormal. The presence of fine râles may be all that is found.

The essentials of treatment are to maintain oxygenation, which may require an oxygen tent, to ensure an adequate fluid intake, and to give an appropriate antibiotic. Nose and throat swabs are taken to discover the offending organism and its sensitivities.

Mouth. Infection of the buccal mucosa and tongue by *Candida albicans* is not infrequent in bottle-fed or debilitated infants. It may also occur during delivery if the mother has vaginal thrush. There are greyish-white plaques which resemble milk curds but which cannot be wiped off. The constitutional upset is slight, but the soreness of the mouth may cause the baby to refuse feeds. Rarely, thrush spreads down the gastro-intestinal tract to cause oesophagitis, gastritis or enteritis. Sore buttocks may be caused by thrush. During antibiotic therapy the lungs may be invaded by the fungus which multiplies under cover of the antibiotic which inhibits the normal bacterial flora.

Treatment is by local application of nystatin 100 000 units in 1 ml of fluid, which is swabbed around the mouth 4 times daily for 1 week. The application of gentian violet 1 per cent in aqueous solution is probably just as effective, but aesthetically it is less pleasant. Perianal infection is treated with nystatin ointment.

Gastro-enteritis. See p. 494.

Infection of the urinary tract. This is as common in the male newborn infant as in the female. Symptoms suggestive of infection without physical signs should always call for investigation of the renal tract. Renal tenderness is seldom found, and the predominant symptoms may be vomiting, diarrhoea and reluctance to feed. The temperature may be only slightly raised. Culture of a clean specimen of urine often shows coliforms, *Streptococcus faecalis* and infrequently *B.pyocyaneus* or *B. proteus*. This finding should not be taken as evidence of renal infection unless pus cells are also found in the urine. The discovery of 5 to 10 leucocytes in each high power field or 10^5 organisms per ml are highly suggestive of renal infection. In doubtful cases it may be necessary to culture a specimen obtained by suprapubic aspiration.

Many infants with pyelonephritis suffer from a congenital malformation of the renal tract causing some degree of obstruction or ureteric reflux. Such infections are resistant to treatment, and intravenous pyelography is often indicated.

Treatment demands a full course of the appropriate antibiotic.

Septicaemia.   This is not uncommon in the newborn infant, following cutaneous or umbilical infection. The general symptoms of infection with fever and splenic enlargement suggest the diagnosis, and blood culture is carried out at the least suspicion.

Osteomyelitis.   Infection of a long bone or the maxilla may be a complication of staphylococcal infection, usually of the skin or umbilicus. Three to 6 weeks after the initial infection there is general malaise with low grade fever, followed by reluctance to use a limb. Redness and swelling and occasionally the development of septic arthritis in a contiguous joint may follow. Full antibiotic treatment and orthopaedic advice about the drainage of pus are essential.

Meningitis.   Coliform bacteria are often responsible for meningitis at this age, but any of the common bacteria may be found. The disease seldom presents in classical form and there may be no definite physical signs. Lumbar puncture is always justified when signs of infection are present without localizing signs.

Skin infection.   The most common skin infection is an eruption of small pustules caused by staphylococci. The soft skin of the infant is easily traumatized by clothing or rubbing with the towel after the bath. The infecting organism may be present in the nose or on the skin of nurses or doctors, or may be transferred from other infected babies. The umbilicus is often colonized, and the infection spreads from there.

Pemphigus neonatorum is a bullous or vesicular eruption caused by streptococcal or staphylococcal infection. It is now rarely seen. Large fluid-containing blisters raise the outer skin layers, which are easily rubbed off to leave raw areas which become secondarily infected. If the lesions are widespread there is a high mortality.

(Another unrelated variety of pemphigus occurs in cases of congenital syphilis, in which bullae appear on the palms and soles).

Any infant with a skin infection should be isolated. An appropriate antibiotic is given systemically; local application is not used as it may cause sensitivity reactions. Gentian violet in 1 per cent aqueous solution may be applied.

Conjunctivitis.   If gonococcal conjunctivitis is a possibility, (and any severe conjunctivitis, especially if it is bilateral, gives rise to anxiety), the help of the laboratory should be sought in taking bacterial swabs which are plated directly onto warm blood agar. Smears are also immediately examined. Penicillin eye-drops are instilled every 15 minutes for the first 6 hours, and then 6-hourly; and penicillin is also injected intramuscularly until the bacterial report is received.

In many mild cases routine bacterial swabs only show a growth of staphylococci or diphtheroids, or there may be no growth. *Staphylococcus epidermidis* may only be a secondary invader following chemical conjunctivitis caused by antiseptics such as chlorhexidine used during labour. In cases with only mild conjunctivitis and no ground for suspicion of gonococcal infection it is common practice to start with instillation of chloramphenicol eye drops until the bacterial report is received. If the conjunctivitis persists for more than a week the possibility of infection with *Chlamydia trachomatis* must be considered. If it is found both parents should be referred to a genito-urinary physician. Infection in the mother's genital tract may produce few if any symptoms, but this organism may cause urethritis in the male.

Dacrocystitis. The nasolachrymal duct may be blocked by a congenital septum. Infection often follows and pus can be expressed by pressure in the angle between the inner canthus and the nose. The help of an ophthalmic surgeon must be sought, with a view to probing of the duct.

Umbilical infection. The stump of the umbilical cord desiccates and separates, usually by the 7th day, leaving a raw area which heals by granulation. Until healing is complete this is a warm moist region that provides an excellent site for colonization by bacteria. Not only may these organisms cause mild local infection, but they may be carried to other infants in whom they cause serious infections. Chlorhexidine in spirit (BPC) should be applied to the area, followed by hexochlorophane dusting powder (BPC).

Infection with a virulent organism may be followed by spread of infection along the umbilical vein to the blood stream and liver, with septicaemia, jaundice and haemolytic anaemia. The infant becomes ill with general signs of infection, and often enlargement of the liver. A swab from the navel and a blood culture to establish the nature and sensitivities of the infecting organism is followed at once by full antibiotic treatment. The prognosis is grave.

General treatment of infection in the newborn

Four main principles of treatment must be observed:

1. The general condition of the infant must be maintained. Alterations may have to be made in the feeding routine. A change to a more dilute or more easily digested feed may be necessary. In severe infections expressed breast milk is of great value if it can be obtained. If the infant tires easily feeds may be given in smaller amounts at shorter intervals. The total daily intake must be sufficient for the infant's needs and must compensate for any unusual losses from diarrhoea. If the infant cannot take adequate fluid by mouth intravenous infusion or tube feeding may be necessary.

2. If the lungs are involved or there is cardiovascular failure oxygenation

must be maintained. If anaemia occurs great benefit may be derived from a small transfusion of 50 to 100 ml of fresh blood.

3. The temperature must be kept within reasonable limits by the application of warmth, or by cooling if hyperpyrexia is present.

4. The infection must be controlled by an appropriate antibiotic. The range of bactericidal drugs is very wide, and if the organism causing the infection is known and its sensitivities have been determined the correct drug for the case can be employed. The newborn infant may show responses to antibiotics which do not occur in older patients, and care to give the correct dose may be very important. Certain drugs have special disadvantages for neonatal use.

Long-acting sulphonamides replace bilirubin on the binding sites on plasma albumin, and may therefore free the bilirubin and increase any risk of kernicterus.

Chloramphenicol is cleared from the body after conjugation as glycuronide. Since glycuronide conjugation is at a low level in the early days of life the drug may accumulate in the body. Newborn or premature babies may show collapse and hypothermia after treatment with this drug—the 'grey-baby syndrome'. It must be used with great discretion.

Table 44.1

Drug	Route of administration	Dose (mg/kg/24 hours)	
Ampicillin	oral, i.m., i.v.	100	
Cephaloridine	i.m.	35	
Chloramphenicol	oral, i.m., i.v.	25–50	To be avoided if there is an alternative
Cloxacillin	oral, i.m., i.v.	100	
Erythromycin	oral, i.v.	25–40	Oral, 10 i.v.
Fusidic acid	oral	20–40	
Gentamycin	i.m.	6	Blood levels must be checked
Kanamycin	i.m.	15	
Nitrofurantoin	oral	8	To be avoided if there is an alternative
Neomycin	oral	50	
Penicillin G	i.m.	150	(240 000 units)
Penicillin V	oral	60	
Nystatin	oral	100 000 units per dose, 4-hourly	

Apart from nystatin these drugs are usually given orally or intramuscularly at 8-hourly intervals, or intravenously by slow bolus injection every 4 hours. It may be possible to obtain estimations of the blood levels of the commonly used antibiotics, so that it is possible to adjust the dose to the best therapeutic range.

Tetracycline given to premature or newborn infants may cause yellow staining of the deciduous teeth, and interfere with bone growth. Since there are safer alternative antibiotics available, the use of tetracyclines for babies is not longer advised.

In the newborn infant it is not desirable to await the results of the laboratory investigations, which may take 48 hours, before starting treatment. Empirical treatment is begun as soon as the signs of infection have been detected, using the antibiotic which is thought most likely to overcome the infection.

Some of the antibiotics commonly used during the neonatal period and their usual dosage are shown in Table 44.1.

Infection with Group B streptococcus. This organism requires special mention because in recent years it has been shown to be an important pathogen for the newborn baby. The infection is acquired from the maternal genital tract. There may be fulminating infection with rapidly progressive septicaemia and pneumonia within a few hours of birth, with a clinical picture hardly distinguishable from that of respiratory distress syndrome. The respiration rate is raised with cyanosis, and x-ray examination shows extensive consolidation in both lungs. The organism may be found in ear, throat and umbilical swabs, gastric aspirate and in the blood. Gentamycin is given intramuscularly with large doses of penicillin intravenously. The mortality is high.

A delayed type of infection also occurs, in which the infant presents with meningitis at about the 7th day. With vigorous antibiotic treatment these babies usually recover fully.

Metabolic disturbances in the newborn infant

Hypoglycaemia. Hypoglycaemia in the newborn is present when the true plasma glucose concentration is below 1.1 mmol/l (20 mg/100 ml). It is particularly likely to occur in the first 72 hours of life in babies who are small for gestational age, but it may develop in any baby under stress, as for example in the respiratory distress syndrome, in congestive cardiac failure or following exchange transfusion. It may be found in infants of diabetic mothers (see p. 225) and in other infants who are large for gestational age. The diagnosis should be considered in any baby who exhibits a sudden fall in temperature, twitching, convulsions, eye-rolling, apathy, refusal to feed, apnoeic spells or, in extreme cases, coma. Consideration of the likely cause is important in management.

In the light-for dates baby, or the baby who has suffered from placental insufficiency, there has been depletion of the glycogen stores and the aim must be to replenish them. In these babies although they have no symptoms 3-hourly Dextrostix tests on blood from a heel stab may reveal low levels of glucose. Such asymptomatic hypoglycaemia has an excellent prognosis and symptoms can be prevented by early feeding. The most certain way of achieving this is by continuous feeding through a nasogastric tube for 24 to 48 hours, starting with 60 ml of feed per kg per day and increasing progressively. If symptoms have already occurred nasogastric feeding is started at once without waiting for laboratory confirmation of the plasma glucose level. *If there have been convulsions* glucose solution, 3 ml per kg of 20 per cent solution, is given *immediately*. In other cases the laboratory estimation can be awaited before giving the glucose. Thereafter Dextrostix tests are carried out to confirm that the hypoglycaemia has been relieved. Only in few resistant cases is it necessary to administer 10 per cent glucose solution intravenously. The advantage of intragastric infusion is the ease of administration, and the avoidance of the risk of reactive hypoglycaemia if the intravenous infusion stops for one reason or another. The baby is also receiving valuable nutrients.

The problem in the large-for-dates babies or the babies of diabetic mothers is different. In them the liver is likely to be full of glycogen, but hyperplasia of the islet cells in the pancreas results in high blood insulin levels, particularly in response to glucose administration. The widespread practice of giving intermittent glucose drinks to these babies can sometimes provoke hypoglycaemia. In practice early milk feeding has proved most successful. Glucose can be released from glycogen stores by administering glucagon, but it is more practical to give small doses of hydrocortisone (5 mg 6-hourly) if hypoglycaemia proves to be persistent in these babies.

Hypocalcaemia.   Some preterm or small-for-dates babies develop symptoms from hypocalcaemia (tetany) soon after birth. Tetany may also occur in babies fed on high-solute artificial feeds, usually between the 7th and 10th days. These infants show twitching and neuromuscular irritability, increased muscular tone, and often vomiting. If the plasma calcium level is lower than 1.8 mmol/l (7 mg/100 ml) treatment will depend on whether convulsions are continuing. If they have ceased it is sufficient to add 3 ml of 10 per cent calcium gluconate solution to each feed (which should be of human or low-solute milk). The total daily dose of calcium gluconate solution should not exceed 20 ml, otherwise diarrhoea may occur. If convulsions are continuing the calcium gluconate solution is diluted to 2.5 per cent concentration with 5 per cent glucose solution and injected *slowly* intravenously until the convulsions cease. Not more than 4 ml/kg body weight of this solution should be given at one time. The heart rate is monitored during the injection, which is stopped if bradycardia occurs. Thereafter calcium gluconate is added to the feeds until the plasma calcium concentration rises to normal.

Inborn errors of metabolism.   Many of these are not detected until after the neonatal period. Phenylketonuria and galactosaemia deserve mention as their early detection will lead to dietary measures which will reduce their ill effects.

Phenylketonuria is inherited as a recessive condition. There is inability to convert phenylalanine to tyrosine. Phenylalanine accumulates in the body fluids, and when the blood level rises to a dangerous point alternative metabolic pathways convert it to phenylpyruvic acid and other substances which are excreted in the urine.

The infant appears normal, and is often strikingly blond with blue eyes. Deterioration occurs as the child grows, with progressive neurological disease and mental retardation. Phenylalanine is not excreted in the urine until the blood level reaches 1.8 mmol/l (30 mg per 100 ml) which is a toxic level, but the renal threshold for phenyl ketones is about half this. However, testing for phenylpyruvic acid in the urine with ferric chloride has not proved to be a satisfactory screening test in newborn infants, and the Guthrie microbiological test for the blood level of phenylalanine must be performed. For the test one drop of blood is taken on the 7th day (i.e. after at least 6 days of milk feeds). The test gives early warning of the disease, and if treatment with a diet low in phenylalanine is started in early infancy mental retardation may be prevented.

Galactosaemia is inherited as a recessive trait. There is a defect in the metabolism of galactose, which is derived from the lactose in milk. Enzyme lack prevents the conversion of galactose to glucose-1-phosphate, which is necessary if galactose is to be utilized by the tissues. Galactose accumulates in the body and appears in the urine. The infant appears normal at birth, but listlessness, vomiting, anorexia and weight loss soon appear, with jaundice and hepatomegaly. Cataracts, mental retardation and cirrhosis of the liver develop in untreated cases.

Galactose in the urine is detected by Clinitest strips, but not by Clinistix. Routine testing of the urine of babies with jaundice, especially those with hepatomegaly, will detect the condition. The diagnosis is confirmed by urine chromatography, and deficiency of the enzyme (galactose-1-phosphate uridyl transferase) can be confirmed by testing the infant's red blood corpuscles. Treatment consists in withdrawing all dietary lactose and feeding synthetic galactose-free milk.

Neonatal cold injury. Babies are sometimes admitted after cold injury. They are cold to touch, apathetic and immobile. They may refuse to feed. The colour may be pink, but there is oedema of the hands and feet, and a firm texture to the subcutaneous fat. The rectal temperature may be 27–32°C, the respiration and pulse rate are slow. They must be warmed very gradually to a normal temperature while glucose solution is given intravenously. Antibiotic cover should be given. See also p. 513

Premature and 'special care' babies

Infants who have suffered birth trauma, those with congenital abnormalities, haemolytic disease or infection, and those who are premature, immature or dysmature (including infants of diabetic mothers) require special care in paediatric units. The terms premature, immature and dysmature have led to much misunderstanding. The old definition of 'prematurity' has been retained by the World Health Organization, and includes any baby that weighs 2.5 kg (5½ pounds) or less at birth, irrespective of gestational age. This definition fails to take into consideration the variations in birth weight in different races or in multiple births, nor does it distinguish between preterm births and babies who are born near term but are small-for-dates. There are also some babies who weigh more than 2.5 kg but are manifestly immature because they are born prematurely. We should try to separate three important groups of babies at special risk:

1. Preterm babies, born before 37 weeks gestation but with weight appropriate for their gestational age.
2. Small-for-dates babies, or small for their gestational age.
3. Large-for-dates babies, or large for their gestational age.

About 30 per cent of babies who are born early (preterm) are also small for gestational age. There is often uncertainty about gestational age. Methods of attempting to assess fetal maturity are discussed on p. 52.

After the baby is born gestational age may be assessed by using tables which include such factors as body proportions, presence or absence of lanugo hair, genital development, auricular cartilage formation and neonatal reflexes, and these are claimed to be accurate within two weeks. A rapid and almost equally accurate assessment can be made from the time of appearance of certain neonatal reflexes.

When intrauterine malnutrition starts early in pregnancy the head circumference and weight are in their normal proportions, but when the onset is late in pregnancy the head is disproportionately large because of relatively normal growth of the brain at the expense of the rest of the body. It is particularly important to recognize the latter type of case in which there is depletion of glycogen stores in the liver and heart, and depletion of fat stores, because these depletions make such babies more susceptible to intranatal hypoxia, hypothermia and hypoglycaemia.

In general, if the birth weight of the baby falls below the 10th centile of the expected weight for the gestational age he is assumed to be small-for-gestational age, but the baby's appearance is often characteristic, with dry folds of lax skin. A graph constructed from the weight in kg and the head circumference in cm has proved to be of practical value. The ratio of the 50th centile weight to the 50th centile head circumference is plotted against the gestational age, and this gives a curve which falls from a ratio of 26:1 at 28 weeks to 10:1 at term. When the observed ratio for the baby lies above this line he is small-for-gestational age and will need special care.

The aetiology of intrauterine malnutrition is not well understood, and may be multifactorial. Placental insufficiency, including cases of maternal hypertension and proteinuria, is generally accepted as the most important single factor, although infections, endocrine and chromosomal aberrations have been incriminated, especially when growth is affected throughout pregnancy. Excessive smoking is an important cause of growth failure. Excessive consumption of alcohol and drug addiction affect the growth and

development of the fetus and produce recognizable neonatal syndromes.
The following table summarizes some of the more important considerations relating to small babies.

Table 44.2

	Preterm (weight appropriate for gestational age)	Light-for-dates (small for gestational age)
Cause	Short gestation	Intrauterine malnutrition (placental insufficiency)
Hazards	Respiratory distress syndrome Hypothermia Infection Anaemia Hyperbilirubinaemia Intraventricular or sub-arachnoid haemorrhage	Hypoglycaemia Hypocalcaemia Hypothermia Hyperbilirubinaemia
Crown-heel length	Less than 45 cm	Usually more than 45 cm
Head circumference	Less than 33 cm	Often more than 33 cm
General appearance	Tendency to lie with frog-like posture Skin thin and red	Position variable Skin dry and may be shiny with loose folds around thighs and buttocks from loss of subcutaneous tissue

(Modified from *Practical Neonatal Paediatrics*, Blackwell Scientific Publications.)

Principles of special care

The purpose of special care is to control the environment according to the special needs of the baby, to monitor all the important bodily functions in order to detect any signs of illness immediately and to treat them without delay, and to use special feeding techniques if necessary. It is important to remember that premature infants have contributed largely to the number of 'battered babies' (30 per cent in recorded series) so that it is essential to involve the mother as closely as possible with the care of her baby, including handling him under supervision. Prematurity is rarely a bar to breast feeding. In several maternity units it has been shown that with encouragement breast feeding can be established with most low birth weight babies, and this is the best way of keeping the mother closely integrated with her child.

Temperature. Small infants become hypothermic very quickly. They have a large surface area relative to their weight which permits rapid heat loss, and there is deficiency of subcutaneous fat for insulation. There is also a deficiency of brown adipose tissue which is present in significant amounts in term infants, and which can metabolise rapidly to produce heat. It is therefore necessary to provide a high and constant environmental temperature. If it is decided to nurse the baby naked in an incubator to improve observation, excessive heat loss by radiation can be reduced by placing a Perspex heat shield (with one end closed to prevent a cooling through draught) over the baby. However, there is a tendency to return to the old tradition of clothing the infant. The covering provided by a thin cotton gown and a stockinette hat incorporating a layer of gamgee is sufficient to make it much easier to maintain the body temperature. Heat loss is also minimized by maintaining a high environmental temperature. With the room temperature at 27°C the infant's rectal temperature should remain at about 37°C if the incubator temperature is as follows:

Table 44.3

Weight of infant	Temperature of incubator
1 kg	35°C
2 kg	34°C
3 kg	33°C

The temperature of the incubator is reduced by 1°C weekly. The larger babies stabilize their temperatures quite quickly and can soon be transferred to a cot and then to a cooler room (24°C). For infants weighing less than 1 kg it may be necessary to make special adjustments to the incubator to raise the temperature further. The use of humidifiers in incubators is no longer recommended because of the increased risk of infection. It must be remembered that infants can lose heat during resuscitative procedures so that these are best carried out under a heat shield or canopy of approved make. When transferring a baby to hospital it should be well wrapped in gamgee, or preferably transferred in a special ready warmed portable incubator. Swaddlers made of aluminium foil are effective in retaining the baby's own heat, but can prevent heat reaching a baby which is cold.

Infection. Low birth weight babies are particularly susceptible to infection, which can be carried from one baby to another on the hands of an attendant or doctor. The most scrupulous care must be taken with hand washing, using special washing solutions containing a suitable antiseptic such as chlorhexidine. It is not necessary to wear masks, but any member of the staff with a respiratory infection should be excluded from the unit.

Feeding. Preterm infants have poor swallowing and coughing reflexes and methods of feeding must prevent aspiration into the lungs. At first it will be necessary to give tube feeds. Small frequent feeds will not lead to overdistension of the stomach, and therefore there will be less risk of aspiration and of apnoea due to embarrassment of respiration. The present consensus opinion is that an attempt should be made to keep up with the rapid rate of weight gain which normally occurs *in utero*. With milk feeds this entails giving quite largely large volumes throughout the 24 hours. This can be safely achieved by continuous infusion through a nasogastric tube. The method is safe and trouble-free, provided that certain basic rules are followed.

The infant is nursed prone on a firm mattress covered by absorbent material; two thicknesses of soft paper are ideal. It is an advantage to have the head raised by tipping the mattress to an angle of 20°; this reduces regurgitation and makes sure that no regurgitated milk is aspirated. A moderately fine PVC tube is passed through the nose into the stomach. The correct distance is gauged by measuring the distance from the tip of the nose to the lower end of the sternum—usually about 20 cm. The part of the tube adjacent to the nose is then marked with strapping. Fluid is withdrawn with a syringe, and if it is colourless and acid to litmus the tube is in the correct position and is then taped firmly to the cheek. If green fluid is obtained the tube is withdrawn 2 cm and aspiration is repeated. Once the infusion has been started aspiration is performed at least 3 times in each 24 hours, and the tube is changed every third day. The milk may be given through a disposable intravenous giving set, the bottle containing the milk being hung about 1 m above the infant, and the rate of infusion carefully controlled. An alternative method is to use a constant infusion pump, especially when very small volumes are being given. A disadvantage with these methods of feeding is that fat in the milk tends to be lost as it may become layered on the sides of the apparatus.

One hour after birth, feeding is started with 5 per cent glucose solution, followed by milk after 2 hours. If expressed breast milk is not available a low-solute cow's milk preparation is used. The initial volume of feed is 60 ml/kg/24 hours, which is increased by 30 ml/kg/24 hours up to a maximum of 240 ml/kg/24 hours provided that it is well tolerated. If breast milk is used the maximum may be increased to 270 ml/kg/24 hours. A careful watch is kept on the baby's abdomen and if this is unduly distended the infusion is discontinued to allow the distension to subside, and the daily rate is put back to that of the previous day for 24 hours. By using the technique described these large volumes of feed have not been associated with aspiration pneumonia or an increased tendency to necrotising enterocolitis.

Continuous infusion is usually continued until the infant's weight reaches 2 kg before changing to intermittent feeding, but if the mother intends to breast feed, the baby can be put to the breast for short periods while the infusion is temporarily stopped, thereby providing a stimulus to lactation. When intermittent feeding is started the feeds are given frequently at first and then gradually the intervals are increased to a 3-hourly regime.

Intravenous feeding with glucose, amino acids and lipid may have a place in the management of infants with necrotizing entercolitis or after intestinal resection, but there is no convincing evidence that it improves the prognosis for infants of low birth weight.

Early and adequate feeding prevents hypoglycaemia (see p. 509) and reduces the maximum serum bilirubin level.

From the second week vitamin supplements are added, such as Abidec 0.6 ml daily, which would provide vitamin A 4000 units, vitamin D 400 units and vitamin C 50 mg, with small amounts of vitamin B complex. In addition iron is given as ferrous fumarate or ferrous sulphate in a dose to provide approximately 10 mg of elemental iron daily.

Apnoeic spells with cyanosis.   Preterm infants are especially susceptible to prolonged periods of apnoea which may be life-threatening, but if the baby is stimulated to breathe within 15 seconds from the onset, normal respiration is re-established without much difficulty. Longer periods of apnoea may not respond to simple methods of stimulation, and the baby may then require resuscitation by intubation. It is therefore advisable to use an apnoea monitor, and set the alarm to go off after 10 seconds of apnoea. If apnoeic spells become frequent oral theophylline cholate in small doses has proved to be of value, but the drug is dangerously toxic if the dose is exceeded, so that its use cannot be recommended unreservedly if facilities are not available for checking blood levels.

The possibility of hypoglycaemia or of intraventricular haemorrhage has to be considered when apnoeic attacks are severe and fail to respond to treatment.

Other hazards.   *Respiratory distress syndrome.* (p. 466), *hyperbilirubinaemia* (p. 449), *hypoglycaemia* (p. 509) and *hypocalcaemia* (p. 510) are special hazards in low birth weight babies that have already been described.

45

Vital statistics

Vital statistics are essential for the planning of health services, and also allow doctors or hospitals to compare their work with that of others, so as to show where progress might be made or where failures have occurred. Because childbirth is usually normal and any one person has limited experience of abnormal cases, pooling of results is necessary if false impressions are to be avoided.

The collection of obstetric statistics

The following account relates to England and Wales, but to a greater or less extent vital statistics are collected in most other countries.

In England and Wales a national census is taken every 10 years. All births, marriages and deaths are notified to the Registrars, and from these notifications statistics are compiled and regularly published. Many maternity hospitals compile their own statistics and prepare an annual summary, but even when this information is not published it is of interest to those concerned and may help them to improve their practice.

Birth rate. In this country the average number of children per family is less than 2.3; this no longer replaces the population, which is falling. From the Registrars' returns the birth rate is calculated. The *crude birth rate* is the number of live births per 1000 total population. Since this population includes men, children and women beyond childbearing age it is more informative to relate the number of live births to the number of women aged between 15 and 44. This gives the *fertility rate*, which is expressed as the number of live births per 1000 women of these ages.

There was a fall in the total annual number of births in the years 1944 to 1955, then there was an increase each year until 1964, after which the annual number has been falling again. The decline stopped in 1978.

In unsophisticated areas of the world where little contraception is practised the crude birth rate is of the order of 50, against which the rate of 11.5 for England and Wales is small. Yet in the developing countries the total population may not rise much, because with lack of development go high stillbirth and infant mortality rates, and a high death rate. When these fall because of better medical services and greater wealth, the community reaction is often a wider use of contraception, in the knowledge that most children born alive will survive.

Obstetric statistics.   From the obstetrician's point of view the Maternal Mortality Rate and Perinatal Mortality Rate are of obvious importance, as they give some indication of the standard of practice and of the health of women. The number of deaths during infancy is an index of the work of paediatricians and also of public health measures directed against infectious diseases but, as will be shown later, the death of an infant in the first week after delivery often has an obstetric cause.

Maternal mortality

In the nineteenth century the number of deaths of women from childbearing was appalling, chiefly from sepsis but also from eclampsia, from disproportion and other complications of labour, and from haemorrhage. Even in 1928, long after the introduction of aseptic surgery, for every 1000 births 4.28 women died; that is to say that any woman embarking on pregnancy had a 1 in 250 chance of dying. With such results it is not surprising that the first task of obstetricians was to make childbearing safer for the mother, and the fate of the fetus was of lesser consideration. In recent years the maternal mortality has fallen to such low levels that it is no longer so useful as an index of obstetric failure or success, and now more attention is given to fetal mortality. Nevertheless every maternal death is a major tragedy, and maternal mortality studies are of great importance for everyone who practises obstetrics.

In the 50 years since 1928 the maternal mortality has fallen from over 4 to 0.12 per 1000 total births. This has largely been due to two groups of factors: (1) the control of infection, blood transfusion, and a readier recourse to operative treatment which has been made safer by advances in anaesthesia and resuscitation, and (2) to improvement in the health and nutrition of the whole population, so that women are in better health when they become pregnant. Nevertheless there is still room for improvement, as a closer look at the causes of death will show.

Statistical data about maternal mortality based on death certification is published annually by the Registrar-General. In England and Wales much

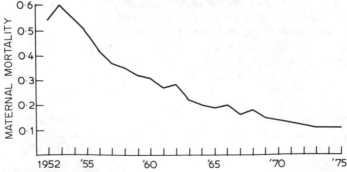

Fig. 45.1   Maternal mortality per 1000 total births (excluding abortion) for the years 1952–1975.

additional information about maternal deaths is derived from the *Reports on Confidential Enquiries into Maternal Deaths*. When a woman dies who is, or has recently been, pregnant the Area Medical Officer sends a detailed form to be filled in by the doctor who was in charge of the patient. Any midwives or nurses who have knowledge of the case may also write reports. At no time is the identity of the person connected with the medical or nursing care of the patient disclosed, and because of this each person giving evidence may be completely frank and unbiased, and nobody filling in the form need fear recriminations of any kind from anybody. After the form is filled in it is sent to an assessor who is a senior obstetrician of standing in the Region who gives his opinion about the cause of death. If the patient had an anaesthetic the opinion of an anaesthetist may also be sought. In giving his report the assessor tries to judge whether the death was 'avoidable' or 'unavoidable'. These terms are not meant to imply criticism of those concerned with the case, but to ask whether the patient, her family, the doctor and the midwife, and anyone else concerned, had made the fullest possible use of all available services and help. If there had been shortcomings in the use of services and administration, or if the standard of professional care had been lower than should be expected, then the death would be classified as 'avoidable'. This is not to say that it could necessarily have been avoided, but only that some factor was present which if foreseen might have made the outcome different. The results of these enquiries are published at three-yearly intervals.

Table 45.1 summarizes some of the conclusions of the last Report.

Table 45.1 Causes of maternal deaths elicited by confidential enquiries 1973–5 (England and Wales)

	Number of cases reported	Rate per 10^6 maternities
Deaths directly due to pregnancy or childbirth		
Hypertensive diseases of pregnancy	39	20.3
Pulmonary embolism	35	18.2
Abortion (including sepsis)	29	15.1
Haemorrhage	21	10.9
Ectopic pregnancy	21	10.9
Sepsis (excluding abortion)	21	10.9
Amniotic fluid embolism	14	7.3
Ruptured uterus	11	5.7
Other deaths directly due to pregnancy and childbirth, including a number of cases related to anaesthesia or Caesarean section, for such indications as prolonged labour, disproportion or malpresentation	44	22.9
Deaths due to associated medical or surgical disorders, and accidents		
Cardiac disease	20	10.4
Other conditions	135	70.1

Hypertensive diseases of pregnancy, including eclampsia and pre-eclampsia. The incidence of these conditions has been falling slowly during the last thirty years in Britain, but they are still the greatest single cause of maternal death. (Table 45.2.) The slow improvement may have resulted from improved antenatal care, but probably also from better living standards and better general health. One of the major aims of antenatal care from the earliest days has been the prevention of eclampsia by early recognition and treatment of pre-eclampsia.

In the last Report deaths from eclampsia and pre-eclampsia were associated with an avoidable factor in three-quarters of the cases. The commonest group were patients who refused antenatal care or who would not cooperate by accepting advice about admission to hospital. Doctors were sometimes at fault by delay in acting on signs of severe pre-eclampsia and instituting efficient treatment. These patients must be under the care of a consultant obstetrician and not in general practitioner units.

Table 45.2 Deaths from hypertensive diseases of pregnancy elicited by confidential enquiries

Numbers of deaths in triennia starting							
1952	1955	1958	1961	1964	1967	1970	1973
200	171	118	104	67	53	47	29

Pulmonary embolism. This is a sudden and dramatic cause of maternal death. In the Reports from 1964 onwards 25 per cent of the deaths occurred during pregnancy, 66 per cent followed delivery, and the remainder followed abortion or ectopic pregnancy. Of the postpartum deaths one-third followed Caesarean section, although only one-twentieth of all the women were delivered by this method, so that the risk of pulmonary embolism is much greater after section than after vaginal delivery. The risk of pulmonary embolism is higher in women aged over 34 years, in those who are overweight, and in those who have an operative delivery of any kind. Most of the deaths during pregnancy occurred suddenly and unexpectedly, and it is difficult at present to see how they could be prevented. After delivery warning signs of deep venous thrombosis were seldom present. Possibly more women in high risk categories should be given prophylactic anticoagulant treatment.

Recently the use of oestrogens to inhibit lactation has been suspected to be one cause of venous thrombosis and pulmonary embolism, and their use for this purpose has been largely abandoned.

Abortion. In 1968 a major change in practice occurred when the Abortion Act of 1967 came into operation. Table 45.3 shows that there has recently been a steady fall in the number of deaths following abortion, without any great rise in the number of deaths following therapeutic termination of pregnancy, despite over 100 000 terminations being notified each year among women resident in England and Wales.

Table 45.3 Deaths after abortion in England and Wales

	1964	1966	1968	1970	1972	1974	1976
Abortions induced for therapeutic reasons	2	4	5	10	10	6	1
Spontaneous abortions	} 60	} 49	12	7	2	0	2
Other abortions, including illegal abortions			33	15	14	5	4
Total	62	53	50	32	26	11	7

In the three years covered by the latest Report on Confidential Enquiries into Maternal Deaths abortion was no longer the most common single cause of death, but it still accounted for 12 per cent of all deaths. Data collected by the Office of Population and Census Studies shows that since that time the number of deaths associated with abortion are continuing to fall. In 1976 abortion accounted for 8.1 per cent of deaths.

Haemorrhage. Maternal deaths associated with both antepartum and postpartum haemorrhage have fallen steadily since 1950. Placental abruption remains one of the most serious complications of pregnancy. For these cases monitoring of the central venous pressure is essential, and large amounts of blood are required to treat hypovolaemia. A third of the deaths from haemorrhage occur in cases of placenta praevia, but these have been greatly reduced since the introduction of conservative management and better diagnosis by radiological, isotopic and now ultrasonic methods of examination. (Table 45.4.)

Table 45.4 Deaths from haemorrhage elicited by confidential enquiries

	Numbers of deaths in triennia starting							
	1952	1955	1958	1961	1964	1967	1970	1973
Antepartum haemorrhage	107	68	69	48	43	25	12	8
Postpartum haemorrhage	113	70	61	44	25	16	15	13
Total	220	138	130	92	68	41	27	21

The number of deaths from postpartum haemorrhage was sharply reduced in the 1950s by the prophylactic use of ergometrine in the third stage of labour. A woman who has had a postpartum haemorrhage is at risk of having another in a subsequent pregnancy; she must always be booked for delivery at a hospital with a blood bank and facilities for immediate transfusion. The existence of a 'flying squad' must not be an excuse for delivering such a patient outside a consultant unit. A grand multipara must also be delivered in a consultant unit.

Ectopic pregnancy. Deaths from this cause have been reduced but not at the same rate as deaths from other causes. The number of deaths in each triennial Report has fallen from 59 in 1952−4 to 21 in 1973−5. A third of the women who died were Afro-Asian. Almost half the patients died at home or in the ambulance before admission to hospital, and another quarter died in hospital before operation. It is essential to operate immediately the diagnosis of ectopic pregnancy has been made. The operation should not wait for resuscitative measures; these should proceed while the operation is being performed, for once the bleeding vessels are secured improvement usually follows quickly.

Infection. Before 1936 puerperal sepsis was the largest single cause of maternal mortality. Since the introduction of sulphonamides and antibiotics, and with better understanding of the mode of spread of infection, it has become a much less common cause of death, but it is often an associated factor in fatal cases. In the 1973−5 Report there was as high a death rate from sepsis as from haemorrhage, and vigilance must be maintained if sepsis is not again to become an important cause of maternal death.

Until recently sepsis contributed to many deaths after abortion, especially after illegal operations. In the 1973−5 Report there were only 6 deaths from septic abortion, of which 5 followed illegal operations.

The septic deaths after surgical procedures mostly followed Caesarean section.

Amniotic fluid embolism. In the three years covered by the 1973−5 Report there were 22 deaths from this cause, and about half of these patients had an associated coagulation disorder. The common symptoms were sudden collapse soon after rupture of the membranes, particularly when the uterine contractions were strong. The collapse was often accompanied by a fit, and the patient was usually dyspnoeic and cyanosed, with frothy blood-stained sputum. Confirmation of the diagnosis is possible if amniotic cells are recognized in the sputum. This condition should be kept in mind in cases of sudden collapse, for it is a difficult diagnosis to make. Treatment with oxygen and steroids can save some of the patients, whilst the ensuing coagulation disorder needs correction (see p. 431).

Uterine rupture. In the last Report there were 11 deaths from this cause. With persisting haemorrhage and shock the uterine cavity should always be examined if there is any possibility of uterine rupture, and laparotomy should not be delayed.

Apart from the causes of maternal death which have been mentioned above, two other factors which operate in many obstetric cases require special mention, anaesthesia and Caesarean section.

Anaesthesia. In the Reports on Confidential Enquiries into Maternal Deaths the deaths associated with anaesthesia are classified under the headings of the conditions for which treatment was required. However, in the Report for 1973−5 it is stated that 31 deaths were directly due to anaesthesia, with avoidable factors in 28 of these, and the death rate from this cause does not seem to be falling. Several women died from inhalation of gastric contents during general anaesthesia. In other cases there was difficulty in intubation, injudicious use of drugs, or incorrect administration of epidural anaesthesia by inexpert doctors. Cardiac arrest occurred in some cases, but there was usually some other discernible cause.

For general anaesthesia during labour a skilled and experienced anaesthetist is required. Patients may be dehydrated after a long labour, and although they may not have been given food for some hours the stomach may still contain food taken before that, and gastric juice will still have been produced. Such women should be intubated in the head-up position, with controlled pressure over the cricoid. A wider use of pudendal block for vaginal procedures will help to reduce mortality.

Caesarean section. In the Report for 1973−5 there were 81 deaths after Caesarean section. From information obtained separately from the Hospital In-patient Enquiry of the Department of Health and Social Services it is estimated that these deaths occurred among 100 870 sections, giving a mortality rate of 0.8 per 1000 operations. This shows that the mortality of section is about seven times greater than that of vaginal delivery but, of course, the conditions calling for treatment by Caesarean section may themselves be dangerous.

Among the 81 cases the immediate causes of death were an anaesthetic complication in 17, haemorrhage in 8, pulmonary embolism in 6, and sepsis or paralytic ileus in 8 cases. In the rest a variety of factors were involved, including the diseases which made the operations necessary.

Deaths from associated and intercurrent conditions. There has been a fall in the number of deaths from cardiac disease in each triennial Report. That for 1952−4 included 121 deaths, whereas the Report for 1973−5 included only 20.

A wide variety of medical and surgical disorders and accidents caused the remaining deaths, but in most of them there was no avoidable obstetric factor.

Stillbirths and neonatal deaths: perinatal mortality

Stillbirths and neonatal deaths are notifiable in Britain, and for statistical accuracy it is essential to use correct definitions.

Stillbirth rate. The term stillbirth refers to any child delivered after

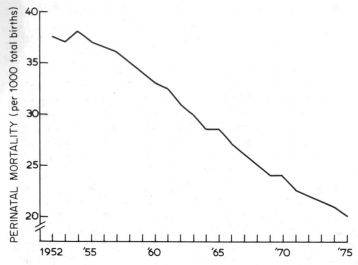

Fig. 45.2   Perinatal mortality per 1000 total births for the years 1952–1975.

the 28th week of pregnancy that does not afterwards breathe or show any sign of life. If the heart is beating after delivery, although there is no sign of respiration, the death should not be recorded as a stillbirth but as a neonatal death. A child born dead before 28 weeks gestation should not be recorded as a stillbirth, in spite of the fact that some babies born before this time have survived. The stillbirth rate is defined as the number of stillbirths per 1000 total births.

Neonatal death rate.   The neonatal period is defined as the first 28 days of life, and the neonatal death rate as the number of infants dying in that period per 1000 *live* births.

Infant mortality rate.   This is defined as the number of infants dying in the first year of life per 1000 *live* births.

Perinatal mortality rate.   As a measure of obstetric success or failure another rate is often preferred to any of the foregoing. The perinatal mortality rate is defined as the number of stillbirths (born after 28 weeks) together with the number of neonatal deaths in the first week of life per 1000 total births. This is a more useful index for obstetric purposes because deaths in the first week are often related to factors occurring during pregnancy or delivery, whereas deaths in the rest of the neonatal period are more often due to paediatric causes.

In the last thirty years the stillbirth rate has fallen from about 19 to about 10 per 1000 total births; the perinatal mortality rate from about 39 to about 17 total births; and the infant mortality rate from about 34 to about 15 per 1000 live births.

Causes of perinatal deaths

In determining the cause of a stillbirth or neonatal death the clinical events and the postmortem findings must both be considered. In about 25 per cent of stillbirths the fetus is macerated and, because of autolysis of the tissues, the autopsy may give very incomplete information about the cause of death. In many cases the final cause of death is asphyxia, but postmortem examination may not be able to distinguish between the various obstetric causes of this, such as placental insufficiency, antepartum haemorrhage, long labour or cord compression. Asphyxia is a mode of death rather than a cause of death, and the obstetric history may be the only clue to the basic cause.

On the other hand postmortem examination may reveal unsuspected congenital abnormalities or intracranial lesions.

The chief cause of death varies according to the time of death. *Antepartum fetal death* is usually due to asphyxia from placental insufficiency or placental separation, a cord accident, haemolytic disease or maternal diabetes. In *intrapartum deaths* asphyxia is again the usual final event, and may result from interference with placental blood flow during uterine contractions, but any preceding cause of placental insufficiency will increase the risk. In addition intracranial haemorrhage or other injuries may occur during labour. A few severe congenital abnormalities are incompatible with survival during delivery, but in many such cases that are recorded as stillbirths the fetal heart is beating at delivery and they should be recorded as neonatal deaths.

Table 45.5 shows the necropsy findings in cases studied during the British Perinatal mortality survey of 1958.

Table 45.5 Primary necropsy finding; percentage indices

	Stillbirths (1407)	Early neonatal deaths (781)
Congenital malformation	17.5	21.6
Iso-immunization	4.4	4.2
Antepartum death	34.4	—
Intrapartum anoxia	30.8	8.7
anoxia and cerebral trauma	7.8	5.3
cerebral trauma	1.7	5.6
Respiratory distress and pulmonary complications	—	34.2
Intraventricular haemorrhage	—	6.4
Remainder	3.4	14.0
	100.0	100.0

Neonatal death may occur as a sequel of complications of pregnancy or labour. Asphyxia or cerebral heamorrhage before or during birth may leave such metabolic or physical injury that the infant dies soon after delivery. In addition respiratory distress may occur after delivery from hyaline membrane formation, pulmonary haemorrhage, pneumonia or other intra-thoracic lesions. Severe malformations may also cause early neonatal death.

Fetal maturity at delivery. Whatever the cause of fetal hazard the maturity of the fetus has a great effect on the outcome. About 50 per cent of all infants who suffer perinatal death weigh less than 2500 g at birth, and about half of these babies are delivered before the 38th week. The old definition of 'prematurity' was a baby weighing less than 2500 g at birth.

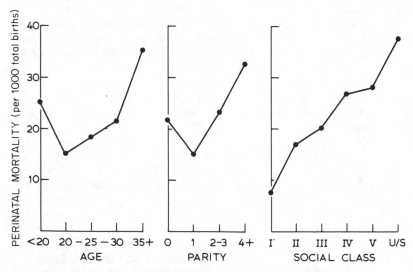

Fig. 45.3 Effects of age, parity and social class on perinatal mortality. (Derived from *British Births,* 1970.)

This definition had the great advantage of simplicity, and the weight was usually accurate, but it included two groups of babies. First were those delivered after pre-term labour but were of appropriate birth-weight for their gestation; for example, a baby born at the 34th week would be expec-ted to weigh about 2000 g. Secondly there were those who were born underweight for their period of gestation; for example a baby born weighing 2000 g after a proven gestation of 39 weeks would be light-for-dates. The first group are born early because of myometrial action or early rupture of the membranes. The second group have suffered from intra-uterine malnutrition from placental insufficiency and have a higher risk of hypoxia during labour; they have a higher mortality and morbidity rate than the first group.

It is probable that the international differences in perinatal mortality can be largely explained by differences in birth weight distribution. Sweden, which has the lowest perinatal mortality rate in the world, has only 4 per cent of babies born weighing less than 2500 g, whereas in England and Wales the proportion is 7 per cent. Japan is a country where the proportion of babies of low birth weight has fallen in the last 20 years, and with this fall there has been a sharp improvement in perinatal mortality.

The aetiology of low birth weight is partly related to the mother's background, including her genetic disposition, nutrition in early childhood, past disease and social upbringing, but also to placental function. The chief cause of death in immature babies are hyaline membrane disease, atelectasis and intraventricular haemorrhage.

Another group of pre-term babies must be considered. Induction of labour is not infrequently necessary to remove the fetus from a hostile intrauterine environment. In such conditions as rhesus disease, pre-eclampsia and diabetes the obstetrician may judge that life outside the uterus may be safer than inside, and this is an iatrogenic cause of prematurity.

Environmental and social background of the mother. The perinatal death rate has been used as a measure of the quality of obstetric services, but it also assays the total health of women in a country. Three major factors affect a woman's performance in pregnancy: her age, her parity and her social class. (Fig. 45.3.) The first two factors often go together, but girls under 20 and women above the age of 35 have the highest risk at any parity. The first baby and those born fourth or later in the family have a higher perinatal mortality rate than do the second or third babies in any particular age group. The social class of a married woman is adjudged from her husband's occupation as classified in an index of occupations prepared by the Registrar-General. The husband's occupation is considered because there is greater differentiation in male than in female occupations, some 80 per cent of women being either housewives or engaged in clerical work. This classification reflects the socio-economic background of married women, but leaves about 9 per cent of women unclassified because they are unwed, and these women cluster at the worst end of the spectrum of perinatal mortality. The classification partly reflects the mother's past nutrition and health, and her education and attitudes. Perinatal mortality is lowest in Social Class I (the professional group) and highest in Social Class V (unskilled) and the unmarried.

Social class is related to other factors; for example maternal height, for that is derived from genetic inheritance and nutrition during childhood. The composition of the population varies from the south-east to the north-west of Britain, the proportion of Social Classes IV and V rising towards the north. The perinatal mortality in different regions of Britain is affected by this, but multifactorial analysis shows that geographical differences are not just the result of social class, but also reflect the obstetric facilities available, and the use the women make of them.

To summarize, the perinatal mortality will usually be lowest in mothers of ages between 20 and 30, whose height is over 165 cm, of Social Class I or II, having their second or third babies. The results will be worst in small women over 35, of Social Class IV or V, having a fourth or subsequent baby.

It follows, therefore, that at least the following groups of women should be booked for antenatal care and delivery in hospital consultant units:

1. Women with obstetric abnormalities, or a history of past abnormalities which are likely to recur.
2. Mothers under 20 or over 30 years of age.
3. Women having their first, or their fourth or subsequent babies.
4. Women under 160 cm (63 inches) in height.
5. Women of Social Class IV or V, and women who are unsupported.

The reduction of perinatal mortality

The three major causes of perinatal mortality are congenital abnormality, prematurity and hypoxia, and these account for about 75 per cent of all perinatal deaths. The remaining causes include birth injuries, haemolytic disease and infection. Deaths from all these causes are being reduced as obstetric care and skill improve, but to an uneven degree.

Congenital abnormalities. The incidence of congenital abnormalities varies from one population to another, implying that there are genetic or environmental causative factors which need to be identified, and may need to be treated by measures wider than those of conventional therapy. For example, in 1974 in England and Wales 1.88 babies per 1000 live births died from congenital malformations, while during the same year in Sweden the figure was only 1.47 per 1000. The difference may seem small, but the higher rate represents 200 more deaths in England and Wales each year.

At present the management of congenital abnormalities involves their detection early enough in pregnancy to allow termination of the pregnancy. The abnormal fetus is removed from the perinatal mortality figures, but of course this is not treatment of the basic problem. The two abnormalities most easily detected are Down's syndrome (p. 502) and defects of the neural tube (p. 501).

Some reduction in perinatal mortality from congenital defects may be achieved by providing protection against known teratogens, for example by rubella vaccination before pregnancy and the avoidance of harmful radiation and certain drugs (p. 63) during pregnancy.

Perinatal mortality may also be reduced by dealing promptly with such lesions as can be relieved by neonatal surgery.

Prematurity. As stated above, this heading includes two groups of babies; those expelled from the uterus too early but of correct size for gestational age, and those lighter-for-dates than the 10th centile for their maturity.

In the first group mortality might be reduced by identifying those who are at higher risk for premature labour, for example women who have had vaginal termination or pre-term labour in a previous pregnancy. Cervical incompetence may be treated by an encirclage stitch. If uterine contractions occur they may be checked with a β mimetic drug (p. 345). If labour is imminent or actually proceeding the mother should be taken to a hospital with a special care unit for the newborn. This may mean moving her by ambulance in early labour. The fetal lung surfactant system may be made more mature by giving the mother steroids.

The second group of babies are protected by careful monitoring of fetal growth. This is done roughly by clinical examination, but more precisely by repeated ultrasonic estimations of the biparietal diameter or other fetal dimensions. Rest in bed may improve uterine blood flow, but if fetal growth is not progressing adequately the fetus is best removed from the adverse uterine environment by induction of labour or sometimes Caesarean section.

Both groups of infants benefit enormously if they are delivered in a fully-equipped hospital, with expert obstetric and paediatric staff. The fetus is then monitored carefully during labour, resuscitation is immediate and skilful, and the newborn infant is looked after in a special care unit with experienced paediatric staff.

Hypoxia. This is one of the major causes of perinatal mortality. Death can occur during labour from placental failure, or during labour if the uterine contractions are so prolonged or frequent that they progressively overcome the natural resistance of the fetus to stress. The fetus that has already suffered from relative placental insufficiency during pregnancy is at special risk if hypoxia is added during labour. Reduction of perinatal mortality will result from identification of fetuses at high risk by recognizing impaired fetal growth during pregnancy, with the aid of placental function tests (see p. 56). Any fetus thought to be at high risk requires special care during labour, with continuous monitoring of the fetal heart rate and intermittent checks of the pH (see p. 352). Again, such care can only be given in adequately equipped hospitals with experienced obstetric staff, and also facilities for neonatal resuscitation.

Such care will not only reduce perinatal mortality but also diminish perinatal morbidity. It is hard to measure morbidity in economic terms, but the cost to the family and to the community of caring for a handicapped child is enormous, and the emotional distress to the parents is beyond computation.

Index